AF566680

FUNDAMENTALS OF

GASTROENTEROLOGY

WITH SELF-ASSESSMENT WORKBOOK

SIXTH EDITION

FUNDAMENTALS OF

GASTROENTEROLOGY

WITH SELF-ASSESSMENT WORKBOOK

SIXTH EDITION

Edited by

Lawrie W. Powell
AC, MD, PhD, FRCP(Lon.), FRACP
Professor of Medicine, The University of Queensland
Physician, Royal Brisbane Hospital, Brisbane
Director, Queensland Institute of Medical Research, Brisbane

Douglas W. Piper
AM, MD, FRCP, FRACP
Professor of Medicine (Emeritus), University of Sydney
Consulting Gastroenterologist, Royal North Shore Hospital, Sydney

McGRAW-HILL BOOK COMPANY Sydney
New York San Francisco Auckland Bogotá
Caracas Lisbon London Madrid Mexico City Milan
Montreal New Delhi San Juan Singapore Tokyo Toronto

NOTICE

Medicine is an ever-changing science. As new research and clinical experience broaden our knowledge, changes in treatment and drug therapy are required. The editors and the publisher of this work have checked with sources believed to be reliable in their efforts to provide information that is complete and generally in accord with the standards accepted at the time of publication. However, in view of the possibility of human error or changes in medical sciences, neither the editor, nor the publisher, nor any other party who has been involved in the preparation or publication of this work warrants that the information contained herein is in every respect accurate or complete and they are not responsible for any errors or omissions or for the results obtained from use of such information. Readers are encouraged to confirm the information contained herein with other sources. For example and in particular, readers are advised to check the product information sheet included in the package of each drug they plan to administer to be certain that the information contained in this book is accurate and that changes have not been made in the recommended dose or in the contraindications for administration. This recommendation is of particular importance in connection with new or infrequently used drugs.

First published 1975 by ADIS Health Science Press, Second edition 1978, Reprinted 1979, Third edition 1980, Spanish edition 1980, Fourth edition 1984, Indonesian edition 1988, Fifth edition 1991 by McGraw-Hill Book Company Australia Pty Limited, Spanish edition 1993, Fifth edition, Sixth edition, 1995 by McGraw-Hill Book Company Australia Pty Limited

---

National Library of Australia Cataloguing-in-Publication data:

Fundamentals of gastroenterology, with self-assessment workbook

6th ed.
Bibliography.
Includes index.
ISBN 0 07 470192 4.

1. Gastroenterology. I. Powell, Lawrie W. (Lawrie William), 1934– . II. Piper, Douglas W. (Douglas William), 1925– .

616.33

Published in Australia by
McGraw-Hill Book Company Australia Pty Limited
4 Barcoo Street, Roseville NSW 2069, Australia

Publisher	John Rowe
Production editors	Sarah Baker, Sybil Kesteven
Designer	George Sirett (Asymmetric Typography Pty Ltd)
Illustrators	Lorenzo Lucia, Rod Semple (Trade Wind-Creations)

Typeset in Australia by Midland Typesetters Pty Ltd
Printed in Australia by McPherson's Printing Group

Foreword to the sixth edition

In this sixth edition of *Fundamentals of Gastroenterology*, Powell and Piper, together with their co-authors, have again succeeded in updating the text by substantial revisions of all chapters as well as the workbook. This has ensured that the text remains at the forefront of knowledge of gastroenterology and liver disease.

With contributors who are all active in research as well as clinical practice in their special fields, the reader can be assured that the material is both up to date and authoritative. As with prior editions, the workbook section effectively complements and reinforces the excellent text.

After twenty years and six editions since it first appeared, *Fundamentals of Gastroenterology* clearly fulfils a need and its continued popularity is assured.

Kurt J. Isselbacher, MD
Harvard Medical School, and
Massachusetts General Hospital
Boston, Massachusetts, USA.

Boston, January 1995

Foreword to the first edition

In current curriculum terms this is a 'core' text rather than an 'options' one. It deals with those aspects of gastroenterology which might be required knowledge of all graduating students rather than those sought after by students wishing to go deeply into gastroenterology.

The reader is introduced to the important basic concepts underlying gastroenterology and, at the same time, to the more important gastroenterological disorders. In an introductory text the importance of basic concepts lies in their application to the maintenance of human wellbeing and must therefore be emphasised, but not to the exclusion of discussion of less understood but equally important disease states. Is peptic ulcer less important because much is still not known about it? Are the concepts underlying the recognised gastrointestinal hormonal disorders less important because we recognise few patients with them?

Experts will differ in detail about what constitutes 'core' material, but the group of gastroenterologists assembled by Lawrie Powell and Douglas Piper has provided a good balance, and those who consider that some aspect has been inadequately covered can get more by using the reference lists provided. By providing a brief text the authors have provided not only the reader with a short text but also themselves with chapters that can easily be updated and avoid the major criticism of students—that a textbook is out of date when it appears.

The provision of a workbook section, a small self-assessment program, is valuable and could well be a regular feature of most or all 'core' texts to facilitate learning at different rates.

C. R. B. Blackburn

Department of Medicine
University of Sydney

Sydney, 1975

Contents

Foreword to the sixth edition v
Foreword to the first edition vi
Preface to the sixth edition xi
Preface to the first edition xii
Contributors xiii

CHAPTER 1 MOUTH, PHARYNX AND OESOPHAGUS
D. J. de Carle
Anatomy and physiology of the oesophagus 1
Oral manifestations of systemic disease 3
Stomatitis 4
Dysphagia 4
Suggested further reading 16

CHAPTER 2 STOMACH AND DUODENUM
S. K. Lam, J. Y. Kang and D. W. Piper
Anatomy and physiology of the stomach 17
Gastric emptying 18
Reaction of tissues to acid and pepsin 19
Gastric mucosal defence mechanisms 19
Gastric secretory abnormalities and disease 20
Peptic ulcer 21
Gastric outlet obstruction 31
Perforation 32
Special types of ulcers 32
Gastritis 33
Gastric carcinoma 35
Suggested further reading 37

CHAPTER 3 SMALL INTESTINE
W. Doe
Anatomy 38
Physiology 39
Malabsorption 46
Chronic secretory diarrhoea of endocrine origin 64
Suggested further reading 65

CHAPTER 4 COLON, RECTUM AND ANUS
D. J. B. St John, G. P. Young and I. T. Jones

Anatomy, physiology and pathophysiology 66
Congenital anomalies 71
Ulcerative colitis 72
Crohn's disease of the colon 79
Diverticular disease of the colon 81
Ischaemic colitis 85
Uncommon causes of colitis 87
Pathogenesis of colorectal neoplasia 88
Carcinoma of the colon and rectum 91
Other colonic diseases 97
Rectal and anal disorders 98
Suggested further reading 102

CHAPTER 5 PANCREAS
J. S. Wilson

Anatomy and developmental anatomy 103
Physiology of pancreatic exocrine secretion 104
Pancreatitis 108
Carcinoma of the pancreas 120
Islet cell tumours of the pancreas 124
Suggested further reading 126

CHAPTER 6 LIVER AND BILIARY TRACT
L. W. Powell and E. E. Powell

Relevant anatomy 127
Physiology 131
Acute viral hepatitis 132
Chronic hepatitis 142
Fulminant hepatic failure (FHF) 147
Cirrhosis of the liver 148
Portal hypertension 154
Ascites 159
Functional renal failure in cirrhosis ('hepatorenal syndrome') 161
Special types of cirrhosis 161
Alcoholic liver disease 165
Cholestasis 167
Drug-induced liver damage 168
Benign hepatic neoplasms 171
Malignant hepatic neoplasms 172
Congenital hyperbilirubinaemia 173
Diseases of the gallbladder and bile ducts 174

Diagnostic techniques in liver disease 177
Suggested further reading 182

CHAPTER 7 INFECTIOUS DISEASES OF THE GASTROINTESTINAL TRACT
T. C. Sorrell

Acute enteritis and enterocolitis 183
Causative agents of non-inflammatory infectious diarrhoea 187
Causative agents of inflammatory diarrhoea 191
Causative agents of non-inflammatory diarrhoea containing blood 199
Helminth infestation of the gastrointestinal tract 204
Neurotoxin-associated food poisoning 209
Suggested further reading 210

CHAPTER 8 MOTILITY AND FUNCTIONAL DISORDERS OF THE GASTROINTESTINAL TRACT
J. E. Kellow

Gastrointestinal motor physiology and pathophysiology 211
Functional gastrointestinal disorders 214
Suggested further reading 221

CHAPTER 9 COMMON SYMPTOMS
N. D. Yeomans

Oesophageal symptoms 222
Abdominal symptoms 223
Miscellaneous symptoms 230
Jaundice 231
Suggested further reading 233

Self-assessment workbook: questions 234

Self-assessment workbook: answers 267

Index 269

Preface to the sixth edition

Gastroenterology continues to be one of the most rapidly developing subdivisions of medical science and practice. This is due to the spectacular advances in molecular and cell biology, molecular genetics, immunology, physical techniques such as magnetic resonance, and the continued rapid progress in endoscopic techniques. No part of the gastrointestinal tract, including the biliary tree, is unable to be illuminated, visualised and photographed by direct endoscopy or by ultrasonography. Surgical advances have also been breathtaking, with liver transplantation becoming commonplace and small bowel and pancreas transplants a reality.

This continued profusion of gastroenterology knowledge has created an even greater need, in our opinion, for a textbook which provides basic concepts and *core* knowledge in an easily readable form for undergraduate and postgraduate students as well as for busy practitioners in medicine and the paramedical professions. A multi-authored book has become essential if all aspects are to be covered concisely and expertly. Accordingly, all chapters have been completely revised, including the figures and tables.

The workbook section has also been extensively revised and updated to provide a ready self-assessment program for all sections of the text, with appropriate emphasis on common and important diseases. We would emphasise that, if intelligently used in conjunction with the text, this section should significantly aid retention of the material, as it is knowledge gained by reading in response to the stimulus provided by clinical problems that is better retained. The exercise is also a more enjoyable one!

We are indebted to the contributors and many other colleagues for their assistance in updating the book and for freely offering advice and constructive criticism. We are also indebted to John Rowe and Sybil Kesteven, and all those involved in the various processes of editing and production at McGraw-Hill Book Company Australia Pty Limited for their expert handling of both manuscript and proofs in minimum time.

The authors and publisher would like to thank individuals and organisations for permission to reproduce material.

January 1995

Lawrie W. Powell
Douglas W. Piper

Preface to the first edition

Gastroenterology is probably the most rapidly progressive of all subdivisions of medicine. This is partly due to the better understanding of many diseases through the exploitation of biochemical and physiological techniques, the improved investigative procedures of endoscopy and biopsy, and through the increasing recognition of the role of surgery. The profusion of gastroenterological knowledge is revealed by the increasing number of monographs that deal with this topic, and consequently the need for another textbook could be queried. We believe there is a need for a basic textbook dealing with this section of medicine which would provide core material in an easily readable form and which would serve therefore as an introductory text for undergraduate students as well as a source of revision for early postgraduate students and practitioners. It is not intended to replace the standard reference books for senior students and postgraduates.

The book is written by a series of authors whose major interests centre on various subdivisions of gastroenterology. It is the only comparable book on this subject of multiauthor origin, which we feel is essential in view of the increasing complexity of the subject. We firmly believe that it is the expert in a particular area who is most likely to write a clear and concise account of his subject, just as it is logically impossible for a single author to cover with accuracy all branches of medicine.

A further advantage of this book is the incorporation in the same volume of a workbook. This includes brief case histories illustrating common clinical problems as well as questions demanding simple factual recall. If properly used by the student in conjunction with the text, the workbook should aid retention of the material substantially, since knowledge gained by reading in response to the stimulus provided by clinical problems tends to be better retained.

August, 1975

L. W. Powell
D. W. Piper

Contributors

D. J. de Carle, FRACP Associate Professor of Medicine, University of New South Wales; Gastroenterologist, The St George Hospital, Kogarah, NSW

W. Doe, MSc, FRCP, FRACP Professor of Medicine and Clinical Science, John Curtin School of Medical Research, Australian National University; Director of Gastroenterology, Woden Valley Hospital, Canberra

I. T. Jones, FRACS Colorectal Surgeon, The Royal Melbourne Hospital, Melbourne

J. Y. Kang, MD, FRCP, FRCP(Ed.), FRACP Associate Professor, National University Hospital, Singapore

J. E. Kellow, MD, FRACP Associate Professor of Medicine, University of Sydney; Visiting Gastroenterologist and Director, Gastrointestinal Motility Research Unit, Royal North Shore Hospital, Sydney

S. K. Lam, MD, FRCP(Ed.), FRCP (Glasg.), FRCP(Lon.), FRACP, Professor of Medicine, University of Hong Kong, Queen Mary Hospital, Hong Kong

D. W. Piper, AM, MD, FRCP, FRACP Professor of Medicine (Emeritus), University of Sydney; Physician, Royal North Shore Hospital, Sydney

E. E. Powell, PhD, FRACP Gastroenterologist, Princess Alexandra Hospital, Brisbane

L. W. Powell, AC, MD, PhD, FRCP(Lon.), FRACP Professor of Medicine, The University of Queensland; Physician, Royal Brisbane Hospital, Brisbane; Director, Queensland Institute of Medical Research, Brisbane

T. C. Sorrell, MD, FRACP Professor of Clinical Infectious Diseases, University of Sydney; Director, Centre for Infectious Diseases and Microbiology, Westmead Hospital, Sydney

D. J. B. St John, FRCP, FRACP Director, Department of Gastroenterology, The Royal Melbourne Hospital; Senior Associate, Department of Medicine, Royal Melbourne Hospital/Western Hospital, University of Melbourne

J. S. Wilson, MD, FRACP Senior Lecturer in Medicine, University of New South Wales; Senior Staff Specialist, Gastrointestinal Unit, Prince of Wales Hospital, Sydney

N. D. Yeomans, MD, FRACP Professor of Medicine, University of Melbourne; Department of Medicine, Western Hospital, Melbourne

G. P. Young, MD, FRACP Associate Professor, Department of Medicine, Royal Melbourne Hospital/Western Hospital, University of Melbourne; Deputy Director, Department of Gastroenterology, The Royal Melbourne Hospital, Melbourne

Read with two objects: first to acquaint yourself with the current knowledge on the subject and the steps by which it has been reached; and secondly, and more important, read to understand and analyse your cases.

SIR WILLIAM OSLER

From 'The Student Life',
in *A Way of Life and Other Selected Writings*,
Dover Publications Inc.,
New York, 1905

CHAPTER 1

Mouth, pharynx and oesophagus

D. J. de Carle

DEFINITION OF TERMS

dyspepsia	any pain, discomfort or nausea referable to the upper abdominal tract, which is not precipitated by exertion or relieved by rest (p.227)
dysphagia	difficulty in swallowing
odynophagia	pain on swallowing food or fluids
oesophageal reflux	reflux of gastric contents into lower oesophagus. This occurs normally but may cause symptoms (dyspepsia) when unduly frequent or if the gastric juice is unduly acid. In a small proportion of cases *oesophagitis* results
regurgitation	regurgitation of gastric contents into the mouth. It occurs frequently but causes no problems

Anatomy and physiology of the oesophagus

The function of the oesophagus is to transport food and fluid from the mouth to the stomach and to prevent the reflux of gastric contents into the oesophagus. This transport is usually facilitated by gravity acting on the bolus of food or fluid, but persons lying flat or even standing on their heads can swallow. The mechanisms involved are complex but co-ordinated, so that normal individuals are not aware of the passage of boluses through the oesophagus.

The oesophagus is a muscular tube with a sphincter at either end. The muscle in the proximal one-third of the oesophagus is striated in type. The upper oesophageal sphincter is formed by the muscles of the distal pharynx and proximal oesophagus. The muscle in the distal two-thirds of the oesophagus and lower oesophageal sphincter is smooth in type. This arrangement of muscle in the oesophageal wall is present in man, other primates and marsupials but not in other mammals, so that many experimental studies on oesophageal function have been carried out using such marsupials as the North American opossum.

The *upper oesophageal sphincter* receives tonic excitatory innervation, and relaxes transiently when a bolus is propelled from the pharynx into the upper oesophagus. Opening of the upper oesophageal sphincter involves both relaxation of the cricopharyngeus and contraction of other surrounding muscles which displace and physically open the sphincter. Once the bolus reaches the oesophagus a contraction which occludes the lumen proximal to the bolus sweeps down the oesophagus, pushing the bolus ahead of it. Peristaltic waves occur in response to either voluntary swallowing efforts or oesophageal distension. The lower oesophageal sphincter is tonically contracted due to intrinsic properties of the muscle. It also receives excitatory cholinergic innervation. When a swallowing effort is made, non-adrenergic, non-cholinergic inhibitory nerves to the lower oesophageal sphincter cause it to relax. The sphincter contracts again when the peristaltic wave reaches it. Primary peristaltic contractions are initiated in the swallowing centre, which is in the brain stem. The vagi are involved in initiating peristaltic waves, and control contractions in the striated muscle part of the oesophagus. The control of contractions in the smooth muscle part of the oesophagus is more complex, and involves the properties of the muscle itself and the local intramural nerve plexuses. Vagal activity may modulate contractions occurring in the smooth muscle part of the oesophagus.

The lower oesophageal sphincter is difficult to identify anatomically, and consequently for many years its existence was questioned. It was thought that mechanical factors such as the acute angle between the oesophagus and the stomach, the compressive effect of the diaphragm, and a mucosal plug prevented gastro-oesophageal reflux. In the past twenty years it has become clear that there is a physiological sphincter at the junction of the oesophagus and stomach which is important in preventing gastro-oesophageal reflux. Studies in experimental animals have shown that there is a short segment of smooth muscle at the oesophagogastic junction which behaves differently from the muscle both above and below. Its metabolic processes are different in that it is much more sensitive to hypoxia. The muscle generates greater tension in response to stretch, and is more sensitive to a variety of excitatory and inhibitory neurotransmitters and hormones. A large number of factors that either increase or decrease lower oesophageal sphincter pressure have been identified, but the role of these agents in precipitating or preventing gastro-oesophageal reflux has not been established.

Table 1.1 *Causes of dysphagia*

1. Oropharyngeal	2. Oesophageal
(a) *Neuromuscular*	(a) *Mechanical obstruction*
Cerebrovascular disease	Carcinoma
Parkinson's disease	Peptic stricture
Cranial neuropathies	Rings and webs
Connective tissue disorders	Post-traumatic stricture (e.g. corrosive injury)
Myasthenia gravis	(b) *Neuromuscular*
Motor neuron disease	Achalasia
(b) *Mechanical obstruction*	Diffuse oesophageal spasm
Carcinoma	Connective tissue disorders
Postcricoid web	(c) *Severe oesophagitis*
Pharyngeal ('Zenkers') pouch	Peptic oesophagitis
Thyroid enlargement	Fungal (monilial) oesophagitis
Cervical osteophyte	Viral oesophagitis

Oral manifestations of systemic disease

Oral lesions, especially if persistent, should alert the astute clinician to the possibility of systemic disorders. Some common examples are:

1. *The gums.* Hyperplastic gingivitis is most frequently caused by chronic phenytoin treatment. In all forms of acute leukaemia, bleeding and ulceration of the gums are common.
2. *Halitosis.* Offensive breath is often caused by poor dental hygiene or cigarette-smoking. Food accumulating in a pharyngeal pouch can give rise to halitosis. Some respiratory tract infections such as sinusitis and bronchiectasis can also be responsible. Acetone may be smelt on the breath of patients with ketosis, which can be a result of starvation but also occurs in diabetic ketoacidosis. A characteristic musty smell, fetor hepaticus, occurs in advanced liver disease.
3. *Glossitis.* A smooth, red and often painful atrophic glossitis can accompany deficiency of iron, folic acid, vitamin B or nicotinic acid. This occurs because of the rapid turnover of epithelial cells of the tongue and gastrointestinal tract, with a consequent high requirement for these compounds.
4. *Xerostomia (dry mouth).* Common causes are persistent mouth-breathing, dehydration (diabetes, uraemia) and drugs, especially those with anticholinergic effects. Sjogren's syndrome (xerostomia, keratoconjunctivitis sicca) should also be considered, especially in women over forty years of age. Patients who are not eating or drinking may develop a 'coated, dirty tongue' due to the absence of the abrasive cleaning action of food on the surface of the tongue.
5. *Pigmentation.* This is an important clinical sign. Apart from reasons of race, Addison's disease, haemochromatosis, drug reactions, malnutrition and Peutz-Jeghers syndrome (hereditary intestinal polyposis) are the major conditions to consider.

6. *Other manifestations.* The characteristic lesions of hereditary haemorrhagic telangiectasia are often visible on the buccal mucosa and lips. Tightening of the skin of the mouth may be an early sign of scleroderma. Stomatitis, associated with ocular lesions such as iritis, genital ulcers and skin rash, should suggest Stevens-Johnson syndrome, a severe form of erythema multiforme often due to drug idiosyncrasy. The triad of oral ulcers, genital ulcers and eye inflammation should also suggest Reiter's or Behcet's syndromes, especially if arthritis and other systemic features are present.

Stomatitis

Inflammation of the oral mucosa has many causes. Correct diagnosis requires awareness of the various aetiological and predisposing conditions, and the identification of causative organisms by culture. The most common causes are:

1. *Recurrent oral ulceration (aphthous ulcers).* These are very common, particularly in the second and third decade. An initial soreness is followed by ulceration, which is very painful for a few days and heals within two weeks. Recurrence is common. The ulcers are shallow with a yellowish base and hyperaemic edges, and occur mostly opposite the molar teeth or inside the lips. The cause of aphthous ulcers is unknown, although they occur more frequently in patients with coeliac disease, Crohn's disease and ulcerative colitis.
2. *Oral candidiasis (moniliasis or 'thrush').* This occurs in debilitated patients and in those on antibiotics or immunosuppressive drugs. Oral and/or oesophageal candidiasis may be a presenting manifestation of acquired immunodeficiency syndrome as well as other gastrointestinal infection. (See also Chapter 7.)
3. *Bacterial and viral stomatitis.* These occur uncommonly. Vincent's angina is the somewhat confusing name given to a mixed infection with *Fusobacterium fusiforme* and indigenous spirochaetes. The symptoms are halitosis, sore throat and bleeding from ulcers. Diagnosis is made by examining a smear for the bacterium from the exudate.
4. *Neoplasia.* This is an important cause of oral ulceration; any suspicious lesion should undergo biopsy.
5. *Poorly fitting dentures.* A common cause of buccal ulceration in the elderly.

Dysphagia

'Dysphagia' means difficulty in swallowing. The vast majority of patients who complain of dysphagia have an identifiable mechanical or motility disorder of the oesophagus to account for the symptom. Dysphagia should be differentiated from the sensation of a lump in the throat (globus hystericus), which does not interfere with swallowing. Occasionally patients will describe a life-long mild difficulty in swallowing specific foods or capsules. Pain on swallowing (odynophagia) usually implies either oesophageal mucosal inflammation or increased tension in the oesophageal wall, due to either smooth muscle spasm or oesophageal distension. The site and characteristics of dysphagia may indicate its cause.

Lesions in the brain stem, cranial nerves and striated muscle of the pharynx give rise to oropharyngeal dysphagia. Patients describe difficulty in initiating swallows, and may cough due to inhalation of food while attempting to eat. Patients may also describe regurgitation of food into the nasopharynx: this syndrome can be due to bulbar or pseudobulbar palsy, Parkinson's disease, myasthenia gravis or cranial neuropathy. It also occurs in elderly patients without any identifiable underlying cause. The diagnosis is usually established by a combination of careful history-taking, the observation of patients attempting to eat and a video barium swallow.

Oropharyngeal dysphagia is an important cause of morbidity in the elderly and debilitated. Swallowing difficulties occur in approximately 30% of hospitalised elderly patients. Patients may be re-trained to swallow by speech pathologists. Changes in posture and dietary modifications often help. A small proportion of patients require long-term feeding by either nasogastric tube or percutaneous endoscopic gastrostomy.

The causes of dysphagia arising in the body of the oesophagus can conveniently be divided into:

1. mechanical obstruction;
2. neuromuscular disturbances of motility; and
3. severe oesophagitis (see Table 1.1).

Mechanical obstruction

Mechanical obstruction can occur at any level in the oesophagus, and the majority of patients can accurately identify the site of the obstruction. About 25% of patients with lesions in the lower third of the oesophagus will identify the obstruction as occurring in the upper oesophagus. The reasons for this are not clear. Mechanical obstruction gives rise to problems with swallowing solid food, particularly meat and bread, but when boluses are impacted in a narrowed segment of the oesophagus, patients are unable to swallow anything, and describe difficulty with liquids (including saliva). Bolus obstruction promptly gives rise to chest discomfort, and repeated retching in an attempt to overcome the obstruction may occur.

The two common and important causes of mechanical obstruction are carcinoma, either arising in the oesophagus or spreading from the gastric fundus, and reflux oesophagitis with or without stricture. The dysphagia in patients with carcinoma is usually more rapidly progressive and associated with weight loss, while patients with oesophagitis and stricture may have a history of recurrent heartburn and regurgitation. Distinguishing between the two conditions can be quite difficult, and endoscopy with biopsy is essential in all patients with dysphagia.

Other causes of mechanical obstruction include webs (Plummer-Vinson syndrome) and lower oesophageal (Schatzki) rings. Compression of the oesophagus by lesions—such as thyroid masses, mediastinal tumour and vascular abnormalities—can also give rise to dysphagia.

Motility disorders

Motility disorders can give rise to dysphagia in several ways. The lower oesophageal sphincter may provide a barrier to emptying if it fails to relax normally, as in patients with achalasia. Failure of propulsion due to abnormalities of peristalsis in the body of the oesophagus may also be associated with difficulty in swallowing. Forceful, non-propagated contractions may transiently obstruct the oesophageal lumen. Motility disorders give rise to difficulties in swallowing both liquids and solids. The problem may be intermittent. If there are forceful contractions or oesophageal distension, the dysphagia may be associated with chest pain which occurs with swallowing but may occur spontaneously and wake patients from sleep. In achalasia the tightly contracted, non-relaxing lower oesophageal sphincter results in accumulation of food in the oesophagus, which then dilates. The food retained in the dilated oesophagus gives rise to recurrent regurgitation and inhalation.

Evaluation of patients complaining of dysphagia

1. *Careful history-taking and physical examination.* The site, frequency, periodicity and food involved in dysphagia are all important in determining the cause. Physical examination, with special emphasis on cranial nerve function, evidence of malignant disease (such as lymphdenopathy or hepatomegaly) and observing the patient swallow, are of great importance.
2. *Endoscopy.* Fibreoptic endoscopy of the oesophagus and stomach is essential in all patients presenting with dysphagia. The gastric fundus should always be examined and any mucosal lesions should be biopsied. Great care is necessary with the introduction of the endoscope, particularly if a pharyngeal pouch or proximal oesophageal web may be present.
3. *Radiology.* Contrast radiography with barium swallow is particularly useful in patients with motility disorders, and in patients with oropharyngeal dysphagia this may be combined with video recording.
4. *Oesophageal manometry.* This is used to establish the presence of abnormal motor activity, and is essential in confirming the diagnosis of disorders such as achalasia and diffuse oesophageal spasm. It is also useful in

documenting oesophageal involvement in systemic disorders, such as scleroderma.

5. *Radioisotope transit studies*. Transit of both solids and liquids through the oesophagus can be quantitated using liquid and solid meals labelled with radioisotopes. Computer analysis of multiple gamma-camera images gives information which may be useful in establishing abnormal oesophageal function in patients with unexplained dysphagia. This technique has also been used to study oesophageal function in patients with a variety of systemic disorders.

Gastro-oesophageal reflux and regurgitation

There is an effective barrier between the stomach and the oesophagus, and under normal circumstances the gastric contents do not enter the oesophagus despite the fact that intragastric pressure may exceed intra-oesophageal pressure. Transient reflux is occasionally seen in normal individuals, but frequent or prolonged episodes of gastro-oesophageal reflux will give rise to symptoms.

The main mechanism preventing gastro-oesophageal reflux is thought to be pressure in the lower oesophageal sphincter. Until fifteen or twenty years ago it was thought that mechanical factors such as the acute angle of entry of the oesophagus into the stomach and the compressive effect of the diaphragm on the lower oesophagus prevented reflux, but recent studies have demonstrated that reflux only occurs when pressure in the lower oesophageal sphincter equals that in the stomach. Oesophageal sphincter pressure may be continuously low, or may relax intermittently in the absence of any swallowing effort. Approximately 80% of reflux episodes occur because of inappropriate lower oesophageal sphincter relaxation. The underlying mechanisms of both constantly reduced sphincter pressure and transient sphincter relaxations are not known. Both myogenic and neurogenic factors may be involved. Although anatomical derangements are not primarily responsible for gastro-oesophageal reflux, pressure within the lower oesophageal sphincter may be augmented by diaphragmatic contractions so that the sphincter functions less well when displaced from its normal site.

Several factors are involved in determining the extent of oesophageal injury associated with gastro-oesophageal reflux. Gastric contents are usually cleared from the oesophagus by peristalsis, induced either by swallowing or oesophageal distension, but in patients with impaired oesophageal function, such as those with connective tissue disorders, gastric contents may remain in the oesophagus for long periods. The concentrations of acid, bile and pancreatic secretions in refluxed fluid influence the extent of injury to the oesophageal mucosa. Delayed gastric emptying may increase the volume of fluid available to reflux. Salivary bicarbonate plays a minor role in neutralising small amounts of acid remaining in the oesophagus after the bulk of gastric content has been cleared from the oesophagus.

Symptoms

Gastro-oesophageal reflux gives rise to burning epigastric and retrosternal discomfort, often associated with frequent belching. The discomfort often follows meals and may be worse when the patient bends, stoops or lies flat. Regurgitation of sour or bitter fluid into the mouth may occur, and this may be associated with salivation.

'Heartburn' is often confused with dyspepsia due to peptic ulceration. It is usually promptly relieved by antacids. Certain foods, such as chocolate and peppermint, or cigarette-smoking and alcohol may precipitate symptoms. It has been suggested that this is because those agents reduce pressure in the lower oesophageal sphincter, but the mechanism has not been clearly established (see p. 222). Although the symptoms are thought to be due to mucosal injury, most patients with symptomatic gastro-oesophageal reflux do not have any mucosal changes that can be documented by endoscopy. The major complication of gastro-oesophageal reflux is reflux (peptic) oesophagitis.

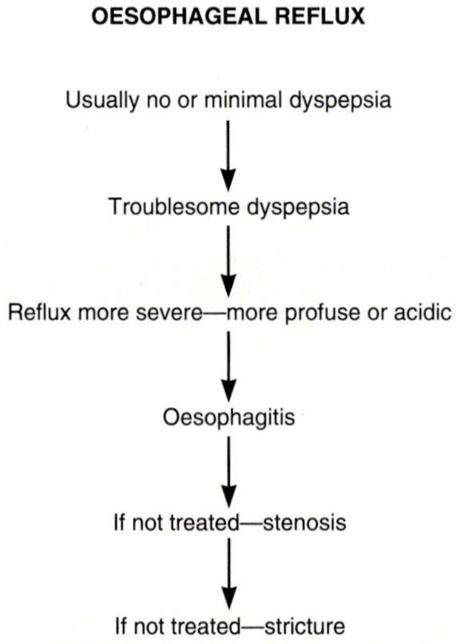

OESOPHAGEAL REFLUX

Usually no or minimal dyspepsia
↓
Troublesome dyspepsia
↓
Reflux more severe—more profuse or acidic
↓
Oesophagitis
↓
If not treated—stenosis
↓
If not treated—stricture

Fig. 1.1 *Sequence of events leading from oesophageal reflux to stricture. Note that stricture may result without symptoms from reflux*

Reflux oesophagitis

This is the reaction of the squamous epithelium of the distal oesophagus to repeated exposure to gastric contents containing acid and bile or pepsin (see p. 17). The earliest macroscopic changes are linear or circular erosions, although erythema of the mucosa and changes in the mucosal vascular pattern have been thought to reflect oesophagitis. The erosions may progress to patchy ulceration which eventually becomes confluent. The inflammation always occurs in the squamous mucosa immediately proximal to the squamocolumnar junction. Severe oesophagitis may lead to fibrosis and stricture. Long-standing reflux oesophagitis leads to metaplastic changes, with this inflamed squamous epithelium being replaced with columnar epithelium (Barrett's oesophagus). The symptoms of reflux oesophagitis are similar to those of gastro-oesophageal reflux, but also include pain on swallowing and dysphagia. Dysphagia may indicate the development of a stricture (fibrous narrowing), but is most commonly due to oedema and other inflammatory changes and motility disturbances.

Complications

1. *Stricture.* This is usually suggested by progressive dysphagia for solids.
2. *Haemorrhage.* Bleeding can be massive and present with haematemesis and/or melaena, or may be occult and lead to iron deficiency. (See Chapter 2, p. 25.)
3. *Development of columnar (Barrett's) epithelium.* Long-standing oesophagitis results in columnar metaplasia with or without inflammation and stricture at the squamocolumnar junction. Patients with Barrett's epithelium are at risk of developing adenocarcinoma in the distal oesophagus. Carcinoma is usually preceded by the development of dysplasia in the columnar epithelium.
4. *Pulmonary aspiration syndrome.* A small proportion of patients with severe gastro-oesophageal reflux develop recurrent inhalation of refluxed gastric contents. These patients may have an abnormality of the upper oesophageal sphincter, which acts as a 'second barrier' to gastric contents entering the lungs. Inhalation usually occurs at night and may lead to pneumonia or lung abscess. Chronic dry cough, laryngitis and asthma are occasionally attributable to recurrent inhalation of gastric contents, especially in children.

The diagnosis of gastro-oesophageal reflux and oesophagitis

This is usually based on a typical clinical history and response to treatment. Barium meal examination has been used to document the presence of gastro-oesophageal reflux, but the patients are studied only for a very brief period and gastro-oesophageal reflux can occur in normal individuals, so that barium meal examination cannot be used to establish that symptoms are due to oesophageal reflux (although it can give indirect evidence of oesophagitis by demonstrating superficial ulceration in the oesophagus). Twenty-four-hour ambulatory intra-oesophageal pH monitoring can be used to quantitate reflux (p. 7)—especially in patients where the diagnosis cannot be established in other ways. Reflux oesophagitis is best diagnosed by fibreoptic endoscopy with mucosal biopsy. Oesophageal manometry is of little help in the diagnosis of gastro-oesophageal reflux and oesophagitis.

Treatment of gastro-oesophageal reflux and oesophagitis

Treatment is aimed at reducing the frequency and duration of reflux episodes and at decreasing the damaging effects of refluxed fluid on oesophageal mucosa. The measures used include:

1. removal of exacerbating factors
   - (a) weight reduction, in obese patients
   - (b) avoidance of large meals
   - (c) avoidance of food or drink for three hours before bedtime
   - (d) avoidance of specific foods, and of smoking or alcohol, if these exacerbate symptoms
2. postural treatment
   - (a) raising of the head of the bed (on bricks) by 15 cm
   - (b) avoidance of any posture, such as bending or stooping, that increases reflux
3. drug treatment: cisapride and metoclopramide hasten the rate of gastric emptying, increase the force of oesophageal contractions, and may raise resting pressure in the lower oesophageal sphincter. These drugs are of most value in patients with evidence of abnormally slow gastric emptying.

Reflux oesophagitis is treated by the measures listed above, but antisecretory agents are also used to reduce the acid output and volume of the refluxed fluid. Cimetidine, ranitidine and famotidine are all effective in controlling the symptoms of reflux oesophagitis, but in the doses commonly used do not result in the healing of erosions or ulcers. Omeprazole is dramatically effective in both controlling symptoms and healing in oesophagitis, but there is a high relapse rate when treatment is ceased. Antacids may provide symptomatic relief, but these need to be taken frequently and do not heal oesophagitis or prevent complications.

In patients resistant to the above measures, particularly in those in whom complications develop, surgery is required: a valve-like mechanism is created at the oesophagogastric junction by wrapping the gastric fundus around the lower part of the oesophagus (fundoplication). The procedure can be performed laparoscopically, although long-term results of this form of surgery have not been established. Other surgical techniques aimed at controlling gastro-oesophageal reflux have also been described. If stricture occurs, regular peroral dilatation may be performed at the time of endoscopy; all such patients should also be on antisecretory agents or should undergo anti-reflux surgery.

Hiatus hernia

A hiatus hernia arises when a part of the stomach herniates through the oesophageal hiatus of the diaphragm.

Classification

There are three types of hiatus hernia (Fig. 1.2):

1. sliding hiatus hernia, in which the gastro-oesophageal junction slides up into the mediastinum (this accounts for about three-quarters of all cases);
2. para-oesophageal or 'rolling' hernia, in which the gastro-oesophageal junction remains in normal position below the diaphragm but a pouch of stomach herniates through the oesophageal hiatus alongside the lower part of the oesophagus; and
3. mixed type, in which sometimes both sliding and rolling types are combined.

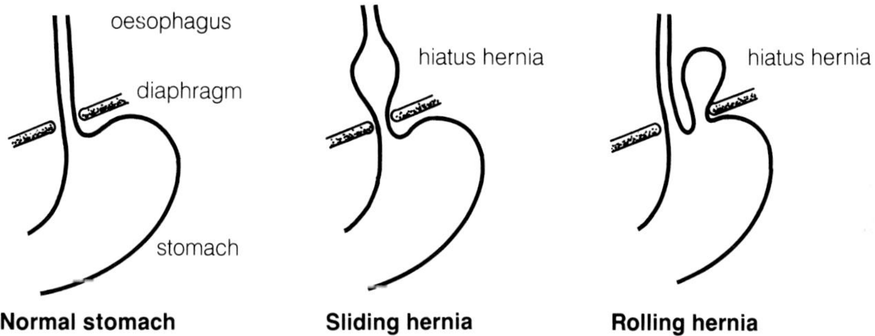

Fig. 1.2 *Anatomical types of hiatus hernia* FROM PIPER, D. W. (ED.), *MEDICINE FOR STUDENTS AND NURSES,* 2ND EDN., McGRAW-HILL, SYDNEY, 1980 WITH PERMISSION

Symptoms and signs

Hiatus hernia is a very common condition, and in the vast majority of cases it is asymptomatic. Symptoms, if present, occur in middle age and are due to:

1. Reflux of the gastric contents into the oesophagus. The relationship of hiatus hernia to oesophageal reflux is not clear, but hiatus hernia probably slightly increases the risk of reflux.
2. Mechanical effects:
   (a) lower restrosternal and epigastric pain fitting no fixed pattern, probably due to intermittent obstruction of the herniated stomach; and
   (b) dyspnoea, if the stomach is predominantly in the chest and reduces the vital capacity.
3. Anaemia: chronic blood loss resulting in iron-deficiency anaemia may occur in patients with otherwise uncomplicated hiatus hernia. Bleeding may be due to linear erosions at the level of the diaphragmatic impression.
4. Volvulus. The intrathoracic part of the stomach in patients with large, rolling hiatus hernias may undergo volvulus. This results in sudden, severe chest pain associated with an inability to swallow.

Diagnosis

This depends on a barium swallow and meal. Endoscopy may not accurately determine the position of the oesophago-gastric junction; however, if dysphagia is present, endoscopy is required to confirm the presence of oesophagitis and to exclude malignancy.

Treatment

The treatment of *sliding* hiatus hernia is basically that for any associated reflux or oesophagitis. In *rolling* hiatus hernia the risk of strangulation is high enough for some to advocate surgery for this indication alone; repair of the hiatus is all that is required. Surgery is essential in patients whose symptoms suggest recurrent gastric volvulus.

Achalasia of the oesophagus

This is an uncommon disease, in which there is abnormal motility in both the body of the oesophagus and the lower oesophageal sphincter. There is failure of both peristalsis in the body of the oesophagus and relaxation of the lower oesophageal sphincter. The tightly closed sphincter will not allow food into the stomach and the atonic oesophagus slowly becomes grossly dilated and tortuous.

Aetiology

There is loss of ganglion cells in the myenteric plexus which is progressive, and the motor disturbances can be explained by denervation, the cause of which is not known.

Symptoms

The disorder may present at any age, but the diagnosis is most frequently made in middle-aged adults. The main symptom is dysphagia, with both liquids and solids equally affected. Dysphagia usually occurs with every meal and is slowly progressive. Many patients do not present until symptoms have been present for months or years. The patients have often become accustomed to eating their food very slowly, 'washing it down' with large amounts of fluid. The condition is chronic and progressive.

Weight loss is common. Pain is not usually a prominent or presenting feature, although many patients report retrosternal discomfort which may be present for months or years before the onset of dysphagia. Regurgitation of undigested food and saliva is a common symptom and usually occurs when the patient bends over or lies flat. The regurgitation may occur when the patient is asleep and be associated with symptoms due to aspiration of oesophageal contents.

Differential diagnosis

This includes benign stricture, oesophageal cancer, diffuse oesophageal spasm and, in South America, Chagas' disease (see opposite).

Diagnosis
The most helpful procedures are:

1. a chest x-ray, which may reveal the dilated oesophagus with or without pulmonary complications;
2. a barium swallow, which shows a dilated oesophagus partially filled with food residue and with an air-fluid level. The lower oesophagus symmetrically tapers to a smooth inverted cone;
3. fibreoptic endoscopy, which confirms the great dilation of the oesophagus; the instrument can also be passed freely through the lower oesophageal sphincter into the stomach. It is important to exclude carcinoma of the oesophagus and cardia, as this can also produce aperistalsis;
4. oesophageal manometry, which confirms the failure of relaxation of the lower oesophageal sphincter in response to swallowing and the failure of peristalsis in the body of the oesophagus;
5. radioisotope transit studies,which can be used to quantitate oesophageal emptying and differentiate achalasia from other causes of dysphagia.

Treatment
The disease process is irreversible, but relief can be provided by destroying the muscular lower oesophageal sphincter, thus allowing food to drain out of the oesophagus by gravity. This can be done by pneumatic dilatation at oesophagoscopy, or by performing a Heller cardiomyotomy operation (in which the lower oesophageal sphincter is divided). Both forms of therapy have a success rate of about 80%.

Chagas' disease

In South American countries a disease identical to achalasia results from infection with *Trypanosoma cruzi*, which damages the myenteric plexus of the gut. Treatment is similar to that for primary achalasia. Megacolon and megaureter also occur.

Diffuse oesophageal spasm

In this type of oesophageal motility disorder, the lower oesophageal sphincter relaxes normally but the peristaltic waves are absent or ineffectual, leading to painful, high-pressure, non-propulsive contractions of the oesophagus on swallowing. The pain may at times simulate ischaemic heart pain and is often induced by swallowing cold fluids. It is an important cause of severe, non-cardiac chest pain. Dysphagia occurs with both fluids and solids.

Diagnosis
Barium swallow can produce normal results, but typically shows failure of peristalsis with the trapping of beads of barium in the oesophagus by segmental

contractions—the so-called 'corkscrew oesophagus'. Manometry also shows that swallowing is accompanied by high-amplitude, non-peristaltic contractions. This is necessary for accurate recognition of the disorder.

Treatment

Adequate control of symptoms is often difficult. Drugs that reduce the vigour of smooth muscle contraction sometimes help (e.g. nitrites, nitrates, calcium antagonists, hydralazine). In a very small proportion of patients with disabling symptoms, long oesophageal myotomy may be necessary.

Oesophageal webs

Epithelial changes resulting in web formation may occur, especially in the postcricoid region, usually in women over fifty years of age. The Plummer-Vinson (or Paterson-Kelly) syndrome is the association of dysphagia due to postcricoid oesophageal webs, iron-deficiency anaemia, glossitis and stomatitis. These disorders may occur independently, however, and up to 50% of patients with webs have no associated anaemia. An association with upper oesophageal cancer is debatable.

Diagnosis

Barium swallow or cineradiology shows a typical, sharply defined filling defect anteriorly in the postcricoid region.

Treatment

Oesophagoscopy usually ruptures the web, and at the same time other possible oesophageal disorders can be excluded. Where iron deficiency is present, it should be treated.

Lower oesophageal (Schatzki) ring

This is a smooth, symmetrical narrowing at the lower oesophagus due to a thin, fibrous diaphragm of mucosa at the squamocolumnar junction. It is probably developmental but usually coexists with a small sliding hiatus hernia. There is no associated inflammation, but reflux oesophagitis has been suggested as a cause. Both sexes are equally affected, usually those over fifty years of age.

Symptoms

The characteristic symptom is episodic, brief dysphagia for both solids and liquids, usually occurring during a hot, hurried meal, usually of meat ('steakhouse syndrome'). Attacks occur at intervals of weeks or months with no symptoms in between.

Diagnosis

The diagnosis is usually made by barium swallow examination. The ring may also be identified at endoscopy.

Treatment

Reassurance and appropriate advice about eating in a relaxed, unhurried fashion is all that is usually required; however, the passage of a large bougie, which fractures the ring, is a simple measure that may relieve symptoms.

Mallory-Weiss tear

This is a postemetic mucosal tear of the lower part of the oesophagus or cardia associated with haemorrhage. The syndrome accounts for 5% of hospital admissions for haematemesis (p. 29).

Symptoms and signs

Classically, non-bloody vomiting is followed by mild to moderate haematemesis. Occasionally there is blood in the first vomit. Many patients are alcoholic.

Diagnosis

Endoscopy is essential for diagnosis, and shows the superficial linear mucosal tears along the lesser curve of the stomach (80%), elsewhere in the stomach (10%) or in the oesophagus (10%) (Boerhaave's syndrome).

Treatment

Active treatment is seldom needed; however:

1. blood transfusion may be necessary;
2. surgery, with suture of the laceration, may be required in patients with continued bleeding or perforation.

Carcinoma of the oesophagus

This occurs in the upper, middle and lower third of the oesophagus in the ratio of 1:2:3. It is usually a squamous cell carcinoma, but at the lower oesophagus it may be an adenocarcinoma, arising either in columnar epithelium lying in the distal oesophagus (Barrett's epithelium) or from the gastric fundus. Alcohol consumption and cigarette-smoking are predisposing factors. There is a marked geographic variation in incidence, the disease being very common in Asia, the Middle East and South Africa.

Symptoms

Dysphagia is the usual presenting symptom. It is rapidly progressive and classically worse with solids.

Diagnosis

Physical examination is usually unrewarding, except occasionally for an enlarged supraclavicular lymph node or, in the late stage, evidence of pulmonary complications or enlargement of the liver due to metastatic involvement. The most helpful diagnostic procedures are those involved in the diagnosis of other lesions of the upper gastrointestinal tract, and include:

1. barium swallow, which characteristically shows an irregular constriction of the lumen of the oesophagus and proximal dilatation;
2. fibreoptic endoscopy with biopsy;
3. computed tomography, which provides useful information about tumour growth and spread;
4. endoscopic ultrasound, which may also be useful in staging of disease.

Treatment and prognosis

The treatment of choice is surgical resection, which offers both palliation and a chance of cure; however, surgery carries high mortality, particularly in patients with lesions in the middle or proximal oesophagus. Cure is seldom possible, with an overall five-year survival of approximately 5%. High-dose radiotherapy may improve survival in patients with squamous cell carcinoma. A number of methods for relieving dysphagia are available in those patients who are unsuitable for surgery. A silicone tube or expanding metal prosthesis can be pushed through the narrowed segment following dilatation at the time of endoscopy. Laser photo-ablation can also be used to relieve dysphagia.

SUGGESTED FURTHER READING

De Caestecker, J. S., Blackwell, J. N., Pryde, A. and Heading, R. C., Daytime gastro-oesophageal reflux is important in oesophagitis, *Gut*, 1987; 28:519–26.

Hendrix, T. R., Schatzki ring, epithelial junction and hiatus hernia—an unresolved controversy, *Gastroenterology*, 1980; 79:584–5.

Hetzel, D., Medical treatment of reflux oesophagitis, *Gullet*, 1993; 3: supp. 60–9.

Kahrilas, P. J., Hiatus hernia causes reflux, Fact or fiction, *Gullet*, 1993; 3: supp. 21–30.

Katz, P. O., Dalton, C. B., Richter, J. E., Wu, W. C. and Castell, D. O., Esophageal testing of patients with noncardiac chest pain or dysphagia, *Ann Intern Med*, 1987; 106:593–7.

Sleisenger, M. H. and Fordtran, J. S. (eds), *Gastrointestinal Disease: Pathophysiology, Diagnosis and Management*, 5th edn, W. B. Saunders, Philadelphia, 1993.

Spechler, S. J., Endoscopic surveillance for patients with Barrett's esophagus: does the cancer risk justify the practice? *Ann Intern Med*, 1987; 106:902–4.

Tobin, R. W. and Pope, C. E., Oesophageal motility, *Current Opinion in Gastroenterology*, 1993; 9:622–8.

Vantrappen, G. et al., Achalasia, diffuse esophageal spasm and related motility disorders, *Gastroenterology*, 1979; 76:450–7.

CHAPTER 2

Stomach and duodenum

S. K. Lam, J. Y. Kang and D. W. Piper

Anatomy and physiology of the stomach

The stomach serves as a storage and secretory organ. The only function essential for life is the secretion of intrinsic factor which is required for the absorption of vitamin B12.

Anatomically the stomach consists of three parts: the body, comprising the middle two-thirds; the antrum, comprising the lower third; and the fundus, which is a small segment above the level of the cardiac orifice (see Fig. 1.2, p. 11). Two types of glands are scattered throughout the stomach, the gastric glands being chiefly in the body and the pyloric glands being situated in the antrum. The surface epithelium secretes mucus and bicarbonate; the gastric glands, as well as containing mucus-secreting cells, contain parietal cells that secrete acid (at a concentration of 160 mmol/L) and intrinsic factor. The pyloric gland area contains cells that secrete pepsinogen (chief cells), cells that secrete gastrin (G cells) and mucus-secreting cells.

Pathway of acid secretion

Receptor sites for histamine, acetylcholine and gastrin are situated on the cell surface, and stimulation on the receptor sites activates a metabolic process within the cell involving adenylcyclase, cyclic-AMP and calcium, with the production of hydrochloric acid. The latter is then transferred by hydrogen-potassium ATPase to the cell canaliculus and subsequently into the lumen of the stomach. In the treatment of ulcer, acid secretion is inhibited by agents that block receptor sites (cimetidine or ranitidine) or inhibit ATPase (omeprazole or lansoprazole).

Control of gastric secretion

Several factors—including the number of parietal cells (parietal cell mass), humoral factors (gastrin), intrinsic nerve reflexes and vagal stimulation—control gastric acid secretion.

Gastrin is produced by the G cells of the antrum and acts on the parietal cells. It is stimulated by gastric distension and by chemical secretagogues in the food. Secretion is inhibited by an acid gastric pH, and at pH2 is totally blocked.

The vagus is a powerful stimulant of acid secretion, and acts by stimulating the effect of gastrin on the parietal cell; the vagus nerve also stimulates gastrin release. Division of the vagus reduces acid secretion and is used in the surgical treatment of duodenal ulcer.

Bicarbonate secretion

Bicarbonate secretion originates in the surface of the epithelium of the stomach and duodenum. It is quantitatively small compared with acid secretion. Its secretion is stimulated by an acid luminal pH, vagal stimulation and gastric distension. Its close association beneath the mucus layer covering the epithelial cells enables a small amount of bicarbonate to protect against a large amount of acid.

Relationship of acid to pepsin

There is a positive correlation of acid and pepsin secretion: patients with high acid tend to have high pepsin secretions. Pepsin is secreted as pepsinogen, the latter being converted to pepsin at a pH below 6. Pepsin is maximally active at pH2 and is inactive at pH levels above 5.

Gastric emptying

This is determined by two opposing forces, namely the peristaltic waves of the gastric antrum (the pyloric pump) and the resistance of the pylorus. The former is the major determinant, and is stimulated by gastric distension and the hormone gastrin. The latter also relaxes the pylorus.

Gastric emptying is partially inhibited by nervous impulses from the duodenum to the stomach—enterogastric reflexes. By this mechanism, gastric emptying is inhibited by gastric irritants such as highly acidic gastric juice, non-isotonic (hypotonic) fluids, and protein and fat breakdown products. By these mechanisms the role of gastric emptying is limited to the amount of gastric content that the small intestine can process (p. 38).

Gastric emptying of liquids differs from that of solids; in general, liquids empty from the stomach more rapidly. The half-life of liquids in the stomach is twenty minutes and that of a mixed meal is 100 minutes.

Reaction of tissues to acid and pepsin

Columnar epithelium

Columnar epithelium is resistant to acid and pepsin digestion. If a lesion does occur it is a punched-out lesion, as is seen in a chronic peptic ulcer. Why the lesion is a localised punched-out lesion when all of the aetiological factors are diffuse (p. 22) is one of the major unsolved problems of ulcer disease.

Squamous epithelium

Squamous epithelium is not resistant to acid and pepsin, and the lesion which results is a diffuse lesion, as is seen in reflux oesophagitis (p. 8).

Gastric mucosal defence mechanisms

Conceptually, whether or not a patient develops an ulcer is expressed in the ulcer equation:

Acid + Pepsin vs Mucosal resistance.

It merely states that some patients with ulcer have normal acid and pepsin secretion and in these we incriminate the ill-defined entity of mucosal resistance.

The gastric mucosa is exposed to acid and pepsin, often at a pH where pepsin is maximally active (pH 1.5–2.0). Several mechanisms have been postulated in protecting the stomach from autodigestion, but a comparative role of each has not been defined. These include:

1. mucus-bicarbonate barrier. The epithelial cells secrete mucus which covers the cell surface; as well, they secrete a small amount of bicarbonate, and together these two secretions form a continuous barrier. The bicarbonate diffuses across the gel and neutralises acid permeating from the gastric lumen (Fig. 2.1). This dual mechanism keeps acid away from the surface of the epithelium, where neither alone could provide this protection. This barrier is broken by non-steroidal anti-inflammatory drugs (NSAIDs). Also, pepsin with its large molecule is retarded in its passage through the gel layer, and is inactivated in the alkaline environment created by bicarbonate secretion;
2. hydrophobic phospholipid, which covers the gastric mucosa;

3. rapid cell turnover, which replaces cell damage; and
4. mucosal blood flow, which removes noxious agents that have penetrated the mucus layer.

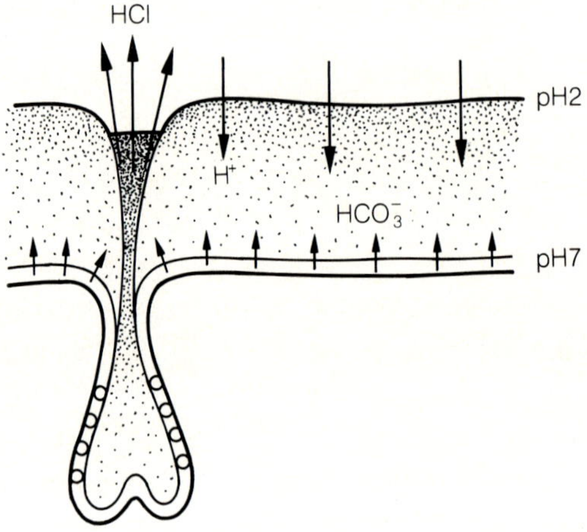

Fig. 2.1 *Diagrammatic representation of the combined 'mucus-bicarbonate' barrier of the gastric mucosa.* MODIFIED FROM FLEMGSTRON, G. AND TURNBERG, L. A. (EDS), ISENBERG, J. I. AND JOHANSSON, C., W. B. SAUNDERS, LONDON, 1984. REPRODUCED WITH PERMISSION

Gastric secretory abnormalities and disease

The secretory abnormalities include hypersecretory and hyposecretory states.

Hypersecretory states

This syndrome is usually due to a gastrin-producing tumour of the pancreas (gastrinoma), and is usually associated with refractory peptic ulcer or oesophagitis.

Hyposecretory states

This syndrome, alternatively called anacidity or achlorhydria, is diagnosed by the failure of the pH of gastric juice to fall below 6 after maximal pentagastrin stimulation. Its clinical relevance relates to:

1. an increased risk of gastric cancer which is increased 3–5 fold in those with pernicious anaemia;
2. an increased risk of gastro-intestinal infections due to the absence of the sterilising effect of acid gastric juice;
3. vitamin B12 deficiency due to lack of intrinsic factor.

It is unlikely therapeutically-induced achlorhydria will cause these complications, as the achlorhydria so induced is not complete or permanent.

The common causes of achlorhydria include:

1. pernicious anaemia;
2. therapeutically-induced achlorhydria as seen in the use of potent ATPase inhibitors;
3. gastric resection or irradiation.

Peptic ulcer

Definition and classification

Peptic ulcer is a benign, localised defect in the mucosa of any part of the gastrointestinal tract which is exposed to acid and pepsin. Peptic ulcer most commonly occurs in the duodenum (duodenal ulcer), stomach (gastric ulcer) and occasionally in the jejunum (post-operative, stomal ulcers or jejunal ulcers).

Peptic ulcers may be chronic or acute. An acute ulcer has a short duration and will not recur if the underlying cause can be removed. A chronic ulcer is a prolonged disease with exacerbations and remissions.

Pathologically, chronic ulcers are at least 5 mm in diameter and have developed fibrosis at their bases; acute ulcers heal with little or no fibrosis. Endoscopically or radiologically, chronicity of the peptic ulcer can sometimes be inferred from surrounding mucosal scarring and sometimes from the ulcer depth but a clear-cut distinction may not always be possible. The term 'erosion' is often used if the lesion is localised to the mucosa, but as depth cannot be determined accurately it is best not to use this term; use ulcer size as an indication of chronicity.

Site

Gastric ulcers most commonly occur in the antrum, just distal to the junction of the body and antral mucosa on the lesser curve. Ninety-five per cent of duodenal ulcers occur in the duodenal bulb, and anterior ulcers outnumber posterior ones by a factor of 2 to 1. Ulcers occur rarely in the jejunum. If they do, they follow the creation of a surgical stoma or the occurrence of the Zollinger-Ellison syndrome.

Epidemiological aspects

It has been estimated that 15–25% of persons would have an ulcer at some stage of their life. The point prevalence of peptic ulcer is 3–5%; if the patient is taking NSAID, the point prevalence may range from 20–30%.

There are marked temporal, geographical and racial variations in the frequency of ulcer disease. In most Western countries its frequency is thought to have fallen over the last few decades. In contrast, the incidence of ulcer complications has increased in Hong Kong and Singapore. Ulcer disease is uncommon in Aboriginal Australians. In Singapore, the Chinese are three times more likely to present with an ulcer than Malays. In those on NSAID therapy, gastric ulcer is more common than duodenal ulcer and women are more commonly involved than men.

In most countries duodenal ulcer is more common than gastric ulcer and both are more common in men than women; however, in Japan, gastric ulcers are more common, while in Australia women are more prone than men to develop gastric ulcer.

The prevalence of both gastric ulcer and duodenal ulcer increases with age; however, patients with gastric ulcer are on average ten years older than those with duodenal ulcer. There is often a positive family history of peptic ulcer, gastric ulcer patients tending to have relatives with gastric ulcer and vice versa for duodenal ulcer.

Aetiology

The aetiology of peptic ulcer has not been completely worked out, but the ulcer equation which was mentioned earlier (p. 19):

Acid + Pepsin vs Mucosal resistance

implies that whether or not a patient develops an ulcer depends upon the opposing forces of peptic digestion and mucosal resistance.

Environmental factors

Most peptic ulcers are due to environmental factors. Aetiological factors relevant in gastric ulcer disease are different from those for duodenal ulcer. For gastric ulcer, smoking, the use of aspirin and non-aspirin and non-steroidal anti-inflammatory drugs are important. The relative risks of gastric ulcer, that is, the frequency of ulcer in those exposed to a particular environmental factor compared to those who are unexposed, varies from 2 for smoking, to 8 for the use of non-aspirin or non-steroidal anti-inflammatory drugs, to 17 for the consumption of more than five tablets of aspirin per day. For duodenal ulcer, smoking confers a relative risk of 7 in the case of men and 2 in the case of women. The use of aspirin does not affect the relative risk of duodenal ulcer disease while non-aspirin, non-steroidal or anti-inflammatory drugs at most marginally increase susceptibility. In contrast, neither alcohol nor the use of paracetamol increases the chances of development of either gastric or duodenal ulcer; alcohol has a protective effect with a relative risk of 0.6. The relative risks of environmental factors and the course of chronic ulcer is shown in Figure 2.2.

Many authors now believe that *Helicobacter pylori* is one cause of peptic ulcer disease. This organism occurs in a large proportion of apparently healthy subjects and is a major cause of histological gastritis. The occurrence of histological gastritis increases the risk of development of peptic ulcer by fourteen times over the next ten years compared to subjects without gastritis. Eradication of *Helicobacter pylori* changes the natural history of peptic ulcer disease and dramatically reduces its recurrence rate. The matter, however, is not totally resolved.

Gastric secretion and peptic ulcer

On average, patients with gastric ulcer have acid secretion rates similar to those of healthy controls. In duodenal ulcer, acid secretion is increased above the normal range in most subjects. One-third of duodenal ulcer patients, however, have normal acid secretion.

Gastric secretory testing is only useful clinically in the extremes of achlorhydria or hyperchlorhydria. Peptic ulcer does not occur in the achlorhydric patient, whereas in the Zollinger-Ellison syndrome there is acid hypersecretion, and the basal acid output usually exceeds 15 mmol/h.

Genetic factors

Duodenal ulcer is more common in those belonging to blood group O (relative risk 1.3), in those with high serum pepsinogen-1 levels, and in those who cannot secrete blood group substances (non-secretors). A slightly increased incidence of gastric ulcer is seen in those who are alpha$_1$-antitrypsin-deficient.

Psychosomatic factors

People with ulcers tend to have a personality that is more neurotic than those without ulcers. The difference is slight, however, and probably of little clinical relevance. Acute life-event stress is not a risk factor for ulcer, but there is reasonable evidence that chronic-difficulty stress persisting for at least six months is a risk factor for both gastric and duodenal ulcer.

Symptoms

The symptoms and signs of peptic ulcer are:

1. Abdominal discomfort or pain

This is usually epigastric or slightly to the right or left of the midline (refer to Fig. 9.1); however, it can occur anywhere from the nipple level to the inguinal ligaments. It tends to occur when the patient is hungry, half an hour to three hours after meals, to be relieved by food, antacids and vomiting and to wake the patient up at night. The pain is initially localised and the patient often points a single finger to the site of the pain; as the pain becomes more severe, it becomes more diffuse and sometimes radiates to the back in the interscapular region. Radiation to the back may be an index of the severity of pain, or it may imply penetration of the ulcer through the stomach or duodenal wall and invasion of other organs. Pancreatic involvement is common and the patient will then complain of back pain at L1 to L2 region. The pain will often be described in fanciful terms, but the only relevant characteristics are that it is deep-seated, related to meals and often nocturnal, and that it exacerbates and remits.

The majority of patients presenting with ulcer-like abdominal pain will turn out not to have ulcer disease. On the other hand, many ulcer patients present with atypical pains, while some do not have pain. It is therefore not possible to diagnose ulcer disease without resorting to special investigations.

Although duodenal ulcer patients typically have hunger pains and pains that arise later after meals, less commonly vomit and have longer remissions and better responses to medical treatment, the nature of the symptoms does not differentiate between gastric and duodenal ulcer.

Ulcer pain is partly due to acid and pepsin acting on nerve fibres in the base of the ulcer. Other factors must be involved since acid perfusion of ulcer craters reproduces pain in only 40% of subjects in exacerbation. Spasm probably plays no part in causing ulcer pain. In the healing of an ulcer, pain relief occurs early—long before radiological or endoscopic examination shows healing.

2. *Vomiting*

The vomiting associated with ulcer may have one of three causes:

(a) it may be induced by the pain, especially in the case of gastric ulcer;
(b) it may be due to gastric outlet obstruction; or
(c) it may be self-induced if the patient's vomiting eases the pain.

3. *Other symptoms*

Other symptoms that may be present, but of less clinical significance, include weight loss, weight gain—especially in the case of duodenal ulcer when the patient eats to ease the pain—nausea, heartburn, acid regurgitation and constipation.

The only physical sign of an uncomplicated ulcer is localised epigastric tenderness. This sign is, however, non-specific.

Complications

Gastrointestinal haemorrhage

This may manifest itself in the form of haemetemesis or melaena and be accompanied by varying degrees of oligemic shock. Occasionally patients may present with iron-deficiency anaemia from chronic blood loss; however, chronic blood loss in an ulcer patient usually means analgesic ingestion or gastrointestinal cancer and not blood loss from the peptic ulcer.

Gastric outlet obstruction

The obstruction is in the duodenum in cases of duodenal ulcer and in the distal antrum in the case of prepyloric gastric ulcer. The stenosis may be due to spasm or oedema around the ulcer, to fibrosis, or both. The distinction is important since oedema and spasm but not fibrosis can resolve with medical treatment.

Clinically there will be obstructive vomiting, weight loss, dehydration, alkalosis and sodium and potassium depletion. A characteristic feature of vomiting due to gastric outlet obstruction is the vomiting of food which can be recognised to have been consumed more than five hours earlier. A distended stomach with a succussion splash and visible peristalsis can sometimes be detected on abdominal examination. The diagnosis is confirmed at barium meal. Endoscopy is not recommended in the acute phase because a good view cannot be obtained in the presence of food residue and because of the risk of aspiration; however, after gastric decompression, endoscopy is useful to determine the case of obstruction.

Perforation

This results in the sudden pouring of acid content into the peritoneal cavity, with severe abdominal pain, shock and vomiting. Marked rigidity is present and x-ray examination of the abdomen usually shows air under the diaphragm. In the frail, sick or elderly patient the features of ulcer perforation may be masked and a high index of suspicion is required to make the correct diagnosis.

Relationship of gastric ulcer to gastric carcinoma

Most believe that the concomitant occurrence of gastric ulcer and gastric cancer represents a chance relationship. However, one-fifth of gastric cancer appears as ulcerated rather than elevated lesions. Conversely, up to 5% of gastric ulcer which look benign on radiological and endoscopic criteria turn out to be malignant. Therefore, all gastric ulcers should be biopsied, then followed up to healing. Occasionally, cancer can be missed at biopsy or an ulcerated cancer can heal, suggesting that a benign ulcer has undergone malignant change when in fact the lesion has been a carcinoma from the outset.

Natural history of peptic ulcer

Refer to Figure 2.2 (p. 27). Peptic ulcer is characterised by remissions and exacerbations. About one-quarter of patients have minimal symptoms, half have moderate symptoms but lead a normal life, while another one-quarter have severe symptoms. Over a lifetime, about 25% of patients develop haemorrhage while 1–2% of ulcers perforate. The ulcer diathesis persists lifelong, with an average of two to three exacerbations each year.

Diagnosis

Symptoms suggest the need for further investigations, but only a minority of patients with ulcer-like pain have ulcer disease. Diagnostic procedures include double-contrast barium meal studies and fibreoptic endoscopy. If duodenal ulcer or oesophagitis is a possible diagnosis, endoscopy is essential. Endoscopy with biopsy enables the diagnosis of malignant ulcer and *H. pylori* infection to be made. In the case of a duodenal ulcer, barium studies may show bulbar deformity: this can be due to a previous ulcer and does not necessarily indicate active ulcer. In the diagnosis of upper gastrointestinal haemorrhage, endoscopy is definitely superior to barium studies because of the ability to determine the bleeding lesion in cases where more than one lesion is found; the ability to prognosticate on the likelihood of rebleeding based on the presence or absence of stigmata of recent haemorrhage; and the ability to render endoscopic haemostasis. On the other hand, barium studies are cheaper than endoscopy in most countries.

Gastric secretory studies have little place in the routine management of peptic ulcer, but they are indicated when the possibility of gastrinoma arises (p. 124).

Treatment

This involves symptomatic relief, initial healing of the ulcer, prevention of ulcer relapse and treatment of complications.

Symptom relief

Ulcer pains are relieved by the use of antacids or H2-receptor antagonists. Even if treatment is not continued and the ulcer unhealed, ulcer pain may not recur. Although not encouraged by physicians because of the possibility of complications, the use of occasional doses of antacid or H2-receptor antagonists for symptom relief is probably widely practised by patients.

Diet: No dietary restrictions are required, although in patients whose pains are brought on by hunger or by specific food items, appropriate dietary changes would be sensible. There is no evidence that avoidance of chillis, citrus fruits or any other foods promote ulcer healing. Although milk relieves ulcer pain by acting as an antacid, it may stimulate further acid secretion and excessive milk ingestion can theoretically be harmful. Smoking and ingestion of anti-inflammatory drugs should be avoided if possible. There is no evidence that stress or hard work has an adverse influence on the course of peptic ulcer, although hospital admission promotes healing. The mechanism of the latter is unknown but bed-rest is not responsible.

Initial healing

A large number of drugs have been shown to accelerate the healing of both gastric and duodenal ulcer. The various histamine H2-receptor antagonists (cimetidine, ranitidine, famotidine and roxatidine) are the most widely used. They are all equally effective in twice daily dosages or in a single nocturnal dosage. Cimetidine affects plasma levels of drugs metabolised by the hepatic P450 system. Theophylline, warfarin and phenytoin levels become elevated when these drugs are used concurrently with cimetidine, which should be avoided in patients who use these medications. This effect is not present with omeprazole and only to a small extent in those on ranitidine. Colloidal bismuth and sucralfate are as effective as H2-receptor antagonists. Omeprazole, a proton pump blocker, is an extremely potent suppressor of acid secretion and, at a dosage of 20–40 mg

SUMMARY OF MANAGEMENT OF CHRONIC PEPTIC ULCER

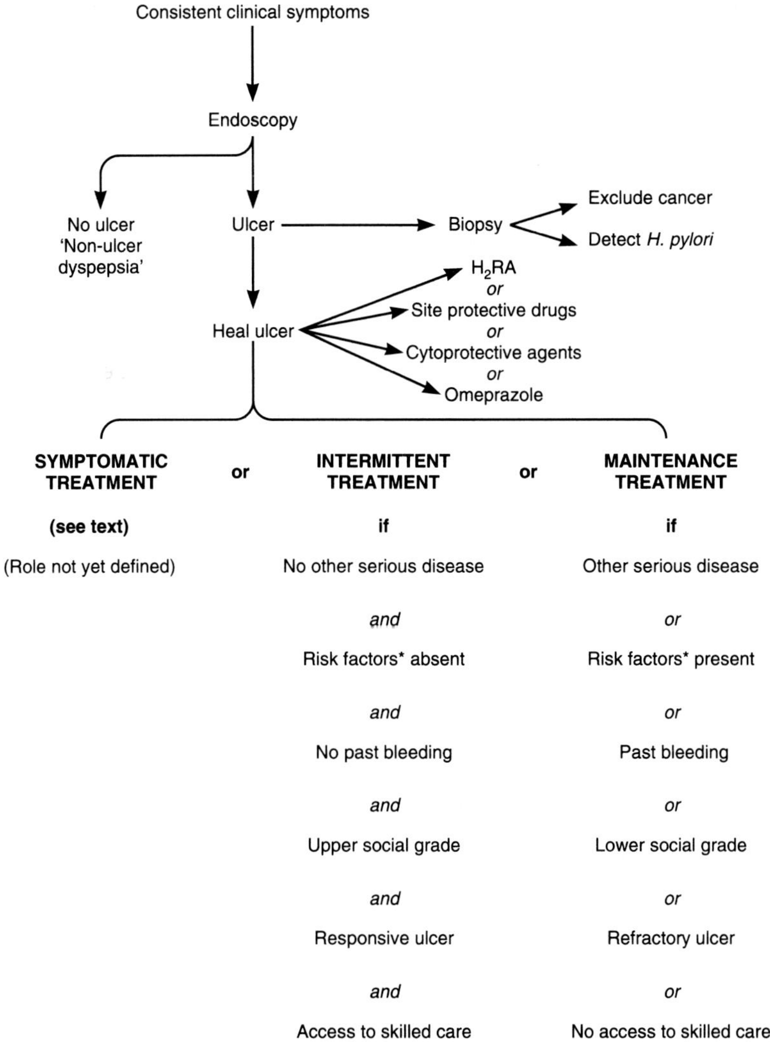

*** Risks and relative risks**

	Gastric Ulcer	Duodenal Ulcer
NSAID	4	1
Aspirin	5	1
Smoking	5	2
Alcohol	0.6	0.6
Paracetamol	1	1
H. pylori	2	4

Fig. 2.2 *Summary of management of chronic peptic ulcer. (H_2RA = H_2 receptor antagonists, NSAID = non-steroidal anti-inflammatory drugs)*

daily, will heal most duodenal ulcers more rapidly than histamine 2 receptor antagonists (H2RA). It is effective in ulcers resistant to other drugs.

It is usually said that high-dose regimes of antacids (420 mEq neutralising capacity daily) have to be used to heal duodenal ulcers, but smaller doses of antacids have recently been shown to be effective also. A large proportion of ulcers will heal on placebo treatment or on no treatment.

The majority of duodenal ulcers will heal after four weeks of treatment. Gastric ulcers are on average larger and take longer to heal. Patients with gastric ulcer should be followed up by endoscopy or radiology and confirmed to be healed, otherwise the occasional malignant ulcer will be missed. For most duodenal ulcer patients it is unnecessary to confirm healing, malignancy not being a problem.

The refractory ulcer

In the majority of patients with peptic ulcer, symptoms will disappear within a few days of starting on effective treatment. Failure of symptoms to respond may indicate:

1. error in diagnosis, the patient's pain being due to irritable colon or to a gastric ulcer being malignant rather than benign;
2. consumption of non-steroidal anti-inflammatory drugs;
3. heavy smoking;
4. gastrinoma.

In some patients symptoms rapidly abate with treatment, but the ulcer crater remains unhealed. This may be due to a large ulcer taking a longer time to heal, to non-compliance with treatment, or to one of the other reasons for continued symptoms listed above. An ulcer refractory to H2-receptor antagonists will almost always respond to ATPase inhibitors.

Long-term treatment

Up to 80% of duodenal ulcers will recur over one year after initial healing once therapy is withdrawn. One of the following options can be followed.

Intermittent therapy

The patient is given no treatment when asymptomatic. Exacerbations are treated with four to six-week courses of medications as used in the initial treatment of ulcer.

Maintenance therapy

A maintenance dose of H2-receptor antagonists, usually half the treatment dose, is given nightly on a long-term basis. This will prevent ulcer recurrence in 70% of cases and is especially indicated in the elderly, those with other serious diseases, those on NSAID, those who have bled and those who have three or more relapses while on intermittent therapy.

Surgery

Elective surgery for uncomplicated ulcers is now uncommon. The usual operation for duodenal ulcer is proximal vagotomy and for gastric ulcer, Billroth gastrectomy.

Management of complications

Acute gastrointestinal haemorrhage

This presents as haematemesis and melaena. Whether one or both occurs depends on the site of the lesion and the severity of bleeding. Lesions beyond the duodenal bulb may not cause haematemesis, while patients with haematemesis tend to have bled more severely compared to those with melaena alone. The black tarry melaenic stools should be distinguished from bright red rectal bleeding more characteristic of colonic or perianal lesions, and from the greyish-greenish stool due to the use of iron supplements. Apart from the haematemesis and melaena, there may be features of hypovolaemic shock, for example, tachycardia, low blood pressure, syncope and cardiac pain. If vital signs are stable in the supine position, a postural drop in blood pressure should be looked for (Fig. 2.3).

Management This includes assessment of severity and resuscitation, diagnosis of the cause of haemorrhage, observation and specific treatment.

Assessment and resuscitation Immediate blood replacement is indicated if there is marked tachycardia (pulse > 110), hypotension (blood pressure < 110 systolic), signs of hypovolaemic shock, or a haemoglobin level below 90 mg/L.

Diagnosis Approximately 40% of patients with upper gastrointestinal haemorrhage have bled from duodenal ulcer: 20% from chronic gastric ulcers, 20% from acute ulcers often associated with analgesic ingestion, 10% from oesophageal varices, 10% from other causes such as Mallory-Weiss lesions, reflux oesophagitis and gastric tumours.

Only when the haemodynamic status of the patient is stable should an attempt be made to diagnose the cause of the bleeding.

Exact diagnosis using endoscopy is essential. Haemorrhage from an acute ulcer not due to other serious disease has a good prognosis (< 1% mortality), whereas bleeding from a chronic peptic ulcer, especially gastric ulcer, is associated with a higher mortality rate (10–15% mortality), particularly in older patients. Bleeding from oesophageal varices has a particularly high mortality and the management strategy is different.

The endoscopic appearance of peptic ulcer is a good indicator of subsequent outcome. Ulcers which are actively spurting or oozing have the greatest chance of rebleeding. Ulcers with a visible vessel have a 50% chance of rebleeding, whereas ulcers with clean bases seldom rebleed.

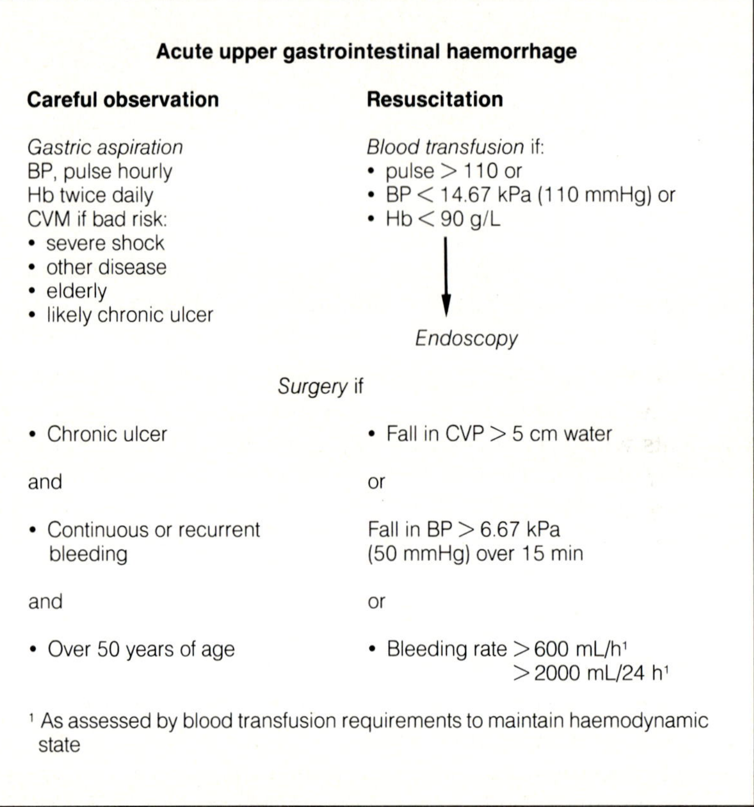

Fig. 2.3 *Plan of management of acute upper gastrointestinal haemorrhage due to ulcer. CVM = central venous monitoring*

Observation All patients with suspected or proven upper gastrointestinal bleeding should be in hospital if a bad risk (over sixty years of age, chronic ulcer, other serious diseases) and should be in an intensive care ward, jointly cared for by the intensivist, a gastroenterologist and a surgeon.

Any further haematemesis or melaena should be noted. Vital signs should be monitored at least hourly and the haemoglobin level estimated twice daily until the patient is stable. Central venous monitoring is indicated in elderly subjects. Continuous gastric aspiration is helpful in detecting continued or recurrent bleeding.

The initial bleed will usually cease spontaneously. Haematemesis, the aspiration of fresh blood from the stomach, significant changes in the pulse, blood pressure or central venous pressure, or a marked drop in haemoglobin level, indicate continued bleeding or rebleeding. The passage of fresh melaena has the same significance. Stale melaena due to the original bleed may continue for several days. Where there is doubt as to whether a patient has rebled, repeat endoscopy may be required.

Specific treatment for bleeding peptic ulcer

There is no evidence that any anti-secretory drug prevents rebleeding.

In cases of active bleeding or ulcer craters with visible vessels in their bases, endoscopy provides an opportunity to render treatment to reduce the chances of rebleeding. Two methods are applicable:

1. injection of a dilute solution of adrenalin with or without a sclerosant. The adrenalin causes vasoconstriction, while the volume of the injection provides a pressure effect and the sclerosant induces local oedema. All these may help to produce thrombosis of the vessels;
2. thermal coagulation can be achieved using a heater probe or NdYag laser.

In patients over sixty years of age with chronic peptic ulcers and continued or recurrent bleeding, surgery is advised, especially if other serious disease is present. Patients with severe bleeding and the signs of oligaemic shock on admission also benefit from surgery, irrespective of their age or the presence of recurrent or continued bleeding. In each case one has to balance the risk of emergency surgery, which is significant especially in the elderly sick person, against the risk of death from exsanguination.

Chronic gastrointestinal bleeding

This presents as iron-deficiency anaemia. In men and post-menopausal women, iron-deficiency anaemia should be assumed to be due to gastrointestinal blood loss, since dietary deficiency and malabsorption rarely presents in this way. Gastrointestinal cancer and colonic polyps have to be considered. Peptic ulcer does not cause chronic blood loss. If both are present, an analgesic associated ulcer is likely, the blood loss being due to microbleeding due to NSAID. Upper and lower gastrointestinal evaluation by endoscopy or radiology is usually required. When there is a need to establish the diagnosis of blood loss, labelling of red cells with radioactive chromium is superior to chemical tests for detection of faecal occult blood which frequently give false positive and false negative results.

Gastric outlet obstruction

There are three causes:

1. para-pyloric stenosis from prepyloric gastric ulcer or duodenal ulcer;
2. carcinoma of the gastric antrum;
3. hypertrophic pyloric stenosis due to hypertrophy of the pyloric antral musculature.

Initial treatment includes fluid and electrolyte replacement. Normal saline supplemented with potassium is given intravenously. Gastric distension is alleviated by nasal gastric suction. If the obstruction is due to ulcer disease, histamine-2 antagonists or omeprazole are given intravenously and antacids can also be instilled into the stomach.

Obstruction due to ulcer disease will often lessen as oedema subsides but severe fibrotic strictures and carcinoma require surgery. In ulcer disease, endoscopic assessment of the severity of obstruction can be misleading. A more reliable assessment is provided by the ability of the stomach to empty barium: 30–40 mL of barium sulphate is given and plain x-ray of the abdomen taken two to four hours later. If delayed emptying persists for three days, surgery is indicated as a matter of urgency. Parenteral nutrition may be required pre- and postoperatively.

Perforation

Treatment is surgical and an operation should be performed as soon as possible after perforation.

Special types of ulcers

Postoperative ulcers (stomal ulcer)

After surgery, an ulcer may occur in the remaining stomach or duodenum, on the stomal anastomosis or in the nearby small intestine (usually efferent loop). Symptoms are similar to those of an ordinary peptic ulcer. Diagnosis is by endoscopy; the possibility of a gastrinoma has to be considered.

Treatment is similar to that of an ordinary peptic ulcer, except that omeprazole is preferred as the anti-secretory drug.

Acute gastric ulcer

Many patients with bleeding or perforated ulcers have a short history of dyspepsia. The absence of marked fibrosis also suggests that such ulcers are acute. Some of these ulcers may be associated with the use of anti-inflammatory drugs.

Patients with major medical illnesses or those who have undergone severe trauma or major surgery sometimes develop acute ulcers. These may be gastric or duodenal, and are frequently multiple. They present with bleeding or perforation. Treatment involves the use of antacids with or without histamine-2 antagonists, the dosage being titrated to maintain gastric pH above 4. Sucralfate has also been used to prevent ulcer development and may be associated with a lower risk of pneumonia. Stress ulcers may carry a high mortality rate because of the associated serious illnesses.

Endocrine ulcers

Less than 1% of duodenal ulcers have a known endocrine origin. The best recognised is the Zollinger-Ellison syndrome, or gastrinoma. This syndrome should be considered if:

1. symptoms are severe and respond poorly to medical or surgical treatment;
2. the ulcers are large or multiple and situated distal to the first part of the duodenum;
3. reflux oesophagitis and diarrhoea are present;
4. ulcers recur following surgery.

Diagnosis is based on a consistent clinical syndrome, markedly elevated serum gastrin level and elevated basal acid output. Provocative tests are available in cases of doubt.

The analgesic-associated ulcer

There are no specific clinical features associated with ulcers related to the use of analgesics; however, these ulcers are often large, painless, occur in elderly subjects—especially females—and are often associated with bleeding or perforation. Response to medical treatment may not be satisfactory, especially if the analgesics are not able to be withdrawn. Omeprazole is often useful in this clinical setting.

A history of analgesic ingestion is important in all patients with peptic ulcers.

Usually the ulcer heals despite continued NSAID ingestion. Omeprazole is the preferred ulcer healing agent. The need for the analgesics should be reviewed.

Helicobacter pylori–associated ulcer

It has recently been reported that eradication of *Helicobacter pylori* in the patient with duodenal ulcer reduces subsequent relapse rates to less than 10%. This treatment can therefore be offered to patients who have suffered previous complications or who frequently experience recurrence.

Whether all ulcer patients who are *H. pylori* positive should have *H. pylori* eradicated is currently being determined. No patient should have elective surgery unless eradication of *H. pylori* has failed to produce long-term ulcer control.

Gastritis

Acute gastritis

This is characterised by anorexia, nausea and vomiting. It can be the result of:

1. infection such as by *Helicobacter pylori*;
2. ingestion of inflammatory agents such as alcohol and non-steroidal anti-inflammatory drugs; and
3. acute stress as occurring in patients who are critically ill, in whom the pathology is that of acute haemorrhagic gastritis and in whom gastrointestinal bleeding can occur.

Patients who are critically ill should be given sucralfate, a gastro-protective agent, or acid-reducing agents such as antacids, as prophylaxis against such 'stress ulcer bleeding'. In practice, similar self-limited symptoms of anorexia, nausea and vomiting may be diagnosed clinically as acute gastritis, but such diagnoses are presumptive.

Chronic gastritis

Chronic gastritis is characterised to varying degrees by mucosal infiltration with mononuclear and polymorphonuclear cells, intestinal metaplasia and glandular atrophy. There is a spectrum of histological appearances. In chronic superficial gastritis, inflammation is marked and glandular atrophy is minimal. In chronic atrophic gastritis, inflammation coexists with glandular atrophy, whereas in gastric atrophy inflammatory cells are few and glandular atrophy extensive. It is most likely that these appearances represent different stages of chronic gastritis: from superficial gastritis to atrophic gastritis to gastric atrophy, a process that has been estimated to take about nineteen years.

There are two important causes and types of chronic gastritis:

1. Type A or autoimmune gastritis involves the body and fundus and spares the antrum. Antibodies to parietal cells are present, and pernicious anaemia may result, with achlorhydria and defective intrinsic factor secretion. There is a four-fold increase in the risk of developing gastric carcinoma.
2. Type B gastritis is mostly associated with *Helicobacter pylori* infection. It occurs in about half the general population, being less frequent in advanced countries and more so in underdeveloped parts of the world. It increases in frequency with age, is often accompanied by intestinal metaplasia, and occurs usually in the antrum but can spread to the body and fundus, particularly with ageing. It is closely associated with duodenal ulcer in the form of a diffuse antral gastritis, as well as with gastric ulcer in the form of multifocal atrophic gastritis; the latter pattern is also associated with gastric carcinoma.

A mixture of these two types can occur. Giant hypertrophic gastritis (Menetrier's disease) is a separate form of chronic gastritis, associated sometimes with excessive protein loss from giant mucosal folds in the gastric body. Recently, two specific forms of gastritis have been recognised: lymphocytic gastritis, which may be related to intestinal malabsorption syndromes; and reflux gastritis, originally described in postgastrectomy specimens and now linked to non-steroidal anti-inflammatory drugs and other chemical injuries.

It is unlikely that chronic gastritis can give rise to clinical symptoms, except in prepyloric gastritis associated with erosions, where ulcer-like pain may be experienced and where H2-receptor antagonists have been shown to be helpful.

Gastritis can be diagnosed by endoscopy and multiple biopsies. Erythema, oedema, petechiae and erosions are commonly seen, but the appearances do not correlate well with the histological changes. The recently introduced 'Sydney System' for the classification of gastritis recommends a descriptive classification, taking into consideration the endoscopic appearance, histological changes, severity grading, anatomical involvement and aetiological factors. (See reference number 4 on page 37.)

Gastric carcinoma

Frequency

Gastric carcinoma (with colonic and pancreatic carcinoma) is one of the three most common cancers of the gastrointestinal tract. There are marked geographical variations in its incidence, up to twenty-fold differences being described between high-risk countries (e.g. China, Costa Rica, Japan) and low-risk countries (e.g. Australia, United States, Western Europe). The risk of gastric carcinoma in Japanese who migrate to the United States is reduced by 25%; the risk is further reduced by 50% in the second-generation Japanese born in the United States. Even within the same country, people in different regions experience different risks of gastric cancer development. For example, northern Chinese are three times more likely to develop gastric cancer than southern Chinese. These differences in the frequency of gastric cancer over place and time suggest that environmental influences are important in the causation.

Pathogenesis and pathology

Two recent studies, one in Europe and one in China, observed that the frequency of gastric cancer correlated with the frequency of *Helicobacter pylori* in the population. Recent studies have also shown that the relative risk of gastric cancer is between 1.6 and 6 in people with *Helicobacter pylori* infection followed for three to fourteen years. Other conditions associated with a several-fold increase in risk of gastric cancer include: pernicious anaemia, atrophic gastritis, adenomatous polyps of the stomach and partial gastrectomy more than fifteen years previously. In these situations, as well as in gastric cancer, acid output tends to be low. Gastric cancer rarely occurs in patients with duodenal ulcer, in whom acid secretion is either normal or high.

Nitrosamines formed by bacterial action on nitrates of dietary origin are thought to be a causal influence. Bacterial proliferation in the achlorhydric stomach has been invoked to explain the increased frequency of gastric cancer in pernicious anaemia. There is evidence that the use of preserved and salty foods confer an increased risk of gastric cancer, while fresh fruits and vegetables have a protective effect.

There are two histological types of gastric carcinoma: intestinal type and diffuse type; the former was previously called adenocarcinoma and the latter anaplastic carcinoma. The former tends to be more common in high-risk countries, older subjects and males, and appears more closely related to atrophic gastritis and possibly intestinal metaplasia, whereas the latter does not have geographical or sexual predilection. Gastric cancer can be early (localised to the mucosa or submucosa) or advanced. Early gastric cancer has a good prognosis after resection, with survival rates approaching that of the control population and can be diagnosed by screening programs in high-risk areas. The outlook of advanced gastric cancer is poor, the five-year survival rate being less than 30%.

Symptoms and signs

Early gastric cancer may be asymptomatic, being detected incidentally or at mass surveys. Other patients may present with dyspepsia or bleeding due to an apparently benign gastric ulcer, carcinoma being diagnosed only on biopsy or after resection.

Advanced gastric cancer may cause the following:

1. epigastric discomfort or pain, anorexia, nausea and weight loss. These symptoms may suggest peptic ulcer but are usually of short duration and without remissions;
2. iron-deficiency anaemia due to chronic blood loss or, uncommonly, haematemesis and melaena;
3. dysphagia if the carcinoma occurs in the cardia, or gastric outlet obstruction if it occurs in the antrum.

Signs of gastric cancer usually appear only in advanced disease and include pallor, abdominal mass, ascites, positive succussion splash and jaundice.

In Japan, mass screening for gastric cancer has increased the proportion of patients diagnosed with early rather than advanced gastric cancer. The survival of patients so diagnosed is also improved. In low-risk populations mass screening is not cost-effective, even among those with an increased risk (e.g. with pernicious anaemia). However, gastric cancer should be considered in any person over forty years of age who develops recent-onset dyspepsia, anorexia or iron-deficiency anaemia that is not otherwise explained.

Diagnosis is by barium meal and/or endoscopy with biopsy. It must be emphasised that the occasional gastric cancer can have all the radiological and endoscopic features of a benign ulcer.

Treatment

This is surgical. Even when curative resection is impossible a palliative resection can prolong survival and improve the quality of remaining life. Obstructive symptoms sometimes require the insertion of an oesophageal prosthesis or the use of laser ablation via an endoscope. Chemotherapy can produce a partial remission in some patients.

SUGGESTED FURTHER READING

Berk, E. J., *Bockus Gastroenterology*, W. B. Saunders, Philadelphia, 1994.

Shearman, D. J. C. and Finlayson, N. D. C., *Diseases of the Gastrointestinal Tract and Liver*, 2nd edn, Churchill-Livingstone, Edinburgh, 1989.

Sleisenger, M. H. and Fordtran, J. S. (eds), *Gastrointestinal Disease: Pathophysiology, Diagnosis and Management*, 5th edn, W. B. Saunders, Philadelphia, 1993.

Working Party Report to the World Congresses of Gastroenterology, Sydney 1990, *J Gastroenterol Hepatal*, 1991; 6:207–8.

CHAPTER 3

Small intestine

W. Doe

Anatomy

The small intestine is approximately 3 m in length and has a vast absorptive surface, the size of a doubles tennis court. The undulating folds of the small intestine—the myriad of slender villi and the microvilli (brush border) which form the external surface of the columnar epithelial cells—all amplify the surface area.

The epithelial cells are highly specialised for digestion and absorption. The microvillous membrane and its outer glycoprotein coat, the glycocalyx, form a critical interface between the potentially toxic contents of the lumen and the carefully regulated internal environment. This microvillous membrane complex displays:

1. digestive enzymes (e.g. saccharidases, peptidases);
2. carrier proteins for nutrient absorption (e.g. sodium, glucose);
3. specific receptors for binding (e.g. the vitamin B12 and bile salt receptors in the terminal ileum);
4. secretory IgA and secretory IgM antibody.

The villous core contains blood vessels, lymphatics for the transport of nutrients from the intestine, and cells involved in mucosal immune responses. The specialised epithelial cells are generated as undifferentiated cells in the crypts of Lieberkuhn, mature into absorptive cells as they ascend the villi, and are shed from the villous tips—a process that takes five to six days.

The epithelium also contains a population of endocrine cells that includes secretin, cholecystokinin, motilin, and somatostatin in the duodenum and jejunum. In the ileum, the mucosal epithelial display of endocrine cells includes those producing enteroglucagon, neurotensin and somatostatin.

Physiology

A clear grasp of the physiology of the small intestine is essential to understanding its diseases and their management.

1. The process of digestion of complex foodstuffs into simple constituents which are non-toxic and non-immunogenic, and their absorption as nutrients, are the major functions of the small intestine.
2. The digestion products of fats, carbohydrate and protein, together with fat-soluble vitamins and most water-soluble vitamins, are absorbed in the jejunum, but there is a large intestinal reserve whereby the ileum can, if required, absorb these nutrients as well.
3. There are regional sites of absorption which are highly specialised for transporting specific substances, including iron, folic acid, vitamin B12 and bile salts (Fig. 3.1).
4. The small intestine is the major site of water and electrolyte absorption.
5. A specially adapted mucosal immune system protects the vulnerable mucosal surface.

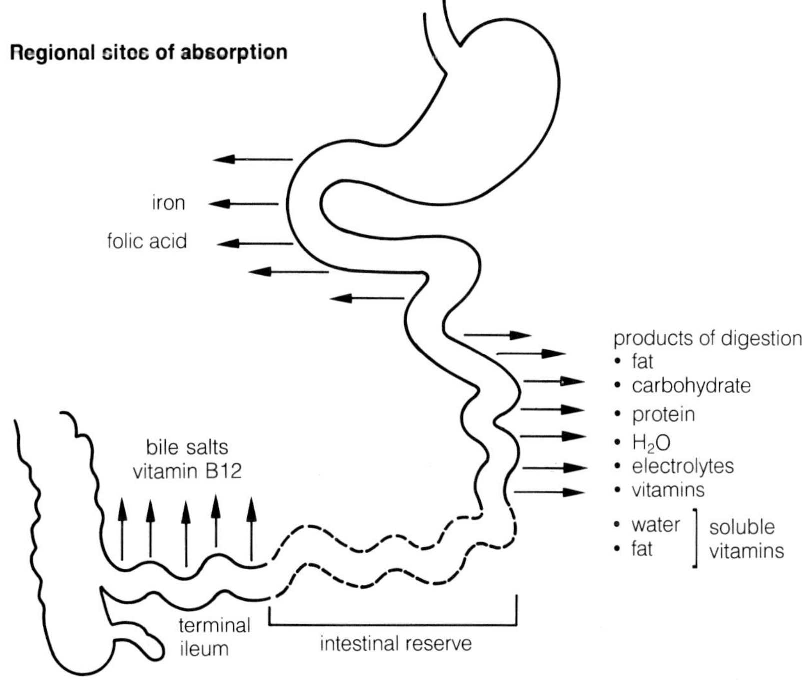

Fig. 3.1 *Regions of the small intestine that are specialised for the transportation of nutrients*

Carbohydrate digestion and absorption

In the typical Western diet, carbohydrates provide the largest source of calories in the form of polysaccharides (about 60%), and disaccharides, sucrose and lactose (about 30%). Salivary amylases begin the luminal digestion of polysaccharides; this mainly occurs in the duodenum, where pancreatic amylase hydrolyses the internal alpha-1, 4-glucose linkages but not the alpha-1, 6 bonds to yield the disaccharide maltose, small oligosaccharides, and the highly branched compounds called alpha-limit dextrins.

Another stage of carbohydrate digestion is necessary before absorption can occur. Oligosaccharidases, displayed on the microvillous membrane, rapidly generate the constituent monosaccharides (lactose yields glucose and galactose, sucrose is split into glucose and fructose), which are actively transported across the microvillous membrane into the enterocyte. Glucose, galactose and D-xylose (a pentose used to test monosaccharide absorption) utilise sodium-coupled transporters—integral membrane proteins that draw their energy from the electrochemical Na^+ gradient created by the sodium pump, Na^+, Ka^+ -ATPase. Fructose is absorbed by facilitated diffusion, a process involving membrane carrier molecules not coupled to any energy source that can also be used by glucose, galactose and D-xylose. Other monosaccharides, such as mannose and the artificial sugar lactulose, are not absorbed in the absence of specific carrier systems. The sugars are therefore osmotically active and draw water into the intestinal lumen. Tests of carbohydrate absorption such as the hydrogen breath test indicate that, while dietary disaccharide absorption is highly efficient, a significant amount of starch reaches the colon where it is fermented by colonic bacteria.

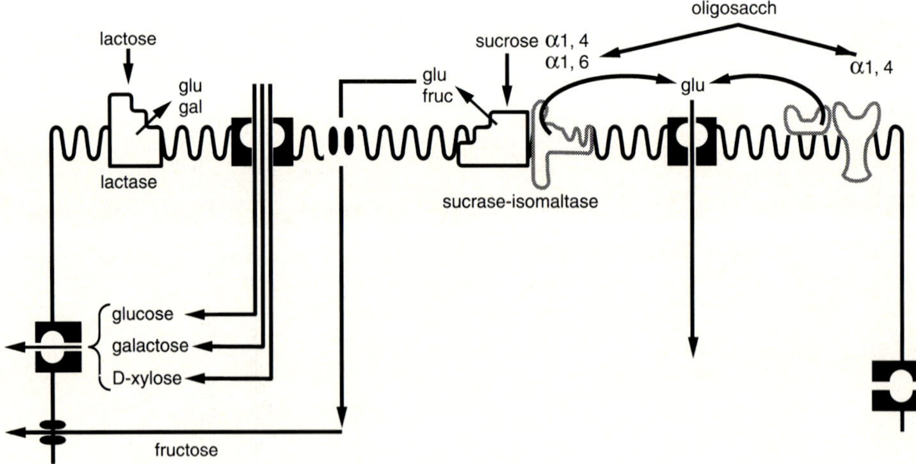

Fig. 3.2 *Carbohydrate absorption*

Protein digestion and absorption

Dietary protein provides 10–20% of the calories in the Western diet and also the essential amino acids required for protein synthesis. Luminal digestion begins in the stomach where the pepsins provide limited proteolysis in acid conditions. The small intestine is the principal site of luminal digestion by the powerful pancreatic proteases—including trypsin, chymotrypsin, elastase and carboxypeptidase—to produce oligopeptides of 2,6-amino acids and a lesser quantity of free amino acids. The pancreatic proteases are secreted as proenzymes, which are activated in the duodenum by a sequence of proteolytic events that begins with the release of enteropeptidase, a product of duodenal enterocytes; this activates trypsinogen to trypsin and thereby initiates the autocatalytic cascade. Brush border peptidases hydrolyse the oligopeptides into amino acids and tri- and dipeptides, which are absorbed by very efficient active transport systems throughout the jejunum and ileum. Dipeptides are more highly absorbed and less osmotically active than amino acid alternatives, and are therefore the preferred source of nitrogen for enteral feeding. Complementary cytoplasmic dipeptidases complete peptide digestion and the amino acids produced are transported across the enterocyte membrane by sodium-coupled active transport, facilitated by simple diffusion to enter the portal vein.

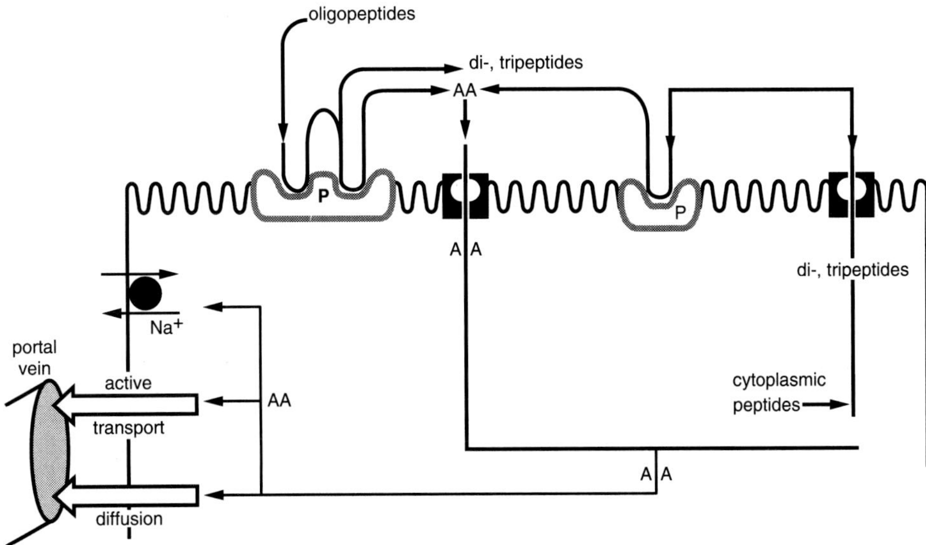

Fig. 3.3 *Protein absorption*

Fat absorption

The 60–100 g of fat ingested daily represents up to 50% of the calorie intake in the Western diet. About 95% of dietary fat consists of long-chain triglycerides

(LCTs), which contain three molecules of long-chain fatty acids esterified to glycerol. The other dietary lipids include cholesterol, other sterols, their esters, complex structural lipids such as phospholipid, and the fat-soluble vitamins (A, D, E and K). Because nearly all dietary fat is insoluble in water, hydrolysis of the LCT ester bonds is essential for their absorption.

Lipolysis begins in the acid milieu of the stomach, where lingual lipase acts with pepsin digestion of associated protein and gastric motility to release a coarse emulsion containing LCTs, products of lipolysis, fatty acids and monoglycerides. At the duodenal pH of 6.5, liberated fatty acids ionise and, together with acid, stimulate the release of cholecystokinin (CCK; also called pancreozymin) and secretin from endocrine cells present in the duodenal and jejunal mucosa. Cholecystokinin induces an enzyme-rich pancreatic secretion and causes the gall-bladder to contract, releasing its bile salts and phospholipids into the duodenum. The LCT emulsion now becomes much more finely dispersed, greatly enlarging the surface area for lipolysis by pancreatic lipase, phospholipase-A_2 and non-specific lipase. Although bile salts are not essential for LCT digestion and absorption, together with biliary phospholipids they stabilise the emulsion, promote lipase activity and help solubilise LCTs. By contrast, cholesterol and the fat-soluble vitamins require bile salts for adequate absorption. Pancreatic co-lipase binds to LCT—displacing absorbed bile salts—and binds pancreatic co-lipase, which hydrolyses LCTs into monoglycerides and fatty acids.

The two primary bile acids (cholic and chenodeoxycholic acid) are synthesised in the liver, where they are conjugated to the amino acids glycine or taurine and secreted into the bile. The conjugated bile acid molecule has detergent properties: it consists of a lipid-soluble (hydrophobic) and a water-soluble (polar) end. When bile salts in solution exceed a critical concentration they spontaneously form macromolecular aggregates called *micelles*. Bile salt molecules orientate so that there is a lipid-soluble core and a water-soluble external surface to the micelle (Fig. 3.4). Fatty acids, monoglyceride fat, soluble vitamins and other lipids are incorporated into the lipid-soluble core of the mixed micelles, which transport these water-insoluble molecules through the water phase of the intestinal lumen and the unstirred water layer to the microvillous membrane, to solubilise in cell membranes and rapidly enter the epithelial cells by passive diffusion (Fig. 3.4). Inside the epithelial cell, the monoglycerides and fatty acids are resynthesised into LCTs and, together with cholesterol, are incorporated into lipoprotein-protein complexes called chylomicrons, which are stabilised by phospholipids and pass into the lymphatic system. The apolipoproteins which are synthesised by enterocytes are essential to chylomicron formation, secretion and metabolism.

Over 95% of the bile salts are reabsorbed, mainly by sodium-coupled active transport at their regional site of absorption in the terminal ileum. Absorbed bile salts are returned to the liver via the portal vein to re-enter the bile (Fig. 3.5). This enterohepatic circulation is essential for normal fat digestion and absorption.

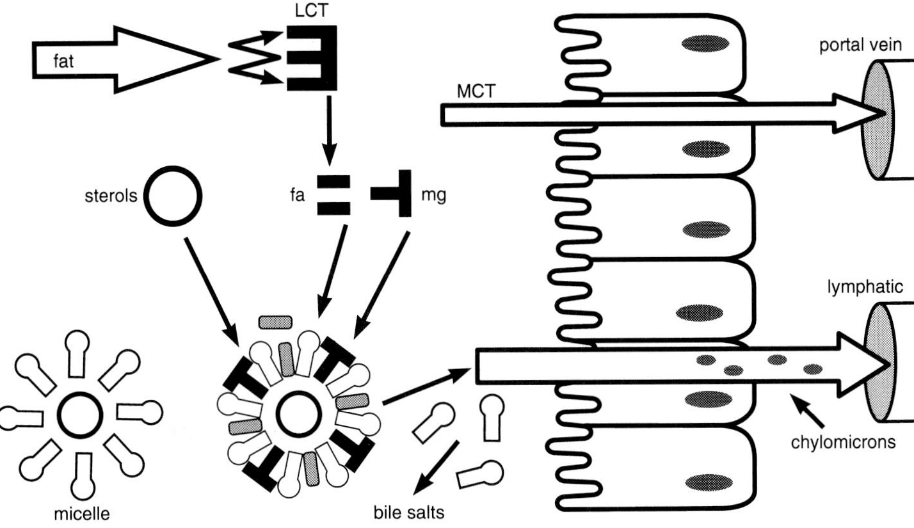

Fig. 3.4 *Mechanisms for fat digestion and absorption, involving lipolysis, micellar solubilisation, absorption, resynthesis for long-chain triglycerides (LCT) and lymphatic transport to the liver as chylomicrons. Medium-chain triglycerides (MCT) are absorbed intact in significant amounts and enter the portal vein*

The total bile salt pool (about 2–4 g) circulates through the enterohepatic circulation four to twelve times a day. Normal fat digestion and absorption therefore depend on the integrity of the enterohepatic circulation of bile salts, the capacity of the terminal ileum to absorb bile salts, and the ability of the liver to replace the 5% of the bile salt pool lost with each enterohepatic circulation. Normally, hepatic synthesis of bile salt replaces the daily faecal losses. When the enterohepatic circulation is compromised, hepatic synthesis of bile salts can be increased five to ten-fold, but substantial interruption of the circulation—for example, resection of more than 100 cm of the terminal ileum—results in bile salt deficiency, because the increased bile acid synthesis cannot compensate for the increased loss.

Although they comprise a very small part of the dietary fat, medium chain triglycerides (MCTs), (8–10 carbon atoms) are important because they are water-soluble and can be absorbed without the need for bile salts or lipases. Medium chain triglycerides are absorbed intact in significant amounts (30%) into the epithelial cell by passive diffusion. They are also readily hydrolysed by pancreatic lipase to medium-chain fatty acids, which are more water-soluble than long-chain fatty acids and are rapidly absorbed by enterocytes. Unlike LCTs, MCTs and medium-chain fatty acids enter the portal system (Fig. 3.5). Medium chain triglycerides are therefore a useful source of fat and calories for patients suffering from some of the diseases discussed later in this chapter.

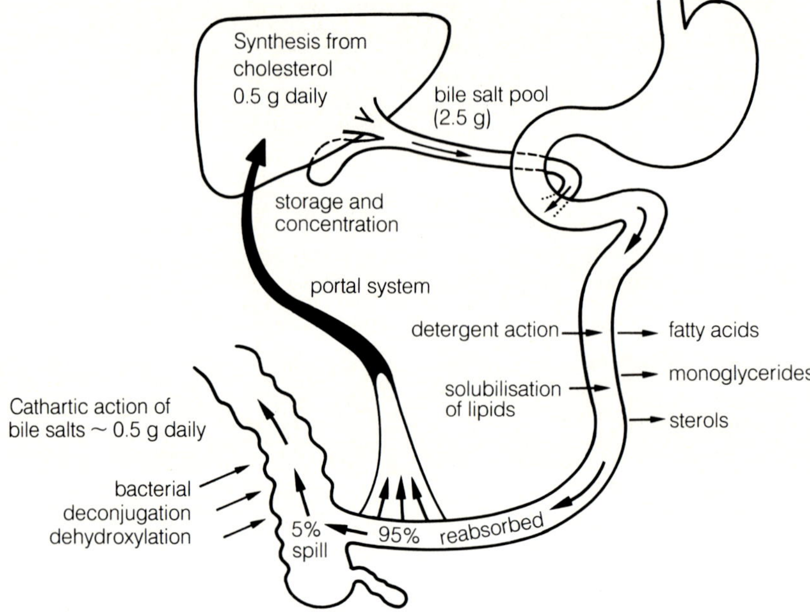

Fig. 3.5 *The enterohepatic circulation of bile salts involving hepatic synthesis, gallbladder storage and concentration, expulsion into the duodenum and reabsorption in the terminal ileum*

Fluid and electrolyte absorption

In healthy subjects the oral fluid intake is 1–2 L/d, but the total fluid load in the small intestine, including the salivary, gastric, biliary and pancreatic secretions, is about 7–10 L/d, of which 75–85% is reabsorbed into the small intestine, leaving an ileocaecal flow into the colon of 1.5–2 L/d (Fig. 3.6). Movement of water is coupled with that of electrolyte, which may move by passive diffusion (leakiness), convection (solvent drag)—in which solute movement is secondary to water flow—or by an active transport system involving Na^+, KA^+ -ATPase, the 'sodium pump' which creates an electrochemical gradient for sodium across the microvillous membrane of the enterocyte. The small intestine also has a mechanism for sodium absorption stimulated by actively transported glucose and amino acids.

In the jejunum, passive water flow created by monosaccharide absorption is the major mechanism for water and sodium absorption, while the glucose-stimulated electrochemical, bicarbonate-stimulated and sodium-hydrogen exchange mechanisms are active to a lesser extent. In the ileum, however, only the latter two mechanisms are significant.

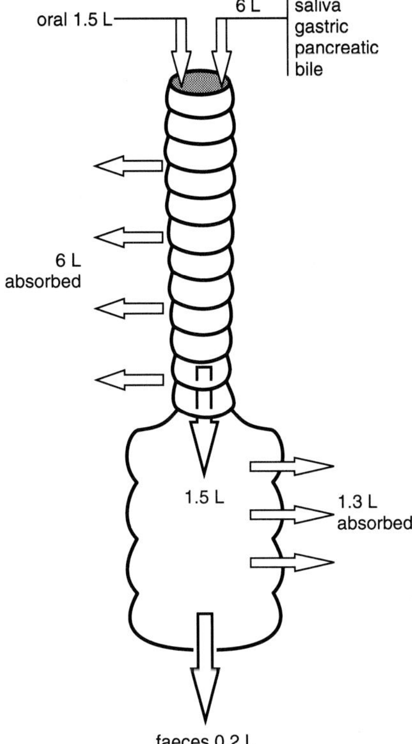

Fig. 3.6 *Fluid balance*

Regional sites of absorption of vitamins and minerals

Although most water-soluble and all fat-soluble vitamins can be absorbed along the length of the small intestine, there are regional sites of absorption specialised for folic acid in the proximal jejunum and for vitamin B12 in the terminal ileum, so that diseases involving these regions have a selective effect on the vitamin involved. Of the minerals, only iron has a regionalised site of absorption which is found in the duodenum (Fig. 3.1).

Folic acid

Folic acid is absorbed by an active transport system in the proximal jejunum. Dietary folate is a polyglutamate which is hydrolysed to pteroylglutamic acid and absorbed by active transport. Folic acid, which is stored principally in the liver, is an essential co-factor for DNA, purine and protein synthesis.

Vitamin B12

Dietary vitamin B12 is released by gastric proteases and complexes with a binding (R) protein. In the duodenum, pancreatic proteases cleave the R protein, liberating the vitamin B12 which binds to intrinsic factor (IF). The vitamin B12-IF complex is resistant to proteolysis and travels to the terminal ileum, where the complex is taken up by a specific receptor-mediated endocytosis and transported via the portal vein to the liver for storage.

Iron

Dietary iron is in the form of haem iron in meat and non-haem iron in vegetables. Haem iron absorption is better than a comparable amount of non-haem iron and is independent of luminal factors, whereas non-haem iron solubility is enhanced by gastric acid and ascorbic acid. Both forms of dietary iron are largely absorbed by active transport in the duodenum and proximal jejunum, where iron complexes with amino acids, citrate or ascorbate. The absorbed iron either enters the portal blood bound to transferrin or is stored in the enterocyte within ferritin and ultimately lost into the lumen. The regulation of iron absorption is unique because there is no physiological excretory process apart from physiological blood loss (e.g. menstruation), so that body iron levels are controlled at the site of absorption. The precise regulatory mechanism is unknown.

Malabsorption

Malabsorption or maldigestion of food may occur in one or more of the three phases in the digestion and absorption process (see Table 3.1), namely the luminal, mucosal and delivery phases.

Luminal phase

The luminal phase involves the hydrolysis of fats and protein by pancreatic enzymes and the solubilisation of fats by bile salts.

Pancreatic exocrine deficiency may result from the causes listed in Table 3.1. Deficiency of pancreatic lipases, proteases and amylase causes marked malabsorption of fats, proteins and, to a lesser extent, polysaccharides. Chronic pancreatitis is the most common pancreatic cause of malabsorption.

Bile salt deficiency may be caused by biliary obstruction, reduced hepatic synthesis, inactivation of bile salts in the lumen of the small intestine, or loss of integrity in the enterohepatic circulation. If the luminal concentration of bile salts falls below the critical concentration needed for micelle formation, malabsorption of fats occurs.

Carbohydrate and protein digestion and absorption are usually unimpaired. In bile salt deficiency MCTs provide a useful source of lipid, as MCTs can be absorbed without the need for micellar solubilisation.

Table 3.1 *Classification of malabsorption*

1. *Luminal*
   - (a) Pancreatic
     - (i) Chronic pancreatitis
     - (ii) Carcinoma of the pancreas
     - (iii) Fibrocystic disease of the pancreas
     - (iv) Pancreatic resection
   - (b) Bile salts
     - (i) Stagnant loop syndrome
     - (ii) Extrahepatic biliary obstruction
     - (iii) Ileitis or ileal resection
     - (iv) Chronic parenchymal liver disease
2. *Mucosal epithelium phase defects*
   - (a) Selective brush border
     - (i) Lactase deficiency
   - (b) Epithelial cell
     - (i) Coeliac disease
     - (ii) Tropical sprue
     - (iii) Small bowel resection or bypass (short bowel syndrome)
     - (iv) Whipple's disease
     - (v) Primary intestinal lymphoma
     - (vi) Hypogammaglobulinaemia
3. *Delivery phase defects*
   - (a) Abetalipoproteinaemia
   - (b) Intestinal lymphangiectasia
4. *Multiple phase defects*
   - (a) Postgastrectomy
   - (b) Crohn's disease
   - (c) Radiation enteritis
   - (d) Diabetes mellitus
   - (e) Endocrinopathies
   - (f) Drugs (e.g. cholestyramine, cathartics)
   - (g) Parasitoses
   - (h) HIV
   - (i) Mycobacterium avium intracellulare
   - (j) Kaposi's sarcoma

Mucosal phase

The mucosal phase involves hydrolysis of carbohydrates and oligopeptides by brush border enzymes, the transport of monosaccharides, dipeptides, amino acids and fats into the enterocyte, and the formation of chylomicrons. Causes of malabsorption at this phase include:

1. inherited deficiency of a disaccharidase, which causes the selective malabsorption of a disaccharide. In these patients, the histology of the microvilli, the epithelial cells and the villi is normal;
2. extensive damage to the epithelial cells of the mucosal surface of the proximal small intestine, seen mainly in coeliac disease (also called gluten-sensitive enteropathy), the related skin disease, dermatitis herpetiformis, and in tropical sprue (see Table 3.1). The mechanisms which contribute to the steatorrhoea caused by the mucosal damage are:
   - (a) *loss of absorptive surface*: the doubles tennis court area may be reduced to that of a ping pong table;
   - (b) *immaturity of the epithelial cells* and damage to the microvilli;
   - (c) *inco-ordination of pancreatic and biliary secretions* during a meal; and
   - (d) *intraluminal bile salt deficiency*, if terminal ileum involvement by the disease process interferes with the enterohepatic circulation of bile salts.

Delivery phase

Malabsorption may also occur when there is an inability to transport fat out of the epithelial cells into the lymphatic system. The defect may be in chylomicron formation, as in abetalipoproteinaemia, or there may be widespread obstruction to the lymphatic drainage of the small bowel, as in intestinal lymphangiectasia.

Investigation of malabsorption

The three main areas which should be considered (see Table 3.2) are:

1. absorption;
2. nutrition; and
3. anatomy.

Table 3.2 *Investigation of malabsorption*

1. *Absorption*	3. *Anatomy*
Faecal fat	Small bowel barium series
D-xylose test	Jejunal biopsy
Schilling test	
^{14}C-glycine breath test	
Pancreatic function tests	
Lactose tolerance test	
2. *Nutrition*	
Haemoglobin, blood film	
Serum folate	
Plasma albumin, calcium, phosphate and alkaline phosphatase	

Absorption tests

Faecal fats

The normal faecal fat excretion is about 5 g/24 h when 100 g of fat are ingested daily. The estimate is based on the daily average of a stool collection performed after at least three days on a standard 100 g fat diet, and assumes regular bowel actions and a complete stool collection. In these circumstances, a faecal fat over 7 g daily indicates steatorrhoea.

More recently, the radio-labelled (^{14}C) triglyceride, triolein, has been used to test fat malabsorption. The metabolism of the unabsorbed ^{14}C-triolein by colonic bacteria produces $^{14}CO_2$, which is absorbed and then excreted in the expired breath, providing a sensitive measure of fat malabsorption.

D-xylose absorption test

D-xylose is a 5-carbon sugar which is absorbed in the small intestine by the same transport mechanism as glucose and galactose. It is poorly metabolised, and over 20% of the oral loading dose of 25 g is normally found in a five-hour urine collection. Measure of the serum level of D-xylose two hours after ingestion eliminates errors caused by factors influencing urinary flow, such as renal impairment and dehydration. The absorption of D-xylose is impaired by mucosal causes of malabsorption and by the presence of bacterial overgrowth in the small intestine. The D-xylose absorption test is therefore a simple test of small intestinal absorption, and is most useful when absorption is otherwise normal in the presence of steatorrhoea, in which case it indicates pancreatic or bile salt insufficiency.

Vitamin B12 absorption (Schilling test)

Because vitamin B12 absorption is localised to the terminal ileum, uptake of an oral dose of radio-labelled vitamin B12 can be used as a test of terminal ileum function. An oral dose of radio-labelled (^{58}Co) vitamin B12 is given, followed by a large intramuscular dose of unlabelled vitamin B12 to ensure that a significant amount of labelled B12 is 'flushed' out in the urine. Normal subjects excrete 5–10% of the labelled vitamin B12 within twenty-four hours. To differentiate deficiency of intrinsic factor (pernicious anaemia), the test includes a vitamin B12-intrinsic factor complex labelled with a different radioisotope (^{57}Co). In pernicious anaemia, the vitamin B12 given with intrinsic factor is normally absorbed. Malabsorption of both types of labelled vitamin B12 occurs in:

1. diseases involving the terminal ileum (e.g. Crohn's disease), or ileal resection;
2. when there is bacterial overgrowth in the small intestine, the stagnant loop syndrome; or
3. pancreatic insufficiency, where the R protein is not released from vitamin B12 by pancreatic proteases to permit intrinsic factor binding.

Bile acid breath test

The amide bond of glycine-conjugated bile salts is split only by bacterial enzymes. When ^{14}C-cholyglycine is given by mouth to normal subjects, 95% of the dose is reabsorbed by the terminal ileum and enters the enterohepatic circulation. A small amount (5%) of ^{14}C-glycine 'spills' into the colon where bacteria deconjugate the bile acid, liberating the ^{14}C-glycine, which is metabolised in the colon to $^{14}CO_2$ or absorbed intact to be metabolised in the liver. Small amounts of $^{14}CO_2$ can therefore be measured in the breath (Fig. 3.7).

The test can be used to detect malabsorption of bile salts in patients with ileal disease or resection of the terminal ileum. If absorption of the ^{14}C-glycine dose is impaired, a much larger amount of bile salt will enter the colon, and this can be quantitated by measuring the $^{14}CO_2$ and determining the amount of faecal ^{14}C bile acids. The bile acid breath test can also be used to detect bacterial overgrowth in the small bowel where the ^{14}C-glycine is malabsorbed, because it is deconjugated in the small intestine (Fig. 3.4).

Tests for lactase deficiency

The direct method of testing involves enzyme estimation in a fresh small intestinal biopsy, and is therefore available only in large centres.

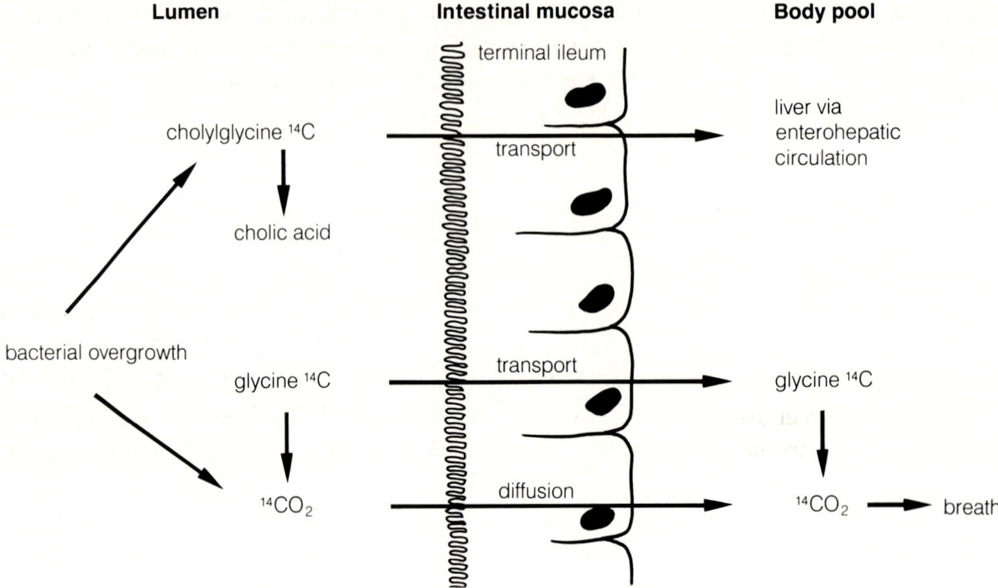

Fig. 3.7 *Cholyglycine* ^{14}C *breath test, showing how it detects bacterial overgrowth in the small intestine. When the small bowel flora are normal this test can be used as a measure of ileal function*

The most widely used indirect method is the lactose tolerance test. After establishing that the glucose tolerance is normal, the patient is given lactose and the blood is collected for glucose estimation as for the glucose tolerance test. A flat blood-glucose curve after lactose suggests lactase deficiency. The test is simple but insensitive and time-consuming.

The most sensitive test for lactase deficiency is the hydrogen breath test. In man, hydrogen production is due exclusively to bacterial fermentation of dietary carbohydrate, and the amount of hydrogen excreted in the breath correlates well with intestinal production. In lactase deficiency, therefore, an oral overload of lactose will not be absorbed and will enter the colon, where its fermentation by colonic bacteria will cause a marked increase in hydrogen production which is then reflected in greatly increased amounts of hydrogen in the breath. No radioactive isotopes are required.

Nutrition

Nutritional tests provide an inexpensive screen for revealing a proximal mucosal cause of malabsorption. The finding of macrocytosis and microcytosis on the same film suggests iron and folic acid deficiency, caused by a proximal lesion such as coeliac disease. The appearance of unexplained iron deficiency on the blood film should also arouse the suspicion of malabsorption, and low serum folate levels are highly suggestive. Malabsorption of fat-soluble vitamins may be revealed in a prolonged prothrombin time (vitamin K) or in evidence of hypocalcaemia or secondary hyperparathyroidism (vitamin D).

Anatomical tests

Jejunal biopsy

The peroral duodenal or jejunal biopsy, often performed through an endoscope, is a simple procedure which yields the most useful information in the differential diagnosis of patients with steatorrhoea (see Fig. 3.5). The surface may be examined by the dissecting microscope for villous structure and then prepared for histological examination. Smears of the fresh biopsy surface can be examined for *Giardia* (p. 188).

Radiology

The small bowel barium examination is used for looking for anatomical abnormalities which may contribute to stasis and the stagnant loop syndrome, or for segmental bowel diseases such as Crohn's disease. It is usually indicated where these lesions are suspected from the history, or when the appearance of the jejunal biopsy specimen in a patient with steatorrhoea is normal, or when a stagnant loop syndrome is suspected.

Intraluminal defects causing malabsorption

There are three major intraluminal defects which can cause malabsorption:

1. pancreatic (see Chapter 5 for details);
2. biliary (loss of bile salts from cholestasis; Chapter 6); and
3. stagnant loop syndrome.

Stagnant loop syndrome

The stagnant (or blind) loop syndrome consists of malabsorption, and of the resulting nutritional deficiencies, in patients who have any small bowel abnormality conducive to the stasis of enteric contents which allows enteric bacteria to proliferate in the lumen of the small intestine.

There are three major causes of stasis in the small intestine:

1. *local causes*, including small bowel diverticulosis, strictures, fistulae;
2. *postabdominal surgery*, including blind pouches, non-functioning Polya (Billroth II) afferent loop, gastrocolic fistula; and
3. *impaired motor function*, including scleroderma, intestinal pseudo-obstruction.

Pathogenesis

Normally the small intestine contains few bacteria except in the terminal ileum, where bacterial concentrations, especially of anaerobes, approach colonic levels. Stasis of the small bowel contents allows the proliferation of anaerobes, resulting in luminal malabsorption. Bacterial overgrowth causes:

1. inactivation of bile salts by deconjugation and dehydroxylation, leading to bile salt deficiency;
2. competition for vitamin B12 binding;

3. formation of hydroxylated fatty acids;
4. fermentation of carbohydrates.

The clinical features are those of malabsorption, usually characterised by diarrhoea with the features of steatorrhoea.

Diagnosis

In a patient suffering from malabsorption, a history of conditions predisposing to stasis in the small intestine and a barium examination of the small intestine showing anatomical abnormality suggest the diagnosis.

The diagnostic test for bacterial overgrowth is an indirect test in which a radio-labelled, conjugated bile salt (^{14}C-glycocholate) is given by mouth and the patient's breath is tested at intervals for $^{14}CO_2$ (see p. 49). If anaerobic bacterial overgrowth is present in the small bowel, the labelled bile salt will be deconjugated and the released labelled glycine absorbed and metabolised to release $^{14}CO_2$, which is measured in the breath (Fig. 3.7).

Treatment

This consists of:

1. surgical correction of the cause of the stasis where possible;
2. replacement of nutrient deficiencies, particularly vitamin B12;
3. long-term intermittent antibiotic therapy, using broad-spectrum antibiotics active against anaerobes.

Defects in the mucosa causing malabsorption

Selective brush border defects

The most common primary deficiency of disaccharidases is lactase. Congenital deficiency is rare in Europeans and, if present, symptoms date from the first feeding. In most racial groups, except Europeans, lactase activity decreases in late childhood, and many adults have alactasia. In Europeans, lactase function persists in adult life.

Clinical features

Most adults with lactase deficiency are asymptomatic, and care should be taken before attributing abdominal symptoms to this cause. The symptoms caused by a lactose load in alactasia are:

1. abdominal cramps, distension and borborygmi due to bacterial fermentation of the unabsorbed lactose in the colon;
2. diarrhoea due to the osmotic effect of the unabsorbed lactose in the small bowel.

The diagnosis may be evident from the history, but tests for lactase deficiency (see p. 49) are often required. Treatment involves excluding milk and milk products from the diet, as milk is the only natural source of lactose.

Coeliac disease (gluten-sensitive enteropathy)

Coeliac disease results from a sensitivity to a peptide derived from the cereal protein gluten, which is found in wheat, rye and barley flour. In patients with coeliac disease, the ingestion of food containing gluten causes a severe, diffuse inflammatory damage to the duodenum and jejunum, resulting in malabsorption. In severe cases the whole of the small intestine may be involved.

Coeliac disease is one of the most common forms of malabsorption in Europeans. It is a familial disease affecting 10% of first-degree relatives, and is strongly associated with histocompatibility serotypes DR3, DR7 and DQw2 at the HLA-D locus.

Pathogenesis

How gluten or its peptide products injure the mucosa is not known. Two mechanisms have been suggested:

1. an aberrant mucosal immune response to gluten peptides, resulting in hypersensitivity and immune-mediated injury to the mucosa;
2. an inherited mucosal peptidase deficiency, resulting in the accumulation of a 'toxic peptide', causing damage to the mucosal epithelium.

Clinical features

Coeliac disease causes symptoms of malabsorption due to diffuse mucosal damage. The time of onset of the symptoms and their severity is widely variable. Commonly, symptoms begin in infancy soon after weaning, when the diagnosis is readily made. In milder cases, however, the onset of symptoms is gradual, and these may become manifest at any stage of adult life. Although a history of childhood coeliac disease may be obtained in some instances, patients presenting in adult life often have had no identifiable symptoms of malabsorption in childhood.

Patients present with feelings of ill health and anaemia, including fatigue and lassitude. In the more severe cases, abdominal symptoms of malabsorption are present. These include diarrhoea with excess fat in the stool (i.e. steatorrhoea). The stools are typically loose, bulky, pale and tend to be frothy and difficult to flush. In addition, there is often abdominal bloating and poorly localised abdominal pain. Weight loss usually occurs, but in societies in which overeating is common, weight may be maintained.

Malabsorption of folic acid and iron in the duodenum and proximal jejunum give rise to the typical anaemia of coeliac disease, and may cause a sore tongue due to glossitis. Bone pains due to osteomalacia resulting from vitamin D malabsorption may occur, especially in climates with restricted sunlight. Similarly, vitamin K malabsorption may lead to easy bruising.

Because of the considerable reserve in the small intestine for absorption of the digestion products of fats, proteins and carbohydrate, mucosal injury confined to the duodenum and proximal jejunum may not cause abdominal symptoms or steatorrhoea. In this instance, those nutrients which are confined to regional absorption in the duodenum and proximal jejunum (i.e. iron and folic acid) are most affected (Fig. 3.1). The result is a chronic anaemia due to iron and folic acid deficiency—a combination nearly always caused by coeliac disease in a patient on a normal diet.

Clinical signs

Except in severe cases, few clinical signs are evident. Skin pigmentation and aphthous ulceration are commonly seen, and the vesicular lesions of dermatitis herpetiformis are occasionally associated with coeliac disease. Glossitis and bruising may be present. Examination of the stool on the glove after rectal examination is a useful means of detecting gross steatorrhoea.

The mucosal lesion

In untreated coeliac disease, biopsy of the jejunal mucosa reveals a flat mucosal surface, devoid of villi (see Fig. 3.8(c)). The flat surface is studded with pits, representing the mouths of the crypts of Lieberkuhn. Histological examination confirms the obliteration of villous architecture. The epithelial cells are immature, reduced in height, and have damaged brush borders. There is a dense inflammatory cell infiltrate in the lamina propria, the crypts of Lieberkuhn are greatly enlarged, and the crypt cells show many mitoses caused by the markedly increased epithelial cell turnover (Fig. 3.8(c)).

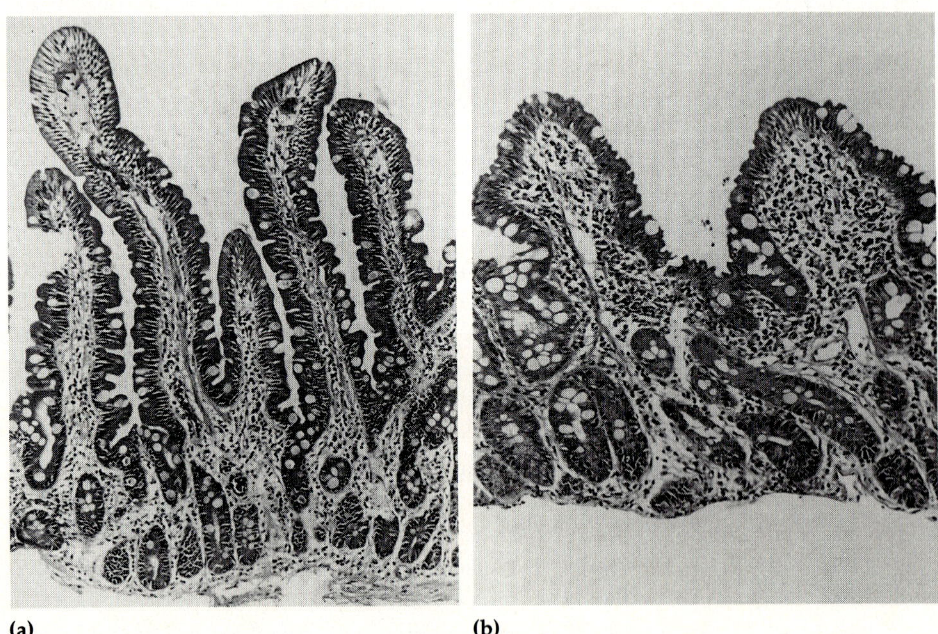

(a) (b)

Fig. 3.8(a) *Normal small bowel mucosa. The villus to crypt ratio is 3:1. H-E stain, original magnification × 40*

Fig. 3.8(b) *Partial villus atrophy. The villus to crypt ratio is 1:1. H-E stain, original magnification × 40*

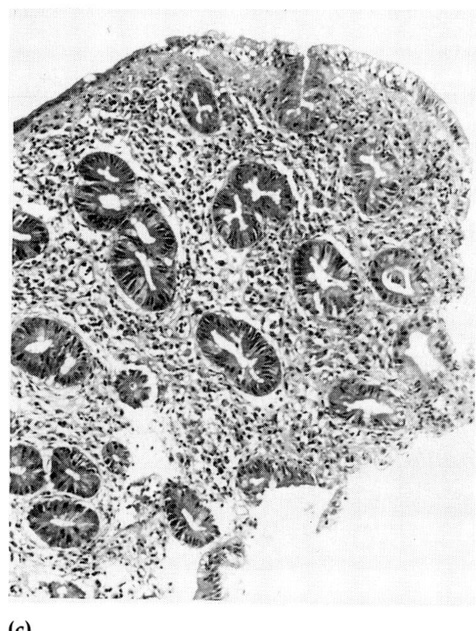

(c)

Fig. 3.8(c) *Total villus atrophy—coeliac disease. There are no villi. The surface epithelial cells are degenerate. The submucosa is widened, and there is a heavy infiltration of mononuclear inflammatory cells. H-E stain, original magnification × 40*

These appearances are characteristic of coeliac disease but are not specific. Other rare disorders such as severe tropical sprue, immunodeficiency and some lymphomas may have similar appearances.

Diagnosis

The criteria for the diagnosis of coeliac disease are:

1. evidence of malabsorption;
2. jejunal histology showing loss of villous architecture;
3. clinical and histological improvement following the exclusion of gluten from the diet.

Occasionally in adults, a gluten challenge may be needed to confirm the diagnosis, especially when a gluten-free diet has been prescribed without prior jejunal biopsy.

Investigation

The approach to investigation in malabsorption is outlined in Table 3.2 (p. 48).

Management

The management of coeliac disease is based on the following principles:

1. provisional diagnosis based on a jejunal biopsy *before* institution of a gluten-free diet;
2. introduction of a gluten-free diet, involving strict exclusion of wheat, rye and barley products from the diet. (Some patients are also sensitive to oats.) Explanation and supervision of the diet by a dietitian;

3. continuation of the gluten-free diet for life;
4. review of the gluten-free diet if symptoms recur (advice concerning access to gluten-free products, especially bread, is available from coeliac societies run by coeliac patients);
5. that, except in severe cases, no other specific treatment is necessary (response of the iron- and folic acid-deficient anaemia, for example, to the gluten-free diet, is good evidence of compliance and of improved mucosal absorption);
6. the mucosal lesion should respond dramatically to the exclusion of gluten from the coeliac patient's diet so that, within about three months of gluten exclusion, the mucosa usually shows more normal villous architecture.

Complications

Rarely, coeliac disease is complicated by:

1. intestinal lymphoma or gastrointestinal carcinoma (usually oesophageal);
2. a state of unresponsiveness to the gluten-free diet, in which malabsorption persists apparently due to irreversibly severe damage to the mucosa.

Tropical sprue

Tropical sprue is a malabsorption syndrome which affects people living in, or visiting, the tropics. The visit need only be brief and the onset of symptoms may occur months or even years afterwards. The condition may be endemic or epidemic, and the cause is unknown. Tolerance to gluten is normal.

Clinical features

Symptoms of anaemia, anorexia, abdominal bloating, steatorrhoea and weight loss are characteristic. Glossitis, pigmentation and dependent oedema also occur.

Diagnosis depends on:

1. nutritional deficiencies (folic acid, iron and vitamin B12);
2. malabsorption of fat and vitamin B12;
3. an abnormal jejunal biopsy, showing shortening or obliteration of the villi and a dense inflammatory cell infiltrate.

Treatment

Tropical sprue responds to folic acid and tetracycline therapy prolonged for six months and repletion of nutritional deficiencies, especially of vitamin B12.

The short bowel syndrome

The factors influencing nutrient absorption after small bowel resection are:

1. *site of resection.* The site of resection may involve one of the regional sites of absorption, that is the duodenum and jejunum proximally (iron and folic acid) or the terminal ileum (bile salts and vitamin B12) (Fig. 3.1);

2. *length of bowel resected.* Because of the large reserve of the small bowel for absorption, resection of up to 40% of the length of small bowel is well tolerated, provided that the regional absorptive sites are not involved;
3. *involvement of the ileocaecal valve.* Resection of the ileocaecal valve impairs the function of the remaining bowel by allowing colonic bacteria to proliferate in the small bowel;
4. *the presence of diseased bowel.* Management of the short bowel syndrome may be complicated by disease of the remaining bowel.

Cause

The short bowel syndrome occurs after surgery for:

1. bowel infarction caused by mesenteric vascular occlusion, volvulus, strangulated hernias or trauma;
2. Crohn's disease, intestinal lymphoma;
3. elective jejunoileal bypass for the treatment of morbid obesity.

Adaptation of the remaining small bowel occurs. The remnant dilates, hyperplasia of intestinal epithelial cells occurs, and an increased absorptive capacity develops.

Clinical features

These can be deduced from the discussion of the function of the small bowel set out earlier in this chapter (p. 39). Points to note are:

1. Ileal resection causes more severe symptoms because bile salt malabsorption leads to an increased likelihood of gallstone formation.
2. Unabsorbed bile salts and fatty acids cause a colonic diarrhoea.
3. Bile salts increase oxalate absorption in the colon, which may result in renal oxalate stones.
4. Huge faecal fluid losses may occur because the small bowel is the major site of water and electrolyte absorption.
5. Transient gastric hypersecretion may cause peptic ulceration.

Management

Total parenteral replacement therapy provides balanced nutrition. Early oral feedings of elemental diets, using frequent small amounts, maximise the use of the small absorptive area and promote adaptation of the bowel remnant. Medium chain triglycerides offer a readily absorbed source of lipids and calories.

When the terminal ileal resection is less than 100 cm, the bile salt-binding resin cholestyramine is helpful in reducing the watery diarrhoea. In more extensive terminal ileal resections, however, cholestyramine is ineffective, and may worsen the steatorrhoea by further depleting the patient's bile salt pool.

Whipple's disease

Whipple's disease is a rare systemic disease which always affects the small intestine, usually resulting in malabsorption. Any other organ system may be affected.

The clinical features are:

1. intestinal malabsorption;
2. fever;
3. skin pigmentation;
4. lymphadenopathy;
5. polyarthralgia and arthritis;
6. serositis.

Involved tissues are infiltrated by large, foamy macrophages which are stuffed with bacterial membrane glycoproteins that can be detected by the periodic acid-Schiff (PAS) stain. The small intestinal lesion shows gross stunting of the villi, with extensive infiltration of the lamina propria by the large, foamy PAS-positive macrophages which are diagnostic of Whipple's disease.

Untreated, Whipple's disease progresses to a fatal outcome. The disease responds dramatically to antibiotic therapy, but long-term follow-up is necessary because relapse may occur.

Defects in delivery phase causing malabsorption

Abetalipoproteinaemia is a rare inherited disease which is characterised by:

1. absence of circulating beta-lipoprotein;
2. malabsorption of fat;
3. acanthocytosis; and
4. ataxic neuropathic disease and retinitis pigmentosa.

The biochemical defect comprises the inability to transport preformed triglyceride from the epithelial cells of the small intestinal mucosa into the lymphatic system. The clinical features are steatorrhoea, abdominal distension and progressively severe neurologic defects. Jejunal biopsies show a striking accumulation of lipid in the epithelial cells.

Low-fat diets, MCT oil, and fat-soluble vitamin supplements ameliorate the steatorrhoea but no effective treatment exists for the neurological disorders, and patients die in early adult life.

Multiple-phase defects causing malabsorption

Surgical causes of malabsorption

Malabsorption commonly results from:

1. gastric surgery;
2. intestinal resection or bypass—the short bowel syndrome (see p. 56).

Gastric surgery

Postgastrectomy steatorrhoea is usually mild, very common, and is rarely clinically significant. The mechanisms include poor mixing of gastric contents with bile salts when there is a gastroenterostomy, and rapid transit due to rapid gastric emptying.

Symptomatic steatorrhoea indicates additional complicating factors, such as stasis due to a non-functioning afferent loop in a Polya-type (Billroth II) gastrectomy or previously undiagnosed coeliac disease. Symptomatic steatorrhoea is managed by:

1. correction of nutritional deficiencies;
2. pancreatic replacement therapy;
3. rarely, revisional surgery; and
4. search for an underlying cause.

Crohn's disease

Crohn's disease is a chronic inflammatory disorder which can affect any portion of the gastrointestinal tract, from the mouth to the anus. In the small bowel it most commonly affects the terminal ileum—hence its synonym 'terminal ileitis'. The colon is the other commonly involved organ (p. 79). In European populations the prevalence of Crohn's disease is about five per 100 000.

Pathogenesis

The aetiology of Crohn's disease is unknown. There is familial predisposition. An underlying immunological abnormality and the presence of a transmissible agent have been suggested, but to date evidence is lacking.

The pathology of the Crohn's lesion is that of a transmural inflammation associated with mucosal ulceration, deep fissuring and the presence of non-caseating granulomas. There are often 'skip' lesions separated by areas of apparently normal bowel. Stricture and fistula formation are common (see Fig. 3.9).

Clinical features

The features most commonly encountered in Crohn's disease are:

1. acute right iliac fossa pain: the clinical picture of acute ileitis may be indistinguishable from acute appendicitis;
2. recurrent lower abdominal pain: frequently worse after meals and due to bowel narrowing and obstruction (bolus colic);
3. weight loss and general ill health;
4. diarrhoea;
5. fistulae, either internal or external.

Less common features include ano-rectal lesions, clubbing of the fingers, 'pyrexia of unknown origin', a malabsorption syndrome, acute perforation and peritonitis, and gastrointestinal bleeding. An abdominal mass, most commonly in the right iliac fossa, is palpable in about one-third of patients; the mass may represent an abscess or loops of thickened or adherent bowel. Anal lesions occur in about 25% of patients with small bowel Crohn's disease.

Crohn's colitis may present as universal colitis, as a segmental colitis or proctitis, or in association with small bowel disease. Differentiation from ulcerative

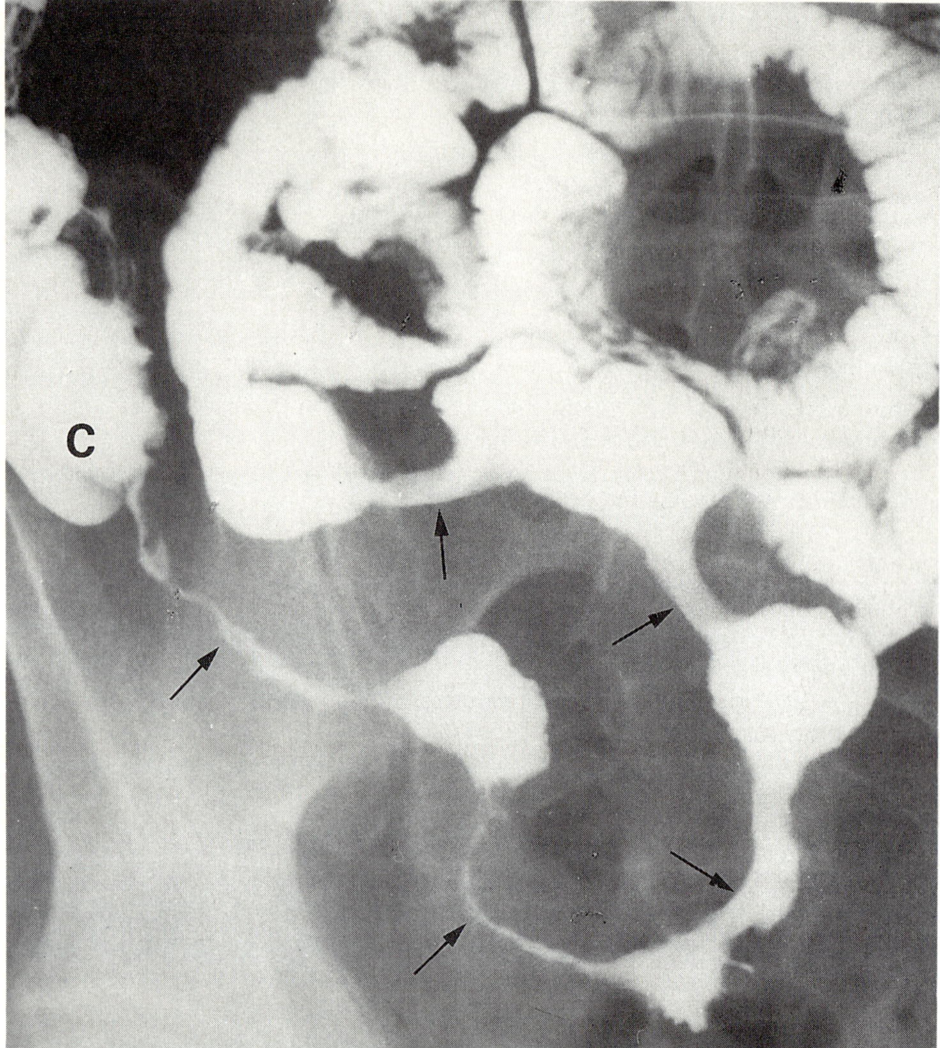

Fig. 3.9 *Crohn's disease of the ileum. Shows classical 'skip' lesions, with narrowed lumen (arrows) and dilated segments of the intervening normal bowel. C=caecum*

colitis may be difficult (see Chapter 4). Diagnosis is based on the following investigations:

1. the non-specific findings of an inflammatory condition, including elevated levels of acute phase proteins and white cell count;
2. anaemia and deficiency of iron, folic acid and, sometimes, of vitamin B12;
3. abnormal ^{14}C-glycocholate breath test results due to ileal involvement;
4. radio-labelled autologous white cell scans, which may be useful for determining the localisation and intensity of active disease. Whenever possible the diagnosis should be confirmed by colonoscopic biopsy of the involved tissue.

Radiology

A barium enema may reveal terminal ileal involvement, but a small bowel series is often required for full assessment of the extent of the disease. Involved areas of the small intestine typically appear rigid and thickened. The lumen may be narrowed and the proximal bowel appear dilated because of obstruction at the site of stricture (Fig. 3.9).

Course and prognosis

Few guides are available to determine the prognosis in the individual patient. Certain generalisations can be made, however:

1. Acute 'regional ileitis' can occur as a self-limited disorder without progression to chronic disease. In some cases, at least, this is due to bacterial infection (e.g. *Yersinia*).
2. Crohn's disease usually presents a chronic problem, giving recurring trouble over many years.
3. Over half of the patients will require surgical treatment at some stage of their illness.
4. The complications of bowel ulceration, fistulae and stenosis may appear at any time.
5. The disease nearly always recurs despite initial surgery to excise all visibly diseased bowel.
6. The extraintestinal manifestations of Crohn's disease include:
   (a) transient acute monoarticular arthritis affecting large joints, especially the knees;
   (b) pericholangitis and fatty infiltration, which may progress to cirrhosis or sclerosing cholangitis;
   (c) conjunctivitis, iritis and episcleritis;
   (d) in HLA-B27 positive patients, sacroileitis and ankylosing spondylitis occur.
7. Growth retardation occurs in children and adolescents.
8. Occasionally, adenocarcinoma develops in a segment of bowel involved by Crohn's disease.

Treatment

Medical treatment involves the following considerations:

1. Bed-rest is often helpful in settling active inflammation.
2. A low-residue diet may reduce bolus colic when there are strictured areas in the small intestine. If malnutrition or growth retardation is present, enteral or parenteral feeding may be required.
3. Patients with extensive terminal ileal disease should receive vitamin B12 supplements. The bile salt-binding resin, cholestyramine, may be helpful if diarrhoea is troublesome (choleric enteropathy) (see p. 57).
4. Metronidazole may be effective, especially in fistulous disease. Sulphasalazine is used mainly when the colon is involved, but new preparations

of 5-aminosalicylic acid (mesalizine) may be useful for terminal ileal disease. Antibiotics are used in managing the purulent complications of Crohn's disease.

5. Corticosteroids usually settle the acute inflammation but have no effect on the natural history of the disease.
6. Immunosuppressive drugs (e.g. azathioprine) are often used as steroid-sparing agents or for long-term therapy.
7. Complete alimentary rest with total parenteral nutrition is used in severe cases which are unresponsive to medical treatment.
8. Surgical treatment is indicated when abdominal or constitutional symptoms occur as a result of structural complications (e.g. intestinal obstruction due to stenosis, abscess formation, internal fistulae and chronic anal lesion). The recurrence rate, however, is very high.

Radiation enteritis

Radiation enteritis may follow radiotherapy given for pelvic or abdominal tumours. Previous abdominal or pelvic surgery, or pelvic inflammatory disease, predisposes to radiation enteritis by causing adhesions which immobilise a normally mobile segment of small bowel.

Pathogenesis

Irradiation causes obliterative changes in the arterioles of the small bowel, and extensive fibrosis can occur.

Clinical features

The onset of symptoms is usually delayed six months to many years after the exposure to radiotherapy. Ileal strictures may present as colicky abdominal pain, and ulceration can cause heavy bleeding.

Symptoms and signs of malabsorption may be present, especially when the terminal ileum is extensively involved and causing bile salt malabsorption. The stagnant loop syndrome may occur because of stricture formation or from the development of enterocolonic fistulae.

Management

The treatment of radiation enteritis includes:

1. careful monitoring of radiotherapy to minimise the risk of radiation enteritis;
2. malabsorption treatment according to whether this is caused by stagnant loop syndrome (see p. 51) or bile salt malabsorption (see p. 49);
3. surgery for enterocolonic fistulae and for progressing strictures causing intestinal obstruction.

Protein-losing enteropathy (PLE)

Excessive gastrointestinal loss of serum proteins frequently contributes to the hypoproteinaemia seen in alimentary disease. Proteins entering the gut lumen are rapidly hydrolysed to oligopeptides and amino acids, and these are re-absorbed. Hypoproteinaemia develops only when protein loss and nitrogen catabolism exceed the body's capacity to synthesise protein.

Hypoproteinaemia due to PLE has been described in many disorders:

1. diseases associated with mucosal ulceration: carcinoma of the stomach or intestine, Crohn's disease, ulcerative colitis;
2. diseases associated with increased lymphatic pressure: congestive heart failure, lymphoma, Whipple's disease, intestinal lymphangiectasia;
3. diseases associated with diffuse mucosal cell damage: coeliac disease, mesenteric vascular insufficiency.

The detection and quantitation of gastrointestinal protein loss involves the measurement of radioactivity excreted in the stool following the intravenous administration of radio-labelled molecules, for example, ^{51}Cr-labelled serum proteins.

Meckel's diverticulum

Meckel's diverticulum is a true diverticulum with smooth muscle in its wall. It is the most common malformation of the gastrointestinal tract representing the persisting proximal end of the vitello-intestinal duct. The remnant persists in about 2% of the population, is usually about 5 cm in length and is situated about 60 cm from the ileocaecal valve. The mucosa of the diverticulum may contain heterotopic epithelium of gastric, colonic or pancreatic tissue.

The vast majority of cases remain asymptomatic throughout life. Complications include severe haemorrhage per rectum due to peptic ulceration in the ileum adjacent to the ectopic gastric mucosa, intussusception, and Meckel's diverticulitis, the symptoms of which mimic those of acute appendicitis. Peritonitis may follow perforation of the sac.

Mesenteric arterial insufficiency

The abdominal viscera are supplied with blood from the coeliac axis, superior mesenteric and inferior mesenteric arteries. When atherosclerotic changes in the abdominal aorta—or in the proximal few centimetres of several of the main arteries—seriously impair arterial flow, the syndrome of 'abdominal angina' can result. Abdominal pain tends to occur one to two hours after meals, and may be so severe that the patient becomes afraid to eat and loses considerable weight.

The diagnosis may be confirmed by mesenteric angiography, but this procedure is not without risk in elderly patients. Progressive arterial occlusion may eventually cause bowel infarction, most commonly in the territory of the superior mesenteric artery (p. 85).

Chronic secretory diarrhoea of endocrine origin

Carcinoid syndrome

Carcinoid syndrome is a disorder characterised by flushing, attacks of wheezing and diarrhoea. It is usually associated with extensive hepatic metastases from a carcinoid tumour of the appendix or ileum, that is the mid-gut, but foregut (including bronchial) and hindgut carcinoids also occur.

Pathophysiology

Carcinoid tumours produce excessive amounts of serotonin, which is excreted in the urine as 5-hydroxyindoleacetic acid (5-HIAA). This provides a useful diagnostic test. In addition to serotonin, carcinoid tumours may also produce excessive amounts of histamine, kallikrein, calcitonin, prostaglandins and substance-P.

Symptoms and signs

Episodic flushing of the face, cyanosis, wheezing, watery diarrhoea, steatorrhoea and pulmonary valve stenosis are the common clinical features. Diagnosis is made by finding elevated levels of 5-HIAA in the urine (over 10 mg/24 h). Prognosis is good because the tumours are slow-growing, and recently octreitide 50 mg twice a day by injection has been shown to control the symptoms.

Medullary carcinoma of the thyroid

Patients with these tumours may present with chronic secretory diarrhoea and hypokalaemia. Elevated levels of calcitonin and prostaglandins have been found and implicated in the syndrome. Treatment is thyroidectomy and, if metastases are present, octreitide may be useful.

Immunology

A wide range of ingested substances and micro-organisms bathe the exposed surface of the small intestine. This vulnerable interface between man and the external environment is protected by the mucosal immune system which is specially adapted to function at this site. Mucosal immune responses are characterised by:

1. processing of antigen in the Peyer's patch, where the B-lymphocytes proliferate and then migrate via the lymphatics and the bloodstream to reach the mucosa as IgA class, antibody-secreting cells;
2. IgA being secreted as a dimer which complexes with a glycoprotein called secretory piece (SP), which is synthesised by the epithelial cell and protects IgA from the digestive proteases so that it can function as an antibody on the epithelial surface. IgM can also bind SP and function as a secretory antibody;
3. secretory IgA antibodies neutralising viruses, preventing access of bacteria or toxins to the epithelial cell or 'blocking' the uptake of food antigens.

Immunodeficiency

Selective *IgA deficiency* is the most common form of immune defect, and affects about one in 600 of the population. Most IgA-deficient people are healthy because 'back-up' immune systems take over. Pernicious anaemia, coeliac disease and non-specific diarrhoea, however, occur with increased frequency in this condition.

Hypogammaglobulinaemia is characterised by deficiency of all the major immunoglobulin classes. Although it occurs less commonly than selective IgA deficiency, hypogammaglobulinaemia usually causes gut symptoms, especially diarrhoea and sometimes steatorrhoea, due to *Giardia lamblia* and bacterial infections, and sometimes to flattening of the intestinal villi. The incidence of pernicious anaemia and of gastrointestinal malignancy is significantly increased.

SUGGESTED FURTHER READING

Doe, W. F., The immunology of the gut, in Lachmann, P. J., Peters, D. K., Rosen, F. S., Walport, M., *Clinical Aspects of Immunology*, 4th edn, Blackwells, 1993; 2079–90.

Fisher, R. L. (ed.), Malabsorption and nutritional status and support, *Gastroenterology Clinics of North America*, 1989; 18.

Sleisenger, M. H. and Fordtran, J. S. (eds), *Gastrointestinal Disease: Pathophysiology, Diagnosis and Management*, 5th edn, W. B. Saunders, Philadelphia, 1993.

CHAPTER 4

Colon, rectum and anus

D. J. B. St John, G. P. Young and I. T. Jones

Anatomy, physiology and pathophysiology

The large bowel (colon, rectum and anus) is the final organ in the digestive process. In a normal person, approximately 2 L of fluid enters the caecum every twenty-four hours, yet only 100–200 mL is passed as faeces. The large bowel thus removes fluid from ileal effluent and controls evacuation of solids to a socially convenient frequency. The luminal environment of the colon is complex and important. It is colonised by billions of bacteria; these ferment dietary fibre and other unabsorbed substances such as carbohydrate and amino acids, and produce short-chain fatty acids which are metabolically important to the epithelium. The luminal environment is a modifying factor in tumorigenesis, large bowel cancer being the most common internal malignancy in many Western countries.

Macroanatomy

The large intestine extends from the ileocaecal valve to the anus and is about 1.5 m long in adults. The appendix attaches to the caecum, the latter not being distinct from the ascending colon in humans. The colon continues distally, turns sharply at the hepatic flexure to form the transverse colon, turning again at the splenic flexure to form the descending colon which continues towards the pelvis. At the entrance to the pelvis it gains a mesentery to form the sigmoid colon of variable length and tortuosity. The sigmoid colon empties into the rectum at the level of the sacral promontory. The rectum is 15–18 cm in length and follows the curvature of the sacrum to end at the anorectal junction, leading to the anal canal (3–4 cm in length).

Muscle coats of the colon comprise inner circular and outer longitudinal layers, the latter being concentrated into three flat bands (taeniae coli). These taeniae shorten the colon and form sacculations (haustra).

The anal canal and rectal musculature are more complex. The upper anal canal possesses longitudinal folds which are separated from one another by sinuses and end distally in small folds called anal valves. The inner layer of rectal smooth muscle thickens at the anus to form the internal sphincter while a circular ring of striated muscle forms the external sphincter. The puborectalis muscle forms a sling-like support to the rectum which maintains an acute angle between the rectum and anus and is the major muscle of continence.

Microanatomy

The four layers of the large bowel are mucosa, submucosa, muscularis externa and serosa. The mucosa, which lines the lumen, consists of columnar epithelial, lamina propria and muscularis mucosae layers. Architecturally, the epithelium and lamina propria are organised such that the epithelium forms pit-like extensions (crypts) into the lamina propria. The lamina propria contains supporting connective tissue, blood vessels, lymphatics and a few nerves and smooth muscle cells. The submucosa is separated from the lamina propria by the muscularis mucosae; the submucosa contains the main nerve plexi and, importantly, blood vessels and lymphatics.

Epithelium

The epithelium consists of three major mature cell types: columnar 'absorptive' cells (or *colonocytes*) with a specialised apical surface consisting of densely packed microvilli; *goblet* cells containing a mass of mucus-containing granules; and *enteroendocrine* cells containing secretory granules and which stain for various gut hormones. All cell types originate from the progenitor cells situated in the lower two-thirds of the crypt. Colonocytes outnumber goblet cells by about two to one, depending on the site in the colon. The colon is capable of producing significant amounts of certain gut hormones, for example, enteroglucagon.

The epithelium undergoes constant and rapid renewal and has one of the highest cell turnover rates for the entire body. The undifferentiated progenitor cells divide in the lower two-thirds of the crypt to provide new cells, which migrate up the crypt to the luminal surface where they are shed. As they migrate, they differentiate into mature cells which cannot divide. Proliferating cells pass through a sequence of phases in the cell renewal cycle. The entire cell cycle lasts one to two days; the synthesis or S-phase about eleven to twenty hours, G_2 (post-synthetic) phase one to six hours and M (mitosis) about one hour. About 8–12% of cells in the proliferation compartment of the normal crypt are in S-phase (i.e. the 'labelling index'). Epithelial cells which migrate up the crypt survive about three to five days before being shed.

Factors which affect colonic structure

These will be discussed under specific diseases; however, a few general physiological and pathophysiological mechanisms will be addressed here to demonstrate the dynamic state of large bowel microanatomy.

Food and nutrients

There is an intimate relationship between intestinal epithelium and the lumen. The intraluminal presence of faecal bulk is important in maintaining cell renewal in the large bowel. Diversion of luminal contents by colonic bypass or colostomy leads to atrophy and reduced proliferation in the colon. During starvation, studies in rodents have shown depression of cell proliferation and decrease in depth of crypts. Atrophy of a lesser degree also occurs in rodents fed on a low-fibre diet or the elemental wholly-absorbed diet 'Vivonex'. These findings are consistent with the recent demonstration that short-chain fatty acids, especially butyrate, produced by microbial fermentation of fibre and unabsorbed carbohydrate in the colon, are the principal metabolic substrates for the colonic epithelium.

Damage to the large bowel epithelium

Both ischaemia and radiation damage, induced experimentally, cause an initial fall in epithelial proliferation, but this is followed within a few days (in the absence of continuing damage) by a marked increase in proliferative activity in an effort to repair the damage. Proliferative parameters then return to normal within a few weeks.

Mucosal disease may cause profound structural changes. For instance, in active ulcerative colitis there is a dense inflammatory infiltrate, a change in the shape of colonocytes to cuboidal, and shortening, branching and loss of crypts. Epithelial proliferation and the size of the proliferative compartment in the crypts increase, but crypts shorten because cells are rapidly exfoliated into the lumen.

There is now increasing evidence that patients with large bowel cancer or adenomas have an increased rate of cell proliferation, a higher labelling index, and an enlarged proliferative zone throughout the large bowel.

Physiology of the large bowel

Approximately 1.5–2.0 L of fluid are delivered from ileum to caecum in every twenty-four-hour period. The fluid is isotonic, of relatively neutral pH and contains a range of unabsorbed dietary substances, especially 'fibre' (i.e. non-starch polysaccharides). The proximal colon is concerned primarily with stasis and mixing of contents to allow bacterial fermentation of fibre and fluid absorption to proceed. The distal colon absorbs less but ensures continent evacuation of the formed stool. The principal determinant of faecal bulk, which is normally less than 200–250 mL per day, is the dietary fibre intake. Recently, it has been recognised that some dietary starches are not fully digested. These ferment in the colon and might also act like dietary fibre.

The majority of normal people pass one bowel action per day, but the normal range extends from three stools per day to three per week. In addition, about 20–25% of the community do not have a regular bowel habit and tend to fluctuate between relative 'constipation' and 'diarrhoea'.

Diarrhoea may be defined in two ways. The objective definition is a twenty-four-hour stool weight of greater than 300 g. The subjective definition is increased stool frequency and/or decreased stool consistency relative to normal for the person. Constipation is less easy to define. Many patients complain of being 'constipated' when they simply have firmer stools which seem more difficult to pass. An objective definition is stool frequency less than once every three days.

Study of the human colon *in vivo* has not been easy: motor activity is complex and still poorly understood; there are significant regional differences in function; and there is a complex interaction with the luminal environment which contains billions of resident micro-organisms. The following discussion is drawn from human data where possible, but occasionally draws on principles established from animal studies.

Absorption and secretion of electrolytes

The major absorptive function of the large bowel is to conserve electrolytes and water, and absorb short-chain fatty acids. Ammonia and other bacterial metabolites are also absorbed, but these do not appear to be nutritionally or metabolically useful. Secretion of fluid is normally more than balanced by absorption, and net secretion is always pathological.

The plasma membranes of epithelial cells pose an effective barrier to hydrophilic substances, unless specialised carrier systems are present. A major site for transepithelial movement of hydrophilic small molecules is between cells, through the 'tight-junctions' linking the cells together. In the colon, passive fluxes of Na^+ or Cl^- through these junctions are small, thus preventing 'leakage'. The active transport of Na^+ across the luminal membrane of the colonocyte results in a transepithelial potential difference of 30–40 mV. This movement is electrogenic and uncoupled. Sodium is then actively pumped out of the cells into the intracellular spaces by Na^+-K^+-ATPase. Neither glucose nor alanine augment transport of Na^+ as they do in the small intestine.

Cl^- ion absorption proceeds in exchange with bicarbonate, and is not coupled with Na^+ movement. Bicarbonate is generated within the cell by carbonic anhydrase.

Microbial digestion of dietary fibre and other unabsorbed carbohydrate generates large amounts of acetate, butyrate and propionate. These are the major anions in faeces in humans and total concentrations are 100–200 mEq/L. They are well absorbed, although the rate depends on the pH (the normal range varies widely from 5.5–8.0) and butyrate, in particular, is preferred as a metabolic substrate for colonocytes, above glucose and glutamine.

Factors which modify the absorption-secretion balance in vivo

Cyclic AMP can stimulate active secretion of Cl^- and is probably the major intracellular mediator for its secretion. Secretion of water follows as a result. Table 4.1 lists some substances which influence the net balance between absorption and secretion, and the probable mechanisms of their action.

Table 4.1 *Substances influencing the net balance between fluid and electrolyte absorption and secretion in the large bowel*

Substance	*Effect*
Hormones (partly active in small intestine)	
Aldosterone	↑Na^+ absorption and K^+ excretion
Glucocorticoids	↑Na^+ absorption and K^+ excretion
Antidiuretic hormone	↓Na^+, Cl^- and water absorption
Vasoactive intestinal peptide (VIP)	Causes Cl^- secretion
Prostaglandins (E_2, F_2)	Causes active Cl^- secretion
Somatostatin	Improves net absorption
Laxatives	
Sodium sulfosuccinate	↑secretion
Diphenolic compounds (e.g. bisacody)	↑secretion
Phenolphthalein	↑secretion
Ricinoleic acid (castor oil)	↑secretion
Osmotic agents ($MgSO_4$, lactulose)	↓absorption
Bile acids and fatty acids	
Dihydroxy bile acids	↑Cl^- secretion[a]
Hydroxylated fatty acids	↑Cl^- secretion[a]
Bacterial toxins (largely active in small intestine)	
Cholera enterotoxin	↑Na^+, Cl^- and water secretion[a]
Certain *E. coli* enterotoxins	↑Na^+, Cl^- and water secretion[a]
Antidiarrhoeal drugs (largely active in small intestine)	
Opiates	Block fluid and electrolyte secretion

[a] Probably act via increasing intracellular cyclic-AMP.

Transit and storage in the large bowel

Human colonic motility depends on factors controlling the electrical activity of the circular layer of smooth muscle, as well as intrinsic and extrinsic nervous activity. Propulsion through the large intestine is slow compared to the small intestine, being measured in days rather than hours. Strong, distally proceeding mass movements are the most propulsive actions. They originate in transverse colon and occur three to four times per day; they are stimulated by food and physical activity and diminish during sleep. Control of these is related in a poorly understood way to intrinsic myoelectric activity. The latter undergoes phasic changes known as the slow wave. The slow wave dictates the time and location of action potentials which cause propulsive contraction. Peristaltic activity occurs on a background of low pressure, segmental, non-propulsive contractions.

The activities of extrinsic, intrinsic and afferent nerves are integrated within the colon, at the prevertebral ganglia and in the spinal cord. The adrenergic system, particularly β-adrenergic nerves, is inhibitory and the parasympathetic is excitatory. The balance is inhibitory such that in paraplegia, constipation is often the result. The gastrocolic reflex, or the desire to defecate after eating, is neurogenic and reduced by anti-cholinergic drugs. The physiologic significance of hormonal interactions with colonic musculature is not clear.

The main role of the ascending and transverse colon is storage, where mixing movements promote absorption of fluid, electrolytes and bacterial fermentation products. Transit proceeds here at only 1 cm/h. The function of the ileocaecal valve is largely to prevent reflux back into ileum and not to regulate flow into caecum. The bacterial count in the caecum is far higher than it is in the terminal ileum. The sigmoid colon also has a short-term storage function.

The rectum accommodates well to distension, for social convenience. The sudden increase in tension in the wall due to distension, is normally short-lived; in the various types of colitis and in constipation, this response is often perturbed. Mechanisms enabling conscious control of defecation are complex. In some subjects defecation empties the rectum only, while in others it empties the entire left side of the large bowel. The urge to defecate originates from sudden tension in the rectal wall. During defecation, there is relaxation of the perineum and puborectalis in association with increased abdominal pressure.

Congenital anomalies

Imperforate anus

Congenital anorectal anomalies occur about once in every 5000 births. A wide variety of anomalies exist, but for practical purposes they may be divided into high and low, depending on their relationship to the levator ani muscle. In low lesions, treatment is usually simple and the child should obtain normal continence. High lesions are more difficult to treat and normal anal continence is less reliably achieved. Imperforate anus and other anomalies in this area should be recognised at birth so that surgical treatment can be planned at an early stage.

Hirschsprung's disease (congenital aganglionosis)

In Hirschsprung's disease, there is absence of the ganglia of the intramural nervous plexuses for varying lengths of the rectum and colon. The aganglionic distal bowel is undilated and poorly distensible (unlike the normal rectum) and obstruction is produced by the absence of peristalsis. The more proximal, normally innervated bowel becomes secondarily dilated and hypertrophied.

Clinical features

Children with Hirschsprung's disease typically have symptoms of constipation which date from infancy, and usually from birth. The condition is more common in males than females. There are three main forms of presentation:

1. low-intestinal obstruction in the neonatal period, requiring colostomy for its relief;
2. constipation and abdominal distension caused by megacolon, presenting in infancy;
3. megacolon presenting later in life, following only mild or no symptoms in infancy.

The most serious complication is acute enterocolitis, the main cause of death in this condition. Ulceration develops in the dilated colon, often progressing to necrosis of the bowel wall, perforation, pericolic abscess or peritonitis and then septicaemia. Decompression of the bowel is an essential part of treatment.

Diagnosis

Hirschsprung's disease must be distinguished from acquired megacolon caused by rectal inertia, which typically presents during or after the second year of life. In acquired megacolon, rectal examination usually reveals anal soiling and a large bolus of faeces lying just above the anal sphincters.

Two investigations provide a specific diagnosis of Hirschsprung's disease. Deep *rectal biopsy* will reveal absence of ganglion cells. *Anal manometry* during balloon distension of the rectum will demonstrate the absence of the normal reflex inhibitory response of the internal anal sphincter.

Treatment

Treatment consists of resection of the aganglionic segment after careful preoperative preparation of the colon. Preliminary colostomy may be necessary in high-grade obstruction in young infants. Bowel continuity is restored by anastomosis of the normal colon to the anorectal junction, with preservation of the anal sphincter muscles. A variety of techniques have been described. The Duhamel procedure places the colon in the presacral plane with a low colo-anal anastomosis being performed. It is the most commonly performed and probably the most successful method of treatment.

Ulcerative colitis

Ulcerative colitis is a diffuse, non-specific, inflammatory disease of the rectal and colonic mucosa of unknown cause; no pathogenic micro-organisms have been identified in the stools. The disease varies greatly in its extent and severity. The typical course consists of repeated episodes of severe diarrhoea, often with blood mixed with the stools, interspersed with periods of freedom from symptoms. Less commonly, the course is chronic with continuous symptoms. In its most dangerous form, ulcerative colitis presents acutely with severe symptoms and the patient rapidly deteriorates unless treatment is instituted without delay.

The net fluid changes in the colon, which are responsible for the diarrhoea, are shown diagrammatically in Figure 4.1. The essential problem is malabsorption of fluid although inflammatory exudate contributes.

Incidence

Females are affected slightly more commonly than males. The disease can occur at any age, but is most common in the fifteen to thirty year age group. Some studies have shown a bimodal age distribution, with a small rise in the number of new cases after the age of fifty-five years. The annual incidence varies from

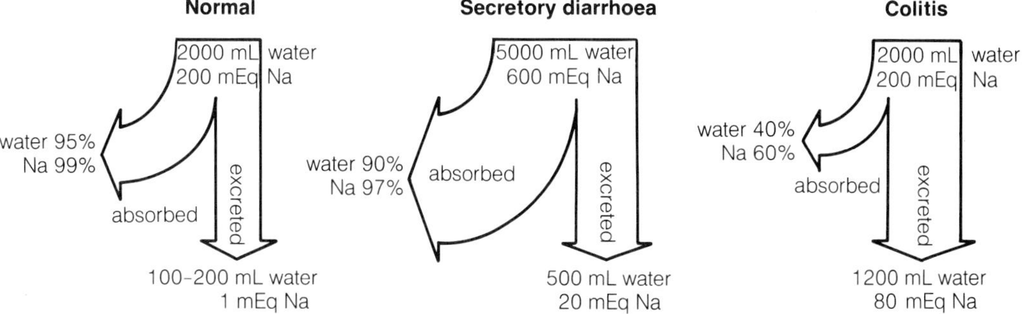

Fig. 4.1 *Net balance of water and electrolytes in the human colon in normal and various disease states. Small bowel secretory diarrhoea—as would occur with* E. coli*-induced toxigenic traveller's diarrhoea. The maximum reabsorption capacity of the colon is about 4.5 L. Colitis: as with conditions such as ulcerative colitis or* Salmonella *infections*

three to eight per 100 000 population. The disease occurs in all races but is more common in white populations than black. In the white population in the United States, Jews are more commonly affected than non-Jews, but the prevalence in Israeli Jews is low.

Aetiology

The cause of ulcerative colitis is unknown, but theories include altered immunity, infection with a transmissible agent (possibly a virus), and a genetic defect (5–10% of patients have a family history of ulcerative colitis). The most popular view is that the disease is autoimmune. This view is based on the observation that lymphocytes from some patients with ulcerative colitis will destroy the patient's colonocytes grown in tissue culture. What induces this state is unknown, although certain strains of *E. coli* from the colon have been shown to have antigenic similarities to colonocytes. Lymphocyte-mediated hypersensitivity reactions might be set in motion by exposure to these bacterial antigens; however, even this explanation of the disease is unsatisfactory in many respects and the changes could be the consequence of the disease rather than its cause. An interesting association has been noted with smoking status. Ulcerative colitis is more common in non-smokers, particularly in ex-smokers. The significance of the association is uncertain.

Classification

The disease is characterised by diffuse mucosal damage, with reduction in the numbers of goblet cells, infiltration of the lamina propria with lymphocytes, plasma cells, eosinophils and neutrophils, and formation of crypt abscesses. Histological differences between acute ulcerative colitis and acute infectious colitis have been described, but biopsies must be obtained early in the illness, preferably within the first four days. With that exception, there are no specific histological features to permit a confident diagnosis of acute ulcerative colitis as opposed to the various types of acute bacterial colitis, and classification by histology is not helpful.

Classifications based on the extent of involvement and on the severity of the disease are useful, both for decisions about treatment and for assessment of prognosis.

Extent of disease can be determined by sigmoidoscopy or colonoscopy, plain abdominal x-ray or barium enema. The disease typically involves the rectum, extending for a variable distance into the colon. There is continuous involvement of the mucosa up to the proximal limit of the disease. Rectal sparing can occur in ulcerative colitis, but is unusual. The extent of the disease may increase with time.

The disease can be classified as:

1. proctitis or proctosigmoiditis (involvement of rectum alone or rectum and sigmoid colon);
2. left-sided colitis (rectum, sigmoid colon and descending colon);
3. extensive or total colitis (rectum and most or all of the colon).

The severity of the disease is determined by the severity of diarrhoea, and the presence or absence of systemic features such as anaemia, dehydration, fever and tachycardia.

1. remission—no symptoms
2. mild—less than four stools per day and no constitutional disturbance
3. moderate—between mild and severe
4. severe—more than six bloody stools per day plus anaemia and leukocytosis, fever, tachycardia and possibly abdominal tenderness and distension. In fulminant ulcerative colitis, the colon may dilate (toxic megacolon) and subsequently perforate. Severe attacks require urgent and intensive treatment as the mortality rate may be as high as 20%

Symptoms and signs

Characteristically, the patients have diarrhoea with blood and mucus mixed with the stools, together with cramping lower abdominal pain. In general, the more severe the rectal and sigmoid inflammatory changes, the more urgent and the more frequent is the diarrhoea. In active proctocolitis, the rectum can be hypersensitive and poorly compliant. Distension of the rectum has been shown to induce prolonged relaxation of the anal sphincter, contributing to the frequent and urgent defecation in acute exacerbations of the disease. When there is only limited involvement of the rectum, patients can present with constipation and rectal bleeding rather than diarrhoea, the inflamed rectum apparently resisting the passage of intestinal contents.

Attacks of colitis in patients with extensive disease are often severe. Dehydration with sodium and potassium loss is common and excessive exudation of protein, combined with poor oral intake, leads to hypoalbuminaemia.

Complications of the disease

1. *Localised to the large bowel.* Complications include megacolon, perforation of the colon, massive haemorrhage, and carcinoma. These complications are very important and mainly occur in patients with extensive colonic disease.
2. *Remote from the large bowel.* These include arthritis, sacro-ileitis, uveitis, sclerosing cholangitis and other hepatobiliary complications, erythema nodosum and a gangrenous lesion of the skin called pyoderma gangrenosum.

Diagnosis

The diagnosis is always one of exclusion, as the symptoms and signs of ulcerative colitis may be mimicked by bacterial or amoebic dysentery. The diagnostic methods used are:

1. *Sigmoidoscopy.* The typical findings are those of a red, oedematous mucosa with mucopus on the mucosal surface and in the lumen. The mucosa is friable (bleeding on contact) and lacks the normally visible vascular pattern, due to mucosal oedema masking the submucosal vessels. Frank mucosal ulceration is relatively uncommon in the rectum. Pseudopolyps may be seen, usually in the upper rectum. Pseudopolyps represent islands of hyperplastic mucosa interspersed with areas of ulceration. The changes in the rectum are usually diffuse. Patchy disease with normal-looking mucosa in between is much more suggestive of Crohn's colitis. Biopsy should be performed to exclude Crohn's disease.
2. *Stool examination and culture.* The search for amoebae should be made by a skilled microbiologist on a fresh stool sample or preferably on material obtained at sigmoidoscopy. Stool microscopy and culture for pathogens such as *Shigella, Campylobacter* and *Clostridium difficile* should be performed on at least three samples. In addition, a search should be made for *Clostridium difficile* toxin, especially in patients treated with antibiotics in the weeks before onset of diarrhoea.
3. *Barium enema.* This provides information about the extent of disease and the severity of mucosal damage; however, barium enema often underestimates the extent of disease and is substantially less reliable than colonoscopy. This examination is contraindicated in severe disease or within ten days of biopsy. If toxic megacolon is suspected, plain abdominal x-ray will confirm the diagnosis. When disease is severe, gas contrast in plain films often shows the presence and extent of colonic ulceration. Barium enema has been superseded by colonoscopy in the diagnosis of ulcerative colitis.
4. *Colonoscopy.* This provides a more accurate assessment of severity and extent of the disease than barium enema and it has an important role in surveillance for dysplasia and colorectal cancer.

Prognosis

In ulcerative colitis, the threat to life is particularly great in three situations:

1. fulminant ulcerative colitis;
2. the elderly patient with ulcerative colitis;
3. long-standing extensive or total colitis.

Medical treatment

Treatment of an acute attack or exacerbation

1. *Diet.* If tolerated, the patient should be given a high-calorie, high-protein diet. A milk-free diet will help control the diarrhoea when coincidental hypolactasia is present. Dietary fibre may worsen the diarrhoea of active ulcerative colitis.
2. *Corticosteroids.* These can be given systemically (as oral prednisolone or intravenous hydrocortisone) or as steroid enemas. Selection of the dose and route of administration depends upon the severity of the attack and the extent of disease. Systemic steroids are usually more effective than topical treatment with steroid enemas, except when the disease is limited to the rectum and distal colon. Most patients can be treated with oral prednisolone, but intravenous administration of hydrocortisone may be required in severe attacks, especially when nausea and vomiting are present. With oral prednisolone, the usual initial dose is 30–40 mg/d given in two divided doses each day. The dose is increased if the disease fails to respond to treatment, and is gradually reduced when the disease comes under control. With severe attacks, prednisolone therapy has to be continued in diminishing dosage for a period of three or four months. Steroid enemas are given daily or twice daily as tolerated.
3. *Sulphasalazine and 5-aminosalicylic acid derivatives.* These drugs are not as effective as corticosteroid therapy for controlling acute attacks but, in contrast to corticosteroids, they do reduce the frequency of relapses of the disease. Because the drug often produces nausea and vomiting, sulphasalazine should not be used in the early stages of treatment of acute colitis until there has been a definite clinical response to steroid therapy. Side-effects of sulphasalazine include drug fever, skin rash, lymphadenopathy and cholestatic hepatitis. A variety of haematological side-effects have been described, including rare but fatal agranulocytosis and aplastic anaemia. Many of the side-effects are due to hypersensitivity to the sulphonamide moiety. New 5-aminosalicylic acid derivatives such as olsalazine and mesalazine, which do not contain sulphonamide, are very effective for patients intolerant to sulphasalazine. Although not readily available in a number of countries, enemas of 5-aminosalicylic acid are effective in many patients with ulcerative proctitis or proctosigmoiditis not responding to treatment with steroid enemas and oral sulphasalazine.

4. *Azathioprine.* Inclusion of azathioprine in the treatment regimen should be considered in patients failing to respond to the combination of corticosteroids with sulphasalazine or one of the 5-aminosalicylic acid derivatives.
5. *Symptomatic treatment.* Antidiarrhoeal agents such as codeine, loperamide and diphenoxylate should not be used in acute attacks because of the risk of precipitating toxic megacolon.

In fulminant colitis, the patient will require blood transfusions, intravenous electrolyte replacement, intravenous steroid therapy and often parenteral nutrition. Patients should be managed jointly by a gastroenterologist and a surgeon, with careful clinical review every few hours to monitor response to medical therapy. Plain abdominal x-rays should be taken at least once each day during the acute phase to follow changes in colonic distension. The decision about the need for, and the timing of, surgical intervention is based on failure to respond to medical therapy, as judged by persistence of abdominal pain, tenderness or distension, continued tachycardia or fever, or other evidence of uncontrolled disease.

Prevention of recurrence

Maintenance therapy with sulphasalazine has been shown to reduce the relapse rate of ulcerative colitis. The standard dose is 2 g/d, given in two divided doses. A lower dose does not appear to be effective in reducing the relapse rate. Some patients require a higher maintenance dose to prevent relapse, doses ranging up to 4 g/d. The drug should be continued indefinitely. Male infertility can occur as a side-effect of long-term treatment with sulphasalazine. The sulphonamide component of sulphasalazine is responsible for a reduction in sperm counts, but the infertility is reversed by changing to olsalazine or mesalazine.

Prevention of cancer

Risk of cancer increases in patients with extensive or total ulcerative colitis after the disease has been present for eight to ten years. Patients with left-sided colitis appear to have an increased cancer risk, although not until a decade later. Most studies have failed to show any increase in risk for colorectal cancer in patients with disease limited to the rectum and distal sigmoid colon.

There is increasing acceptance of the view that regular surveillance for premalignant changes, such as epithelial dysplasia, should be started after eight years in patients with extensive ulcerative colitis and after sixteen to eighteen years in those with left-sided colitis. Colonoscopy with multiple biopsies should be performed every two years and, depending on the patient's views, consideration should be given to the option of obtaining sigmoidoscopic biopsies in the intervals between colonoscopy. The only caveat is that surveillance endoscopies should not be performed during an exacerbation of colitis. Particular attention should be given to mass lesions which frequently harbour an occult cancer. In the absence of any focal abnormality, random biopsies (eight to twelve) should be taken, along the length of the colon and rectum. Decisions about the need for prophylactic colectomy are based on the severity and persistence of dysplasia. Assessment of dysplasia is subject to considerable inter-observer variation and requires expert pathological evaluation.

Surgical treatment

Surgery is indicated for life-threatening complications (severe attack, perforation, haemorrhage or megacolon), for chronic disease with intolerable symptoms or complication of medications, and less frequently for dysplasia, carcinoma or extra-intestinal manifestations.

In the acute situation, total colectomy with ileostomy leaving the rectal stump in situ is the simplest and safest procedure. It averts the acute crisis, avoids the extra morbidity of pelvic dissection and allows the possibility of a later reconstructive procedure when the patient's health has been restored.

In the elective situation, a number of options are available. Proctocolectomy (removal of the entire colon, rectum and anus with a permanent ileostomy) is the traditional procedure of choice. Although it eradicates all diseased bowel and cures the condition, the need for an ileostomy is a major drawback. It is now mainly reserved for the older patient, for those with sphincter dysfunction or a coexistent distal rectal cancer, or for the patient unwilling to embark on more complex reconstructive procedures.

While popular in the 1960s and 1970s, total colectomy with preservation of the rectum and ileorectal anastomosis has become a less commonly performed procedure. The operation should only be employed in carefully selected patients, as persistent disease in the rectum may lead to intolerable diarrhoea and incontinence. Furthermore, long-term surveillance is necessary because of the risk of cancer developing in the diseased rectum.

The operation of choice is the restorative proctocolectomy or 'pouch' operation. Although the entire colon and rectum are removed, a new rectum is constructed from small bowel and anastomosed to the anal canal. The 'pouch' or reservoir is constructed from two or more loops of ileum and is designed to prevent diarrhoea that would follow a direct ileo-anal anastomosis without any reservoir. More than ten years of experience has been obtained with these pelvic reservoir or 'pouch' operations. Despite occasional problems of postoperative sepsis, non-specific inflammation of the reservoir ('pouchitis') and some uncertain functional results, reliable results are achieved in most patients. The combination of eradication of all disease and avoidance of an ileostomy makes restorative proctocolectomy the most desirable procedure for surgical management of ulcerative colitis. These features make it particularly attractive to younger patients.

Crohn's disease of the colon

Crohn's colitis is being recognised more frequently than in the past. In certain countries, its prevalence is similar to that of ulcerative colitis. Increased recognition may be due in part to previous misdiagnosis as ulcerative colitis. The disease shows a familial tendency and is more common in Jews than in other races in the United States.

The disease is characterised by inflammatory changes that extend throughout the wall of the bowel, often with deep fissures penetrating into the submucosa and the muscularis.

Distinguishing between this disease and ulcerative colitis can be difficult and separation is not possible in 10% of all cases; however, making a distinction between the two diseases is important for the following reasons:

1. In contrast to ulcerative colitis, Crohn's disease may involve any part of the gastrointestinal tract from mouth to anus. Recurrent disease in other parts of the intestine is extremely common after surgical ablation of earlier lesions.
2. Although the incidence of colon cancer in Crohn's disease has been shown to be increased substantially in patients who developed their disease before the age of twenty-one years, the risk is much less than in extensive ulcerative colitis. Screening appears to have less to offer in Crohn's disease and is not widely practised at present.
3. Some of the surgical options for ulcerative colitis, notably pelvic reservoir surgery, are contraindicated in patients with Crohn's colitis as the disease may recur in the ileum used to construct the 'pouch', with serious consequences.

A number of features may assist in distinguishing Crohn's colitis from ulcerative colitis:

1. Although Crohn's disease can cause distal or total colitis, the typical distribution is patchy ('skip lesions'), often with sparing of the rectum (Fig. 4.2).
2. The local anorectal complications of stricture, suppuration and fistula are far more common in Crohn's disease.
3. Epithelioid granulomas are found in 75% of patients with Crohn's disease.
4. Bloody diarrhoea is less common than in ulcerative colitis.

The general principles of medical and surgical treatment of Crohn's disease are similar to those of ulcerative colitis. The disease is often persistent and may also involve the small bowel. Corticosteroids and sulphasalazine are useful for treatment of acute exacerbations of Crohn's colitis but, as yet, there is no evidence to indicate that maintenance therapy with either drug reduces the risk of further relapses. Treatment with azathioprine may produce a remission in some patients with Crohn's colitis and permit a reduction in steroid dosage. It can also be effective for treatment of intestinal fistulae. Acute attacks may also respond to a

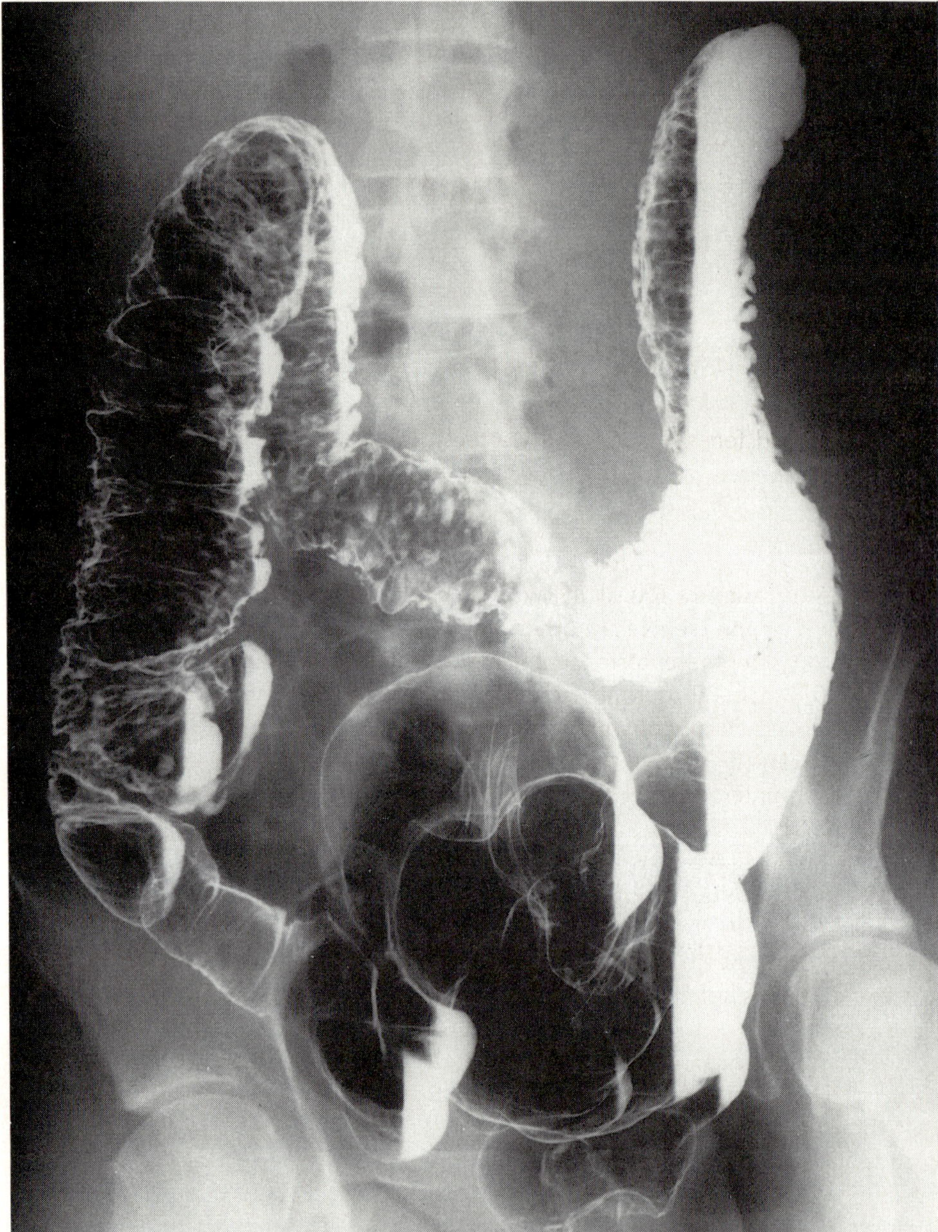

Fig. 4.2 *Crohn's colitis. Air-contrast barium enema showing severe ulceration extending from caecum to descending colon, but with sparing of the sigmoid colon and rectum*

short course of metronidazole. Long-term treatment with metronidazole or tinidazole is often effective in controlling suppurative anorectal disease, although there is a risk of side-effects with these drugs, particularly peripheral neuropathy with metronidazole.

Surgery in Crohn's colitis is required if life becomes intolerable because of chronic ill health or complications. Surgery usually takes the form of total proctocolectomy with ileostomy, or total colectomy and ileorectal anastomosis if the rectum is spared. Segmental resection is rarely performed and has a poor reputation because of early recurrence, even when the rest of the colon appears normal at the time of surgery. When Crohn's disease also involves the small bowel, macroscopically diseased small bowel is resected or, if multiple skip lesions are present, bowel length can be preserved by performing one or more strictureplasties rather than resection.

Diverticular disease of the colon

The sigmoid colon is the most common site for diverticula in the gastrointestinal tract. Males and females are equally affected and it is believed that as many as 30% of people aged over fifty years have colonic diverticula.

Aetiology

Diverticula are mainly found in two rows on the antimesenteric aspect of the colon related to the taeniae. Another row appears within the mesentery itself in relationship to the mesenteric taenia. These rows indicate the site of penetration of the blood vessels through the circular muscle coat adjacent to the taeniae, the weak points where mucous membrane herniation can occur. Each diverticulum is therefore closely related to a colonic blood vessel. This relationship may be important in understanding the aetiology of severe rectal haemorrhage in diverticular disease.

It is now considered that colonic diverticula develop as a result of disordered motility (Fig. 4.3). Segmenting movements normally occur in the colon but in diverticula-bearing segments, abnormal segmenting pressures can be demonstrated in response to such drugs as neostigmine and morphine. The circular muscle of the sigmoid colon in diverticular disease is hypertrophied.

A possible clue to the aetiology of colonic diverticula is its rarity in rural African populations. The rural African diet has a high fibre content and is associated with rapid intestinal transit and increased faecal weight. It is believed that the low-fibre diet of Western society, which is commonly associated with constipation, produces a prolonged transit time and a low faecal weight, which in turn predisposes to abnormal colonic motility. In a recent study, colonic motility returned to normal when patients with diverticular disease changed to a high-fibre diet.

Symptoms and signs

Most people with colonic diverticula have no symptoms at all. A number of others have abdominal pain and change in bowel habit. The underlying mechanism is uncertain. As the symptoms are similar to those of irritable bowel syndrome, it is presumed that the mechanism is similar. All complications of colonic

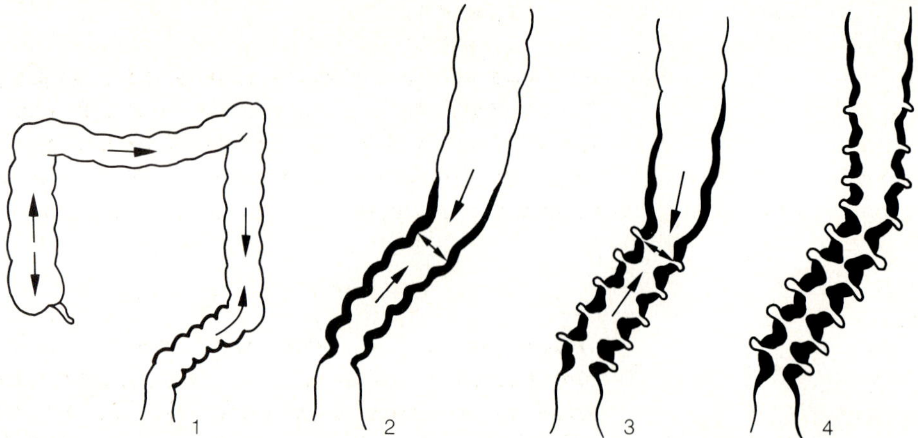

Fig. 4.3 *Steps in the formation of diverticula (after Painter, N. S. et al., Segmentation and the localization of intraluminal pressures in the human colon, with special reference to the pathogenesis of colonic diverticula,* Gastroenterology, *1965; 49:169–77. (**1**) To and fro movements of colon contents during absorption of water to form solid stool which passes into the rectum. (**2**) Abnormal segmenting movements in sigmoid colon with circular muscle hypertrophy. (**3**) and (**4**) Abnormally high pressures during segmentation lead to pulsion diverticula through muscle defects at site of blood vessel penetration*

diverticula probably follow one or more microperforations of the intradiverticular mucosa. The clinical features of complicated diverticular disease are as follows:

Acute diverticulitis

Acute diverticulitis may occur without warning as an acute attack, characterised by constant lower abdominal pain, fever, anorexia and occasional vomiting. Constipation is usual but diarrhoea may occur. The physical signs are those of a local peritonitis, usually in the left iliac fossa but the signs may involve the whole abdomen or pelvis. A mass of thickened colon may be felt abdominally or on rectal examination, although in many patients the guarding or rigidity of the abdominal wall muscles prevents deep palpation.

Pericolic abscess

This complication may follow acute diverticulitis, the abscess frequently being located within the mesentery. Typical clinical features are failure of recovery after an acute attack, with occurrence of an abdominal mass and swinging fever. A paralytic ileus or small bowel obstruction due to adherence of bowel to the abscess may develop.

General peritonitis

Peritonitis may be purulent following rupture of a pericolic abscess or faeculent due to frank rupture of a diverticulum. The latter is frequently lethal and the patient is likely to be shocked and gravely ill.

Intestinal obstruction

Although obstruction to the colon may occur, small intestinal obstruction due to adhesions is probably the most common form of intestinal obstruction in this disease.

Rectal haemorrhage

This is a relatively uncommon complication of diverticular disease. Haemorrhage is often profuse and recognisable by the patient as red blood rather than the black tarry stools of melaena. There are usually no other symptoms or physical signs apart from those of blood loss. Diverticular disease is a common cause of profuse rectal haemorrhage in middle-aged and elderly patients.

Fistula

A fistula is produced by rupture of a pericolic abscess into an adjacent viscus (Fig. 4.4). The most common is vesico-colic fistula which presents as recurrent urinary tract infections, or as passage of gas or faecal material during micturition (pneumaturia, faecaluria). Typically, a fistula develops as the signs of an acute abscess resolve.

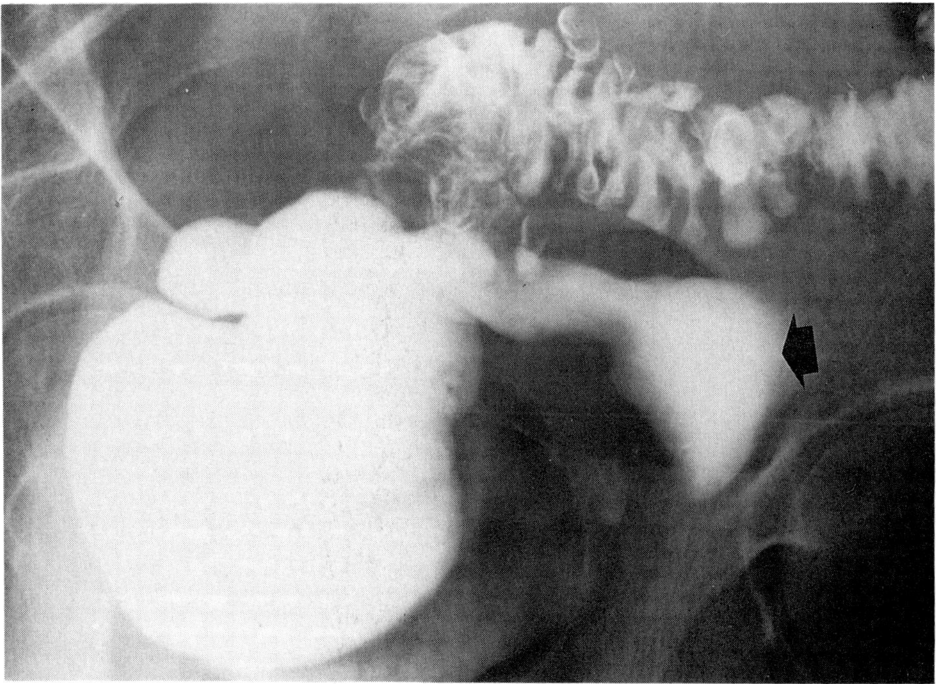

Fig. 4.4 *Diverticular disease of the colon. Air-contrast barium enema showing a fistula into the bladder (arrow)*

Diagnosis

In complicated forms of the disease, it is often easy to be confident about the diagnosis because of the characteristic history and findings on physical examination. Sigmoidoscopy should be performed, but is more useful for excluding cancer of the rectum or sigmoid colon and ulcerative colitis as the causes of symptoms than for making a diagnosis of diverticular disease. In severe diverticular disease, there is often distortion of the lumen at the rectosigmoid junction, making it difficult to pass a rigid sigmoidoscope. The mouths of the diverticula are commonly seen when a flexible endoscope is used.

The mainstay of diagnosis is radiologic examination of the colon by barium enema. The number and extent of the barium-filled diverticula can be seen and any alterations in contour due to spasm or fibrosis are shown. It may be difficult to distinguish narrowing of the colon in this disease from cancer. If any doubt exists, colonoscopy with biopsy should be performed, although distortion of the colon can make colonoscopy technically difficult.

Treatment

Prevention

A change to a high-fibre diet should make it possible to prevent or to arrest the progress of the disease.

Conservative measures

The majority of patients with symptoms can be treated by conservative measures. These are:

1. *Diet.* A diet containing adequate fibre is advised, except during an acute attack. The fibre content of the diet should be steadily increased to produce regular soft stools. Addition of excessive amounts of fibre worsen symptoms in some patients. Until recently, the main emphasis was on addition of unprocessed bran to the diet. As this can produce excessive flatulence and abdominal discomfort, other sources of fibre, particularly fruit and vegetables, should be included in the diet. If constipation remains a problem, hydrophilic granules such as methylcellulose may be given.
2. *Relief of pain.* Dietary measures and relief of constipation are usually sufficient to relieve symptoms such as pain.
3. *Antibiotic therapy.* Antibiotics are used in patients with acute diverticulitis as evidenced by local tenderness and fever. For the patient with mild diverticulitis, who can be managed on an out-patient basis, oral amoxycillin and metronidazole may be used. For more severe attacks—for example, with pericolic abscess or peritonitis, and in patients needing surgery—parenteral antibiotic therapy to cover both aerobic and anaerobic bowel flora—for example, gentamicin, amoxycillin and metronidazole in combination—is usually required.

Surgical treatment

Surgery is required only in the small proportion of patients who have one of the following forms of this disease:

1. repeated attacks of acute diverticulitis
2. intestinal obstruction
3. perforation of pericolic abscess with peritonitis
4. uncontrolled haemorrhage from a diverticulum
5. fistula, for example, to bladder, vagina or small intestine
6. inability to distinguish from cancer of colon, despite colonoscopy

The usual form of surgical treatment involves excision of the segment of colon involved in the inflammatory process, followed by an end-to-end anastomosis to restore continuity. Sufficient colon is removed to excise most of the diverticula, but more particularly the area of hypertrophied smooth muscle. Typically, this involves a sigmoid resection with anastomosis of the descending colon to the upper rectum. In the treatment of perforation, fistula or obstruction, resection of the colon with end-colostomy (Hartmann's operation) and delayed (or staged) reconstruction might be advisable if primary anastomosis is deemed unsafe.

Prognosis

The risks of diverticular disease are those of complications such as perforation, abscess and fistula formation. These complications should be prevented by dietary adjustment in the early stages of the disease. The surgery of diverticular disease and its complications is much safer if done electively rather than at the time of a severe complication.

Ischaemic colitis

Ischaemia of the colon may be present as one of a variety of clinical syndromes which depend on the extent and severity of the interruption of the blood supply.

Aetiology

The rapidly dividing cells of the colonic mucosa are very susceptible to ischaemic injury; other layers of the wall are much more resistant. The lesions occur most commonly at the splenic flexure and the adjacent descending colon; anatomically, this is the 'watershed' area between the areas of supply of the superior and inferior mesenteric arteries.

Ischaemia may be produced by interruption to the arterial supply or to the venous drainage of the colon; however, ischaemia can occur without obvious arterial or venous obstruction. This type of ischaemia is produced by a low flow rate as a result of vasoconstriction, small vessel disease or a fall in cardiac output.

Acute ischaemia of the colon may be a complication of surgery for aortic aneurysm, where interruption of the inferior mesenteric artery can produce a critical ischaemia of the colon when other arteries supplying the colon are obstructed by atheroma. Other predisposing factors include arterial emboli, cardiac disease, atherosclerotic disease and diabetes mellitus.

Clinical features

Acute ischaemic colitis

The patient has lower abdominal pain (commonly on the left side), diarrhoea and passage of blood per rectum. Fever and tachycardia are usually present, with tenderness and guarding over the affected colonic segment.

Gangrenous ischaemic colitis

There is a short history of severe abdominal pain and possibly diarrhoea. Rectal bleeding is unusual. The patient collapses with hypotension, tachycardia, widespread tenderness and abdominal rigidity, indicating the presence of generalised peritonitis.

Post-ischaemic stricture

Acute ischaemic colitis sometimes progresses to stricture formation caused by damage to the muscle coats. The main clinical feature is colicky abdominal pain. Prolonged mucosal ulceration may cause diarrhoea and bleeding. Rarely a patient may present with little or no history of acute ischaemic colitis, but with typical features of large bowel obstruction.

Diagnosis

The most common form of this disease is acute ischaemic colitis.

1. *Plain abdominal x-ray* in the acutely ill patient may suggest the diagnosis. Oedema of the bowel wall and thickening of mucosal folds is often evident, producing a characteristic 'thumb printing' appearance.
2. *Rigid (25 cm) sigmoidoscopy* usually shows no abnormality other than the presence of blood in the lumen.
3. *Barium enema* is often diagnostic. The involved area is narrowed and the normal haustral pattern is lost. 'Thumb printing' (swelling caused by submucosal haemorrhage or oedema which displaces the barium) is seen if the barium enema is performed in the early stages of the illness. Later development of intramural fibrosis can lead to formation of a smooth, funnel-shaped stricture.
4. *Flexible (60 cm) sigmoidoscopy or colonoscopy* is the investigation of choice, showing a patchy 'inflammation', haemorrhagic bullae or mucosal ulceration, usually located in the left side of the colon. Endoscopic examination has the added advantage of being available in intensive care units where these cases are often found.

5. *Doppler ultrasound* is a useful method for examining blood flow in the inferior mesenteric artery. Arteriography may also be helpful when major arterial obstruction is suspected.

Treatment

The treatment of ischaemic colitis is initially conservative. In the acute phase, treatment includes fluid replacement, pain relief and antibiotic therapy. Frequent abdominal examination and monitoring of temperature, blood pressure and pulse rate are essential. If peritonitis is suspected, a laparotomy must be performed to resect the gangrenous colon. Persistent symptoms and stricture formation usually require surgical excision of the lesion, with end-to-end anastomosis. Most patients recover without requiring surgery.

Uncommon causes of colitis

Rare or uncommon causes of colitis include collagenous colitis, radiation colitis and diversion colitis.

Collagenous colitis

The diagnosis of collagenous colitis depends upon demonstration of a subepithelial band of collagen in the colonic mucosa. Most cases occur in middle-aged women, who present with abdominal pain and watery diarrhoea. Findings at barium enema and colonoscopy are usually unremarkable and mucosal biopsies must be taken to establish the diagnosis. Treatment is often unsatisfactory, but sulphasalazine has been helpful in management of some cases.

Radiation colitis

Radiation injury of the colon often occurs in association with radiation injury of the small intestine. A careful history is required, as the exposure to radiation may have taken place up to thirty years before presentation. Investigation may reveal the presence of proctitis, strictures and fistulae. Radiological features can be confused with ischaemic colitis and Crohn's disease. The long-term sequelae of radiation damage to the intestine involve vasculitis.

Other causes of colitis

Other conditions that might be confused with ulcerative colitis, Crohn's colitis or infective colitis include drug-induced colitis (e.g. gold-induced colitis), chemical colitis (e.g. exposure to endoscope cleaning solutions as a result of inadequate cleaning of endoscopes) and diversion colitis. Diversion colitis is produced by surgical diversion of the faecal stream, with change in bowel flora below the diversion. Recognition of this entity is important, as the rectal discharge or diarrhoea promptly responds to treatment with short-chain fatty acid enemas or to surgical restoration of intestinal continuity when that is feasible.

Pathogenesis of colorectal neoplasia

The process of tumorigenesis in the colon consists of multiple steps which are recognisable phenotypically. Over the last few years, the genetic events responsible for change in adenomas and transformation to carcinoma have been steadily defined. The transition from a normal epithelial cell, constrained by normal growth control mechanisms and restricted to a single layer on the basement membrane, to one that has escaped normal control mechanisms and has acquired the ability to invade through the basement membrane, takes five to ten years on average. The process may occur at a faster rate in some of the hereditary colorectal cancer syndromes.

Progress in understanding the pathogenesis of colorectal cancer has been made possible by the ready availability of colonoscopy and the ability to remove precursor lesions. It is now recognised that activation of oncogenes (e.g. *ras* oncogene) and alterations in the expression of tumour suppressor genes (e.g. APC and MCC genes on chromosome 5, p53 gene on chromosome 17 and DCC gene on chromosome 18) each lead to a selective outgrowth of neoplastic cells. With each mutation, a new clone of cells with a different growth pattern emerges. Mutations of the *ras* oncogene and the APC gene often occur early in development of adenomas, while mutation of the p53 gene is often associated with transformation of a benign adenoma to carcinoma. These changes are usually acquired but need not occur in any specific order nor involve all of the common mutations.

Research on the germ-line mutations responsible for the hereditary colorectal cancer syndromes also has proceeded rapidly over the last few years. In 1987, the APC gene for familial adenomatous polyposis was mapped to chromosome 5q21,22; in 1991 the gene was identified and characterised; and since 1991 over 170 different mutations that can cause familial adenomatous polyposis have been described. On clinical grounds, hereditary non-polyposis colorectal cancer (HNPCC) appeared likely to be due to a mutation of a major gene but identification of the gene(s) proved more elusive.

In 1993, however, the gene responsible for many, but not all, HNPCC families was mapped to chromosome 2p. The gene was identified later in the same year and was shown to control mismatch repair in DNA replication. Late in 1993, the gene responsible for some other HNPCC families was mapped to chromosome 3p. An important practical outcome of the research will be development of blood tests to identify those members of cancer families who have inherited the special predisposition to cancer and who need regular surveillance.

Adenomas of the colon and rectum

A polyp is a term used to describe a lump. In the colon, neoplastic polyps or adenomas are the most common and important. Other types of polyp include hyperplastic polyps, juvenile polyps, inflammatory pseudo-polyps, benign lymphoid polyps and, uncommonly, lipomas, neurofibromas and carcinoid tumours.

Adenomas are derived from the glandular epithelium of the intestine. Typical adenomas are polypoid and therefore easily recognisable at sigmoidoscopy or colonoscopy. A number of reports, mostly from Japan, indicate that adenomas may be flat and more difficult for the endoscopist to identify.

Adenomas occur throughout the colon, especially in elderly patients, but large adenomas are more common in the rectum and sigmoid colon. Based on size, adenomas are classified as *small* (less than 10 mm in diameter) and *large* (10 mm or greater in diameter); based on histological appearances, adenomas are classified as *tubular*, *villous* or *tubulovillous*. All adenomas show dysplasia, a very early phenotypic step in the complex process of tumorigenesis in the large bowel.

Small tubular adenomas (<10 mm) rarely cause symptoms or undergo malignant change without enlarging and acquiring a villous component. Large adenomas may bleed intermittently or cause obstruction by intussusception or prolapse through the anus. Areas of malignant change with invasion through the muscularis mucosae may be found in up to 50% of adenomas over 20 mm in diameter. Villous and tubulovillous adenomas are more likely to undergo malignant change.

The important question about adenomatous polyps is whether or not they are premalignant. Adenomas commonly occur in association with colorectal cancer; there is a direct relationship between adenoma size and the likelihood of the presence of cancer; remnants of adenoma are sometimes found in continuity with colorectal cancer; and patients with familial adenomatous polyposis inevitably develop cancer unless they have prophylactic surgery. Furthermore, genetic mutations associated with abnormalities of growth occur with a greater frequency in large, more villous and more dysplastic adenomas. These factors provide the basis for the theory of the 'adenoma-adenocarcinoma sequence'.

It is normal practice to remove all polyps, as it is difficult to predict histology by endoscopic appearance. Polypectomy is usually carried out by excision with a diathermy snare at colonoscopy, and is sufficient treatment as long as the polyp is histologically benign and has been totally removed. When a focus of invasive carcinoma is present within an adenoma, local endoscopic excision can sometimes be adequate treatment if there is a substantial clear margin between the invading malignant cells and the line of resection, and if the carcinoma is well differentiated (Fig. 4.5). Otherwise, bowel resection will be required to ensure total removal of the tumour. If an adenoma is sessile or is greater than 4.0 cm in diameter, operative removal is usually advisable.

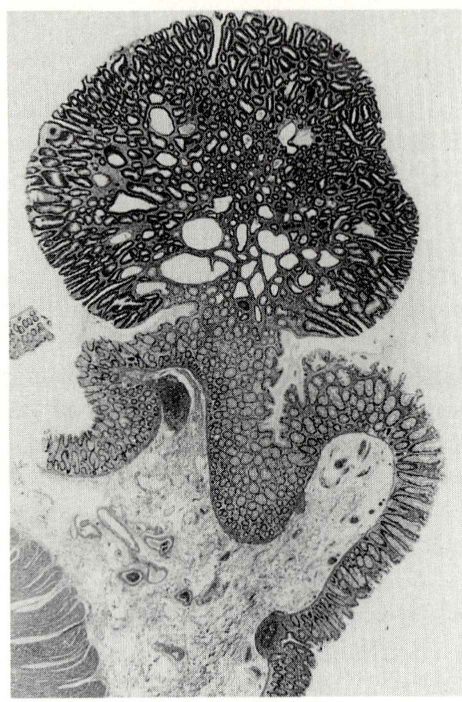

(a)

Fig. 4.5 *(**a**) Benign tubular adenomatous polyp of the colon. The nuclei of the epithelial cells of the polyp are mildly dysplastic and hyperchromatic. H–E stain, original magnification × 4;*
*(**b**) Photomicrograph of a malignant polyp of the colon. The irregular glandular arrangement of the polyp and the hyperchromatic nuclei of the cells can be compared with the normal colonic mucosa on the bottom right of the photograph. Tumour tissue can be seen extending through the muscularis mucosae into the submucosa (arrow). H–E stain, original magnification × 4*

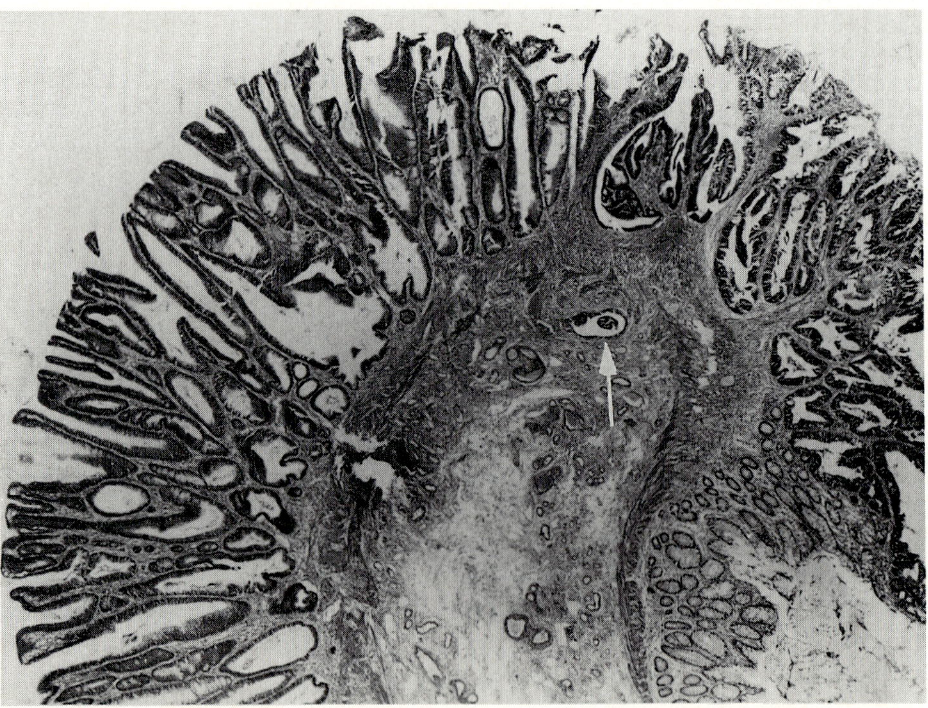

(b)

Patients known to have had adenomas should have periodic colonoscopic surveillance. Current opinion favours three to five-yearly colonoscopy to detect metachronous lesions. Some recent studies suggest that the risk for colorectal cancer is not increased in individuals who have had one or more small (<10 mm) *tubular* adenoma(s) in the rectum, making colonoscopic follow-up less important in that subgroup.

Large villous adenomas, which usually occur in the rectum or sigmoid colon, deserve special consideration. They are sessile, papillomatous, soft and often involve wide areas of mucosa. Most patients with large villous adenomas notice excess mucus in the stools. The major importance of these lesions is their pre-malignant nature, the risk of cancer being very high unless the lesion has been totally excised. Symptoms and signs indicating the development of cancer in a villous adenoma are rectal bleeding and induration or ulceration of the lesion. If these signs are absent, the lesion is treated by local removal; if cancer is present or suspected, the treatment is radical excision as for rectal and colonic cancer.

Carcinoma of the colon and rectum

In many Western countries, colorectal cancer is the most common or the second most common internal cancer. Colorectal cancer is uncommon in patients under forty years of age, but the incidence then rises progressively with advancing age. The level of risk for colorectal cancer is determined by age, personal medical history and family medical history (Table 4.2).

Table 4.2 *Risk categories for colorectal cancer*

Low risk

1. Aged below fifty years
2. No special risk factors present

Standard risk

1. Aged fifty years and older
2. No additional risk factors present

Elevated risk

1. Previous colorectal cancer
2. Previous colorectal adenoma[a]
3. Familial adenomatous polyposis
4. Hereditary non-polyposis colorectal cancer syndrome
5. First-degree relative with common colorectal cancer or adenoma
6. Chronic inflammatory bowel disease
7. Uretero-sigmoidostomy

[a] Some studies indicate that risk for colorectal cancer is not increased for individuals with small (< 1 cm) tubular adenoma(s) of the rectum.

Studies on migrants moving from low incidence to high incidence countries have shown that colorectal cancer incidence rates rise to those of the adopted country within one or two generations. The change indicates that environmental factors, probably dietary in nature, are important in pathogenesis of the disease.

A high total fat intake appears to be the most important predisposing factor, although a low fibre intake and deficiency of other specific micronutrients might be contributory.

Genetic factors also contribute to risk, interacting with environmental factors. Case-control family studies have revealed a two-fold increase in risk for colorectal cancer in first-degree relatives of patients with common colorectal cancer. Age at diagnosis and the number of affected relatives affect risk for other family members, risk being greater when two (or more) family members have had colorectal cancer or with colorectal cancer diagnosed in patients under fifty-five years of age.

Hereditary colorectal cancer syndromes

The risk for colorectal cancer is greatest (50% chance) in several uncommon syndromes where the tendency for colorectal cancer is transmitted in an autosomal dominant manner. Special features are early age of onset and multiple colorectal cancers in affected family members. The two principal syndromes are familial adenomatous polyposis and hereditary non-polyposis colorectal cancer syndrome.

Familial adenomatous polyposis

This genetic disease has a Mendelian-dominant mode of inheritance with complete or almost complete penetrance. The condition is responsible for less than 1% of all colorectal cancer. As described above, the APC gene has been identified on chromosome 5q. After the age of ten years, adenomatous polyps may appear in the colon and rectum in great numbers in affected family members. Cancer of the colon or rectum is inevitable without prophylactic surgery, cancer often occurring in the third or fourth decades of life. Despite the presence of large numbers of adenomas, often many hundreds, patients usually remain symptom-free until bowel cancer develops.

Tests to identify the genetic mutation have been developed and will soon be widely available for clinical application. Until the place of the tests is firmly established, however, all apparently unaffected at-risk members of familial polyposis families should have sigmoidoscopy performed every twelve or twenty-four months from around the age of ten to fifteen years until thirty years. If no adenomas have been detected by thirty years of age, the interval between sigmoidoscopies can then be lengthened. Flexible sigmoidoscopy is an adequate investigation as adenomas almost invariably occur in the rectum when the disease is present. Provision of a reminder service through a central registry for this disease overcomes many of the problems associated with organisation of follow-up.

Affected individuals should have total colectomy performed in early adult life to prevent development of cancer of the colon or rectum. The rectum may be preserved for ileorectal anastomosis, but only if there are few rectal polyps present and regular follow-up by sigmoidoscopy is possible. Total proctocolectomy and ileo-anal anastomosis with pelvic reservoir is an excellent alternative for these patients. Extra-intestinal manifestations, including peri-ampullary carcinoma, desmoid tumours and brain tumours are dangerous possibilities in later life.

Hereditary non-polyposis colorectal cancer (HNPCC)

As with familial adenomatous polyposis, HNPCC or Lynch Syndrome has an autosomal dominant mode of inheritance with a high degree of penetrance. Hereditary non-polyposis colorectal cancer is distinguished from familial polyposis by the absence of more than a few adenomas in the large bowel, by a predominance of cancer in the proximal colon (two-thirds of cancers are proximal to the splenic flexure), and association with cancer of the endometrium, ovary, stomach, small bowel, kidney and other sites in some, if not all, families. It is thought to account for between 1% and 5% of all colorectal cancer, but genetic tests rather than clinical criteria are needed for accurate calculation of the frequency of HNPCC.

Pathology

With rare exceptions, cancers of the large bowel are *adenocarcinomas* with discernible tubular differentiation (classified into well differentiated, moderately differentiated and poorly differentiated according to the architectural features). Tumours often differ macroscopically depending on their site in the colon; right-sided lesions (proximal to the splenic flexure) tend to be fungating and ulcerated, and left-sided lesions stenotic and circumferential. The most common sites for cancer are rectum, sigmoid colon and caecum.

Cancer of the colon or rectum spreads by one or more of the following routes:

1. by direct infiltration through the bowel wall to surrounding tissues or organs;
2. by lymphatics to regional lymph nodes;
3. by the blood stream, with portal venous spread to the liver;
4. peritoneal spread.

The overall five-year survival rate is 40–45%. Careful pathological staging provides an important indication of prognosis. The Dukes' system is the best known pathological classification for staging cancer of the rectum and colon. Other forms of pathological classification are also used, but all are similar to the Dukes' system. The Australian Clinico-Pathological Staging (ACPS) System incorporates a useful clinical component. In the United States, the TNM system is currently promoted as the staging system of choice: T defines the extent of the primary tumour, N the absence or presence of nodal metastases and M distant metastases.

Dukes' classification, with the prognosis for each stage, is as follows:

1. Stage A (confined to bowel wall): five-year survival 90%
2. Stage B (invasion through bowel wall): five-year survival 65%
3. Stage C (lymph node metastases): five-year survival 40–45%

Patients with distant metastases ('Stage D') rarely survive for five years. The overall five-year survival rate is 40–45%. Patients presenting with large bowel obstruction or perforation usually have a poor long-term prognosis, as the lesion is often very advanced locally when these complications occur.

Symptoms and signs

These vary considerably depending on the site and nature of the lesion.

Cancer of the caecum and ascending colon

Fungating, ulcerated cancers in the proximal colon do not usually obstruct the wide lumen of the proximal colon. Symptoms are those of ill health and loss of weight; often the patient complains of vague discomfort and poorly localised abdominal pain. Occult bleeding from the lesions may lead to iron-deficiency anaemia and lesions involving the ileocaecal valve can cause small bowel obstruction. The physical signs are those of anaemia and loss of weight. A mass may be felt if the lesion is large, particularly with cancer of the caecum. It cannot be over emphasised that unexplained iron-deficiency anaemia requires full gastrointestinal workup.

Cancer of the descending colon or sigmoid colon

Patients with cancer of the descending colon or sigmoid colon often recognise dark blood and mucus in the stools. A change in bowel habit is very common, with development of constipation, diarrhoea or alternating bowel habit. Intermittent lower abdominal or left lower quadrant pain is also common and would suggest partial obstruction. The pain may be relieved by defecation. Physical signs may be absent, but a mass is often palpable in the left iliac fossa, or through the rectal wall in the rectovesical or rectovaginal pouch.

Cancer of the rectum

Frank rectal bleeding is the most important symptom. The patient may also notice liquid stools and mucus and complain of inability to empty the rectum (unsatisfied defecation). Pain can occur as tenesmus, but constant localised pain in the anus occurs only if the rectal tumour has invaded the anal canal.

Other forms of clinical presentation

1. *Abdominal mass.* Patients sometimes present with an abdominal mass, produced either by the primary tumour, or by liver or omental metastases.

2. *Intestinal obstruction.* This occurs at the site of the tumour and causes typical symptoms and physical findings. The site of the obstruction is usually close to the rectosigmoid junction, and abdominal distension is often very severe.
3. *Perforation.* Cancer of the colon may be complicated by local abscess formation within the tumour mass, the patient presenting with features of peritonitis.

Diagnosis

With rectal cancer, a clinical diagnosis is made by rectal examination in many patients. An ulcerating, fungating or constricting lesion can usually be palpated if it is situated in the lower 10 cm of the rectum. There may be blood on the examining glove after rectal examination.

A definite diagnosis of cancer is usually made in rectal, rectosigmoid and sigmoid lesions by rigid (25 cm) or flexible (60 cm) sigmoidoscopy with direct biopsy of the lesion. Higher colonic lesions are diagnosed by colonoscopy with biopsy or barium enema. When a cancer is identified within the reach of a sigmoidoscope, colonoscopy should be performed, if technically possible, to check for a synchronous cancer or adenoma(s).

There are two types of lesion that may be difficult for the clinician and the radiologist to diagnose. These are caecal tumours, and tumours at the rectosigmoid junction. Colonoscopy has greatly facilitated the diagnosis of carcinoma at these sites, although the increasing availability of flexible sigmoidoscopy is making diagnosis of rectosigmoid tumours less of a problem.

Early diagnosis

Although the prognosis of colorectal cancer does not appear to be influenced by the duration of the patient's symptoms at the time of treatment, this is likely to reflect the variable growth rate of cancers. In an individual patient, prompt diagnosis after the onset of symptoms should improve prognosis, at least in some patients.

Interest in presymptomatic diagnosis of colorectal cancer has increased considerably in recent years. Colorectal cancer is often at a pathologically advanced stage (Stage C or D) when symptoms first develop. Screening offers the prospect of detection and treatment of adenomas and early, curable Stage A cancers. In standard risk subjects and in patients with one first-degree relative with colorectal cancer, cancer surveillance is usually based on annual faecal occult blood testing, with the option of periodic (e.g. three to five yearly) flexible sigmoidoscopy as well. To date, one randomised controlled trial has shown a significant reduction in mortality associated with screening based on annual faecal occult blood testing. Two case-control studies indicate that screening sigmoidoscopy reduces mortality of rectal and sigmoid colon cancer. In some situations—for example, having one first-degree relative with colorectal cancer before fifty-five years of age or two close relatives with colorectal cancer, periodic colonoscopy rather than sigmoidoscopy is recommended.

Various methods of screening are used for other risk groups. Sigmoidoscopy is the method of choice in familial polyposis families. Colonoscopy is the method of choice in families with HNPCC, in adenoma follow-up and in patients with previous successful treatment of colorectal cancer. In ulcerative colitis, screening is based on two-yearly colonoscopy with multiple biopsies to check for the presence of mucosal dysplasia.

Treatment

Cancer of the colon

The principles of surgical treatment of patients with colonic cancer are as follows:

1. removal of the tumour with a wide margin of normal bowel beyond the macroscopic edge of the tumour
2. excision of all the lymph nodes that are situated in the mesentery along the colonic arterial supply

These principles apply to all colonic growths that are resected along with the mesentery. Bowel continuity is then restored by an end-to-end anastomosis.

Cancer of the rectum

Although cancer clearance is the greatest priority, there has been a growing trend for sphincter preservation in the management of rectal cancer. The need for colostomy has fallen from 80% to 20% over the last forty years because of a better understanding of the pathology of rectal cancer, particularly the fact that distal spread is usually limited (except in very aggressive tumours). This permits a reduction in the distal resection margin and a greater chance for sphincter preservation. The distal margin of resection should be at least 2 cm from the tumour edge. Furthermore, technical advances such as introduction of anastomotic stapling instruments and the development of colo-anal anastomoses, have allowed experienced surgeons to avoid a stoma in many patients. In general, lesions in the upper and middle parts of the rectum are treated by anterior resection (through the abdomen) with primary anastomosis of the bowel. Lesions in the lower part of the rectum may require abdomino-perineal anastomosis and permanent colostomy, although colo-anal anastomosis is an option for some.

Very early, small cancers of the rectum can be treated by local excision if the cancer is well differentiated. In elderly, unfit patients with rectal cancer, diathermy fulguration can be useful for control of symptoms.

There is now increasing evidence that adjuvant therapy has a role to play in the management of colorectal cancer. Early reports of randomised United States studies have indicated a benefit for patients with lymph node positive colon cancer (Dukes' Stage C) receiving a combination of 5 fluorouracil and levamasole for twelve months after surgery. Other regimens, including folinic acid, are being investigated.

In rectal cancer, local recurrence is more common after surgery than for colon cancer. While pelvic radiotherapy has been shown to reduce the incidence of post-operative pelvic recurrence, recent studies indicate that when given in combination with chemotherapy, patient survival is also improved, albeit at the expense of morbidity in some.

Acute large bowel obstruction

Whatever the site, the obstruction has to be relieved, but extracellular fluid depletion must be replenished first.

With obstruction from cancer of the caecum, ascending colon or transverse colon, an immediate resection (hemicolectomy) and anastomosis is performed. The standard treatment of the more common left-sided obstructive cancer is a staged procedure:

1. resection and end-colostomy (Hartmann's operation) with re-anastomosis three to six months later; or
2. the traditional three-stage approach of proximal colostomy to decompress the bowel, followed by resection and anastomosis some two to four weeks later, and finally closure of the proximal stoma after another three to six months;
3. colonic lavage on the operating room table followed by resection and primary anastomosis is advocated by some surgeons.

The immediate mortality of patients presenting with obstructed cancer of the colon is 20–30%.

Perforated cancer of the colon

Perforation is an uncommon complication and may occur at the site of the tumour, or proximal to the tumour, as a result of colonic distention (usually at the caecum). The treatment is resuscitation and immediate operation. If possible, the tumour should be resected immediately and the proximal end brought out as a colostomy. The ends are re-anastomosed at a later date when the patient has fully recovered. The immediate mortality in perforated cancer of the colon approaches 30%.

Other colonic diseases

Angiodysplasia

Although angiodysplastic lesions most commonly occur in the caecum and ascending colon, their distribution includes stomach, small bowel and distal large bowel. These vascular lesions are often multiple, with focal degeneration of arterioles, capillaries and venules within the submucosa.

Angiodysplasia is associated with ageing, aortic stenosis and severe atherosclerotic disease. The clinical manifestations are acute or recurrent gastrointestinal blood loss and iron-deficiency anaemia caused by chronic occult blood loss.

Isotopic technetium (^{99m}Tc) red cell scans, selective mesenteric angiography, and colonoscopy are useful methods for localisation of lesions. Acute bleeding stops spontaneously in most cases; however, if haemorrhage is on-going and the site of bleeding has been localised, segmental resection is curative. When lesions are confined to the colon, endoscopic electrocoagulation should be effective.

Pneumatosis coli

This is an uncommon condition which affects both the small bowel and large bowel. Gas-filled cysts are present in the submucosa and subserosa. They are often discovered incidentally in plain abdominal x-rays or at barium enema. The cause of the condition is unknown, but there is a clinical association with obstructive airways disease and bronchial asthma. The condition is usually symptomless, but some patients have severe chronic diarrhoea or symptoms of obstruction. The cysts and symptoms usually disappear with hyperbaric oxygen therapy.

Rectal and anal disorders

Internal haemorrhoids (piles)

Internal haemorrhoids are composed of collections of specialised arterio-venous communications in the submucosa of the upper half of the anal canal above the dentate line. Mucosa-covered swellings occur mainly in three positions (right anterior, right posterior and left lateral) in the anal canal.

Aetiology

These arterio-venous communications are present in all individuals but become clinically detectable when they bleed or swell and prolapse. They are usually caused by a low-fibre diet leading to constipation and straining at stool. Internal haemorrhoids commonly occur during pregnancy.

Clinical features

The cardinal symptoms are bright rectal bleeding and prolapse at defecation. Occasionally, the piles prolapse and become strangulated with thrombosis and ulceration. It is important to consider other causes of rectal bleeding in patients presenting with piles. Those over forty years of age or with special risk factors for colorectal cancer should have full examination of the sigmoid colon as well as the rectum, preferably by flexible sigmoidoscopy, followed by colonoscopy if there is still doubt about the cause of the bleeding.

Treatment

In all patients, adjustment of the diet with addition of fibre will improve symptoms. If bleeding persists, it can be controlled by submucosal injections with phenol in almond oil or by application of rubber bands to the base of the piles. If prolapse persists, the patient is best treated by haemorrhoidectomy.

Perianal haematoma

These lesions are common and occur suddenly as a painful blue lump, 1 cm in diameter, at the anal verge. The lesion is a small haematoma in the external haemorrhoidal plexus. If the lesion is painful, it may be treated effectively by excision of the haematoma under local anaesthesia. The vast majority resolve spontaneously.

Anal fissure

This extremely painful lesion is usually related to the passage of hard stools. There is a longitudinal split in the anal canal with the internal sphincter muscle in its base. The split is usually in the midline posteriorly or occasionally in the midline anteriorly in females. The symptoms are severe anal pain following defecation, and minor bleeding.

Treatment of anal fissure is by stool softening with a high-fibre diet and the application of a local anaesthetic ointment. If symptoms persist or the fissure is chronic, it is necessary to divide the internal sphincter by a subcutaneous internal sphincterotomy to relieve internal sphincter spasm and allow the fissure to heal.

Patients with inflammatory bowel disease, especially Crohn's disease, may also develop severe fissures, single or multiple, which may occur in any part of the circumference of the anal canal. These fissures are often undermined anal ulcers and are difficult to treat. Anal cancer can masquerade as a fissure.

Anorectal abscess

Anorectal abscesses are usually perianal or ischiorectal. They may occur in association with a fistula-in-ano and many are believed to result from abnormal anal glands which penetrate the internal sphincter muscle. Infection of these glands then leads to an intersphincteric abscess, which extends into the perianal space or into the ischiorectal fossa. The patient has severe perianal pain and swelling and there is an extremely tender swelling on palpation in the affected area.

Treatment is surgical, with incision of the swelling under anaesthesia to release the pus and inspection of the anal canal for an associated fistula.

Anorectal fistula

In most cases fistulae follow the discharge of an anorectal abscess, and are believed to arise from abnormal anal glands and an intersphincteric infection. They also occur commonly in Crohn's disease. The fistulous track usually opens internally at the dentate line, most commonly in the midline posteriorly. Rarely, fistulae are very complex with horseshoe-shaped tracks around the anus or extending into the pelvis. The main symptoms are purulent discharge and occasional spotting of blood on the underclothes.

Treatment of the common low anal fistula is by simple laying open of the track (fistulotomy) and healing by secondary intention. The treatment of the less common high or extensive horseshoe fistulae is more difficult. Staged fistulotomy, seton threads or direct repair of the internal opening (advancement flap) may be necessary to avoid sphincter injury that might otherwise be caused by simple fistulotomy.

Pruritus ani

This unpleasant disorder varies in severity from a mild occasional itch to a severe intolerable itch which profoundly affects the patient's life. Most patients have no associated anal or rectal disorder and it is unusual to discover any specific infection; however, fungal diseases, trichomonas and diabetes must be excluded. Examination in severe chronic cases reveals white thickening of moist perianal skin and associated cracking and excoriation from scratching.

Treatment in the mild case is by careful anal hygiene, the patient bathing or showering after defecation, with careful drying of the perianal skin and cautious application of 1% hydrocortisone ointment or antifungal creams. It is very unusual to have to resort to more radical treatment.

Rectal prolapse

This disease occurs in two forms:

1. *Mucosal prolapse.* There is a circumferential prolapse of 1–2 cm of mucosa on straining. It usually occurs in aged patients and, if symptoms are sufficiently severe, it may be treated by rubber band ligation or an operation similar to haemorrhoidectomy.
2. *Complete rectal prolapse.* Rectal prolapse can occur in infants as well as adults. In this condition, the rectum prolapses on straining through the anal canal for up to 40 cm. There is laxity of the anal sphincters and flattening of the perineum. Ultimately, stretching of the sphincters leads to faecal incontinence. Complete rectal prolapse is produced by an intussusception of the rectum and sigmoid colon, the origin of the intussusception being in the upper third of the rectum.

Treatment of rectal prolapse in infancy is by toilet training and avoidance of constipation and prolonged straining. Occasionally, treatment by injections of phenol in almond oil is necessary to fix the rectum into the pelvis. When the child grows, the normal sacral hollow develops and fixation of the rectum in the pelvis becomes secure.

In adults, treatment of the prolapse is by an abdominal operation which fixes the upper rectum to the sacrum, usually the Ripstein procedure. Faecal incontinence may persist in some cases but improvement is common after rectopexy. For the frail, elderly patient, a perineal operation (e.g. the Delorme procedure) may be preferred as it is less taxing.

Anal incontinence

There are two major groups of faecal incontinence—that due to an injured or torn anal sphincter and that due to a degenerate or denervated sphincter. In the latter, incontinence may be caused by neurological disease affecting the spinal cord or by peripheral neuropathic changes which disrupt the motor or sensory innervation of the anal canal, rectum and pelvic floor. In the absence of an obvious problem as described above, incontinence usually occurs in association with anorectal pathology or secondary to faecal impaction.

Continence is maintained by a complex mechanism. Tone in the puborectalis muscle and the anterior angulation of the anorectal junction are important to continence, as are an intact internal and external sphincter muscle.

Important causes of anal incontinence include:

1. spinal cord lesions (e.g. spinal trauma, spina bifida, spinal tumours);
2. pudendal nerve injury (e.g. repeated straining and perineal descent associated with chronic constipation, injury produced at childbirth as a result of prolonged and multiple vaginal deliveries, rectal prolapse);
3. congenital anorectal anomalies;
4. trauma to the anal sphincter (e.g. obstetric tears, operative anal dilatation for treatment of anal fissure, fistulotomy);
5. destruction of the anal sphincter mechanism by anorectal carcinoma;
6. faecal impaction.

A detailed history and physical examination is essential for evaluation of the severity of the problem and for assessment of the likely cause. Several special investigations are available for investigation of patients where the cause or mechanism is unclear. These include defecating proctograms for demonstration of anatomical abnormalities such as rectal prolapse, anorectal manometry and electromyography to study pudendal nerve function.

Minor incontinence often responds to dietary measures, constipating drugs and pelvic floor exercises.

For severe incontinence, surgery may be required. This has the best results in cases where there is a history of trauma to the sphincters, especially obstetric injury. A direct overlap repair of the defect gives a satisfactory result in most cases. When incontinence is due to degeneration of the sphincter (often secondary to pudendal nerve dysfunction), attempts to buttress the anorectal angle by postanal repair give improvement in perhaps 50% of cases.

Solitary ulcer of the rectum

This condition is more appropriately called benign idiopathic recurrent rectal ulceration, as the lesion may not be solitary. The ulceration is usually localised to the anterior rectal wall, but the lateral rectal wall and posterior rectal wall can be involved. Sometimes there is inflamed hyperaemic mucosa without ulceration which may resemble idiopathic proctitis on sigmoidoscopic examination. The symptoms include increased frequency of defecation, change in bowel habits, rectal bleeding, mucus discharge, tenesmus and a sensation of anal obstruction. Often, a rectal prolapse is found in association with the solitary ulcer. Diagnosis is confirmed by biopsy and treatment involves correction of constipation, avoidance of straining and repair of rectal prolapse if present. Where symptoms are severe and prolapse is absent, local excision of the lesion may be considered.

Descending perineum syndrome

This consists of a sagging of the pelvic floor, with reduced efficiency of the anal sphincter associated with permanent lengthening of perianal muscle fibres. There is often a long history of constipation and straining at stool. The anterior rectal wall descends and can be seen bulging into the rectum on proctoscopy. Treatment consists of exploration of the cause of the symptoms and ensuring soft, normal bowel motions with mild laxatives.

SUGGESTED FURTHER READING

Corman, M. L., *Colon and Rectal Surgery*, 3rd edn, J. B. Lippincott, Philadelphia, 1993.

Fazio, V. W., *Current Therapy in Colon and Rectal Surgery*, B. C. Decker Inc., Toronto, 1990.

MacDermott, R. P. and Stenson, W. F., *Inflammatory Bowel Disease*, Elsevier, New York, 1992.

Morson, B. C., and Dawson, I. M. P., *Morson and Dawson's Gastrointestinal Pathology*, Blackwell, Oxford, 1990.

Sleisenger, M. H. and Fordtran, J. S. (eds), *Gastrointestinal Disease: Pathophysiology, Diagnosis and Management*, 5th edn, W. B. Saunders, Philadelphia, 1993.

Yamada, T., *Textbook of Gastroenterology*, J. B. Lippincott, Philadelphia, 1991.

CHAPTER 5

Pancreas

J. S. Wilson

Anatomy and developmental anatomy

Despite its importance as a digestive and endocrine gland, the adult pancreas is a relatively small intra-abdominal organ with a weight of approximately 100 g and a length between 12 and 15 cm. Macroscopically, the pancreas has a lobulated structure and lies retroperitoneally in the upper abdomen, draped across the spine at the level of the first and second lumbar vertebrae (see Fig. 6.2, p. 129). The head of the pancreas accounts for approximately 30% of its mass and lies within the curve created by the first, second and third parts of the duodenum. The body and tail of the organ cross the upper abdomen in a transverse and slightly cephalad direction and extend to the hilum of the spleen. The splenic artery and vein run along the posterior aspect of the upper part of the body and tail. The superior mesenteric vessels run behind the junction of the head and body of the gland, and it is at this point that the superior mesenteric and splenic veins join to form the portal vein.

Exocrine pancreatic tissue is subdivided into lobules. At the microscopic level, each lobule comprises numerous acini consisting of pyramid-shaped acinar cells grouped around a central lumen. Acini are drained by small ducts known as intercalated ducts. The most proximal cells of these ducts extend into the lumen of the acinus, and are called centroacinar cells. Intercalated ducts empty into intralobular ducts and these in turn empty into interlobular ducts, which then join the main pancreatic duct. In the majority of individuals the main pancreatic duct, together with the common bile duct, enters the duodenum through its medial wall via the ampulla of Vater. Interspersed in the connective tissue of the exocrine pancreas are clusters of endocrine cells called the islets of Langerhans. These endocrine cells are responsible for the production of a variety of peptide hormones including insulin, glucagon, somatostatin, vasoactive intestinal peptide (VIP) and pancreatic polypeptide (PP).

The pancreas begins to develop at four weeks of gestation as ventral and dorsal outpouchings at the junction of the primitive foregut and midgut. The dorsal element emerges rapidly and eventually forms the body and tail of the pancreas. The smaller ventral bud is associated with the developing biliary system. The ventral bud rotates and comes into close proximity with the dorsal bud, with which it fuses at seven weeks of gestation.

Physiology of pancreatic exocrine secretion

Pancreatic juice

In response to stimulation, the pancreas delivers an enzyme-rich, bicarbonate-rich fluid into the second part of the duodenum. The enzymes are responsible for digestion of ingested proteins, lipids and carbohydrates. The bicarbonate component of pancreatic juice neutralises gastric acid, thus providing an optimum pH for enzyme action.

Pancreatic exocrine cells

When stimulated, ductular and centroacinar cells produce a high-volume bicarbonate-rich secretion. Four components appear to be essential for ductular secretion to proceed. These are:

1. an adequate supply of carbon dioxide from the blood;
2. the enzyme carbonic anhydrase;
3. a sodium/hydrogen pump on the basolateral surface of the cell; and
4. the cystic fibrosis transmembrane conductance regulator (CFTR).

The sodium/hydrogen pump actively secretes protons into the interstitial fluid, thereby pulling the carbonic anhydrase reaction in the direction of bicarbonate formation (Fig. 5.1). The recent cloning of the cystic fibrosis gene has enabled identification of the protein which it encodes—the cystic fibrosis transmembrane conductance regulator (CFTR). In pancreatic ductular cells, the CFTR is believed to act as a cAMP sensitive chloride (Cl^-) channel. Its activation results in the secretion of Cl^- into the ductular lumen. Intraluminal Cl^- is then available to exchange with bicarbonate (HCO_3^-) across the apical surface of the ductular cell resulting in HCO_3^- secretion. Water passively follows ion movement (Fig. 5.1).

Acinar cells comprise 80% of pancreatic cells. They are responsible for pancreatic enzyme secretion. The pancreas is an enzyme factory with a protein synthetic capacity rivalled only by the lactating mammary gland. Between 6 and 20 g of enzymic protein are delivered to the duodenum each day. It is estimated that each acinar cell synthesises ten million enzyme molecules a day.

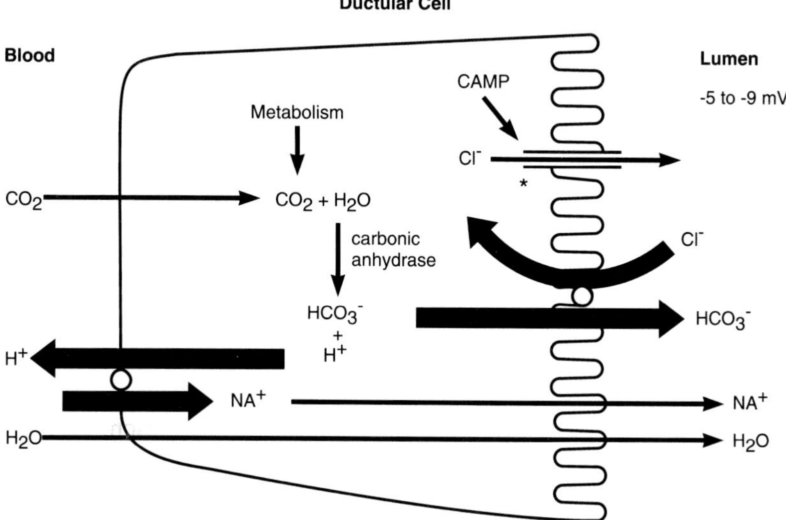

Fig. 5.1 *Electrolyte secretion by pancreatic ductular cells. Thick lines denote active processes. Activation of the cystic fibrosis transmembrane conductance regulator (CFTR)* results in secretion of chloride (Cl^-) into the ductular lumen. Bicarbonate (HCO_3^-) is secreted into the ductular lumen in exchange for Cl. Sodium (Na^+) moves down an electrochemical gradient. Water passively follows ion movement*

Pancreatic enzymes

Some of the diverse enzymes synthesised and secreted by pancreatic acinar cells are listed in Table 5.1. Proteolytic enzymes account for almost 80% of all protein in pancreatic juice. Amylase and lipase, the other major enzymes, are present in small amounts but have very high enzymatic activities. As a protective mechanism against autodigestion, the majority of pancreatic zymogens are secreted as inactive precursors and undergo activation in the duodenum. Trypsinogen is activated by the brush border enzyme enterokinase, and the trypsin so formed is responsible for the activation of the other zymogens. Alpha-amylase is secreted by the pancreas in its active form. It cleaves 1,4-ester linkages between glucose molecules in starch to yield maltose, the trisaccharide isomaltose, and alpha-limit dextrins. The endopeptidases (trypsin, chymotrypsin and elastase) act on peptide bonds in the interior of protein molecules. Carboxypeptidases A and B are exopeptidases which remove amino acids from the C-terminals of polypeptides. The main lipolytic enzyme of the exocrine pancreas is triglyceride lipase, which is secreted in its active form. It cleaves triglycerides at their 1- and 3-ester linkages, yielding free fatty acids and 2-monoglyceride. The pancreas also secretes colipase, a peptide which serves as an anchor for lipase at the fat-droplet surface and prevents inhibition of lipase activity by bile salts.

Table 5.1 *Pancreatic digestive enzymes*

Proteolytic enzymes	*Lipolytic enzymes*	*Amylolytic enzyme*	*Nucleases*
Trypsinogen Chymotrypsinogen Proelastase Procarboxypeptidase A Procarboxypeptidase B	Lipase Procolipase Phospholipase A_2 Carboxylesterase	Alpha-amylase	Ribonuclease Deoxyribonuclease

Synthesis and export of digestive enzymes

The synthesis and export of digestive enzymes by pancreatic acinar cells is a complex process (Fig. 5.2). Amino acids are actively transported across the basolateral membrane of the cell, and polypeptides are assembled from a messenger RNA template on the surface of the rough endoplasmic reticulum (RER). The nascent polypeptide chain is vectorially directed into the cisternae of the RER. Proteins move passively through the RER, and are subsequently transferred to the Golgi apparatus where structural modifications and condensation occur. The precursors of zymogen granules (condensing vacuoles) arise from the Golgi apparatus. Mature zymogen granules are formed from condensing vacuoles by concentration of their contents. The enzymes contained within zymogen granules are extruded from the cell by the process of exocytosis.

Control of pancreatic secretion

The major stimulants of pancreatic exocrine secretion are:

1. secretin,
2. cholecystokinin and
3. acetylcholine.

Secretin is the primary stimulant of bicarbonate secretion by ductular cells. It is released from the mucosa of the proximal duodenum when the ambient pH falls below a threshold of 4.5. Its action is potentiated by cholecystokinin (CCK) and acetylcholine. Secretin is known to stimulate acinar cell secretion in rodents via activation of adenylate cyclase and cAMP generation. The mechanism of its effect on pancreatic ductular cells is probably mediated via the effect of cAMP on the CFTR (see above).

Both *CCK* and *acetylcholine* stimulate enzyme secretion from acinar cells. Cholecystokinin is released from the mucosa of the small intestine in response to intraluminal amino acids, peptides and fatty acids. Acetylcholine is released from nerve endings within the pancreas, following stimulation of vagal nuclei within the central nervous system or the stimulation of volume and osmo-receptors in the stomach and duodenum.

Acinar cells possess specific receptors for CCK and acetylcholine. These secretagogues act via activation of protein kinase enzymes following release of

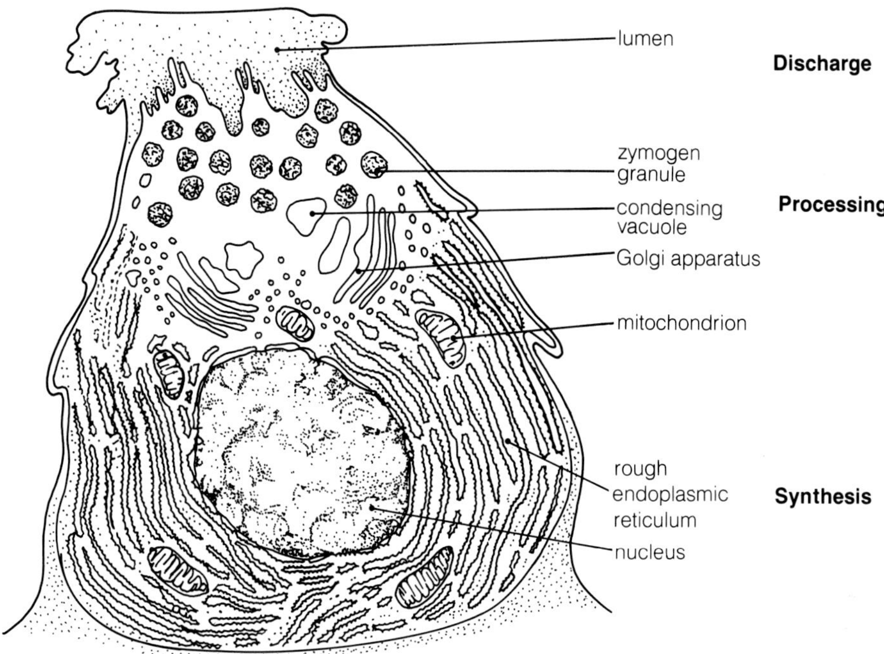

Fig. 5.2 *Diagram of a pancreatic acinar cell. Amino acids are actively transported across the basolateral membrane and polypeptides are assembled on the surface of the rough endoplasmic reticulum (RER). During their synthesis, polypeptides are vectorially transferred into the cisternae of the RER and are then transported to the Golgi apparatus, where they undergo condensation and structural modifications. Condensing vacuoles containing digestive enzymes arise from the Golgi apparatus; further condensation of their contents results in the formation of zymogen granules. Zymogen granules expel their constituent enzymes into the acinar lumen by exocytosis*

calcium from intracellular stores (Fig. 5.3). Protein kinases act to phosphorylate structural and regulatory cellular proteins, resulting in altered configuration and, therefore, activity.

Pancreatic secretion is controlled in a negative feedback fashion via a number of mechanisms, including inhibition of intestinal CCK release (by the presence of pancreatic proteases in the duodenum) and by release of the inhibitory hormone pancreatic polypeptide from the gland.

Patterns of pancreatic secretion

Interdigestive pancreatic secretion is generally minimal in humans; however, every one to two hours there is an increase in secretion coincident with the passage of phase 3 of the migrating myoelectric or motor complex (MMC) (p. 212) through the intestine. This may serve a 'housekeeper' role in digesting debris in the intestinal lumen. The stimulation of pancreatic secretion associated with the ingestion of a meal can be divided into the cephalic, gastric and intestinal phases.

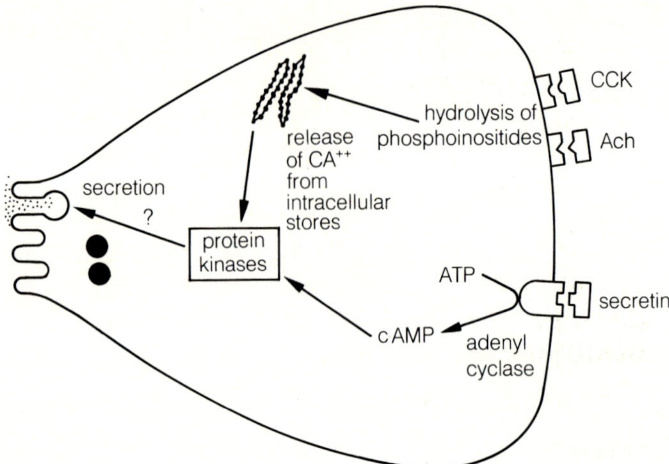

Fig. 5.3 *Stimulus-secretion coupling in the pancreatic acinar cell. Cholecystokinin (CCK) and acetylcholine (Ach) act via the hydrolysis of membrane phosphoinositides, release of calcium (Ca^{++}) from intracellular stores and activation of protein kinase enzymes. Secretin activates protein kinases via the generation of cAMP*

The *cephalic phase* can stimulate the pancreas to 50% of maximal levels. It is initiated by the sight and smell of food and by the act of eating, resulting in the activation of vagal efferent impulses with subsequent stimulation of enzyme secretion and potentiation of bicarbonate secretion in response to intestinal factors.

The *gastric phase* of pancreatic secretion is mediated through vagovagal reflexes initiated by gastric distension. Overall, the gastric phase accounts for only minor stimulation of pancreatic secretion.

The *intestinal phase* of pancreatic secretion is quantitatively the most important, resulting in pancreatic stimulation to between 70% and 100% of maximal levels. The presence of acid, amino acids, peptides, fatty acids and calcium in the intestinal lumen stimulates vagovagal reflexes and the release of secretin and CCK.

Pancreatitis

Pancreatitis is a non-specific term covering a variety of pancreatic pathologies, including necrosis, interstitial inflammation, atrophy, fibrosis and calcification. Pancreatitis is classified as being either acute or chronic. The term *acute* implies functional and morphological restitution of the gland to normal with resolution of the disease process. On the other hand, *chronic* implies irreversible morphological changes in the gland, which may be associated with permanent loss of exocrine and endocrine pancreatic function.

Acute pancreatitis

Associations of acute pancreatitis

Known associations of acute pancreatitis are listed in Table 5.2. Gallstones are the commonest association of acute pancreatitis in Western society. The development of pancreatitis in individuals with gallstones is thought to be related to the migration of gallstones down the biliary tree and into the duodenum. This event results in pancreatic inflammation, probably via blockage of pancreatic secretion and the subsequent intracellular activation of pancreatic digestive enzymes by lysosomal enzymes. Recent evidence suggests that microscopic biliary crystals (in the absence of frank gallstones) can also cause pancreatitis—probably by a similar mechanism.

Table 5.2 *Associations of acute pancreatitis*

Common	*Uncommon*
Gallstones	Hypertriglyceridaemia
Alcohol abuse	Hyperparathyroidism
Unknown cause	Trauma
	Drugs (see Table 5.3)
	Infections (mumps, mycoplasma, Coxsackie virus, Echo virus)
	Connective tissue disorders with vaculitis
	Pancreas divisum
	Obstruction of the ampulla of Vater
	Pancreatic carcinoma
	Penetrating duodenal ulcer

Strictly, alcohol abuse is associated with the development of chronic pancreatitis. Five to fifteen years of heavy drinking usually precede the first attack, and chronic changes have been described in the gland at the time of the first clinical presentation. Nonetheless, alcoholic pancreatitis may be indistinguishable from acute pancreatitis in its early stages.

Marked elevations of serum triglycerides (hyperlipidaemia types I, IV and V) are sometimes associated with pancreatic inflammation. Pancreatic injury may result from the release of fatty acids from triglycerides by lipase in the interstitium of the gland. For reasons that are not clear, serum amylase levels are often normal in the presence of hyperlipidaemia. Thus, the diagnosis of pancreatitis can be difficult to make, but should be entertained in any patient with hypertriglyceridaemia who presents with abdominal pain. Hyperparathyroidism and, less commonly, other hypercalcaemic disorders may result in acute pancreatitis. The mechanisms are unknown.

Most cases of postoperative pancreatitis occur after abdominal operations involving the stomach and biliary tract. Mechanisms proposed for pancreatic injury in this setting include direct pancreatic trauma and interference with pancreatic blood supply. The diagnosis is often difficult and mortality is high.

Endoscopic retrograde cholangio-pancreatography (ERCP) often results in elevations of serum amylase levels. In approximately 1% of examinations, clinically significant pancreatitis develops. It is thought to result from overfilling of the pancreatic ductal system with contrast agent. It may be more common in women. Pancreatitis may also occur following blunt or penetrating abdominal trauma. Blunt trauma to the abdomen may compress the pancreas against the spine, resulting in damage to the head and neck of the gland. Sometimes, complete transection of the gland occurs.

A number of drugs have been associated with the development of pancreatitis (see Table 5.3). A careful drug history should be taken in cases of unexplained pancreatitis.

Table 5.3 *Drug-induced pancreatitis*

Definite association	*Probable association*
Azathioprine	L-asparaginase
Thiazides	Iatrogenic hypercalcaemia
Oestrogens	Chlorthalidone
Frusemide	Corticosteroids
Sulphonamides	Ethacrynic acid
Tetracyclines	Phenformin
Valproic acid	Procainamide

Pancreatic injury may result from disorders associated with a vasculitis and from a number of viral infections, including the viral hepatitides, mumps and infectious mononucleosis. Pancreas divisum results from failure of fusion of the dorsal and ventral duct systems in the developing pancreas (see 'Anatomy and developmental anatomy', p. 103). It is a normal anatomical variant which may occasionally be associated with recurrent acute pancreatitis. The mechanism is thought to be stenosis of the minor papilla through which, in pancreas divisum, the majority of pancreatic secretion drains. A variety of neoplastic and non-neoplastic lesions can lead to obstruction of the pancreatic duct and the development of acute pancreatitis. The mechanism of all these obstructing lesions is thought to relate to increased pressure in the pancreatic ductal system, with subsequent intracellular activation of pancreatic enzymes as described above (p. 109) for gallstone pancreatitis.

Pathology and pathophysiology

It is generally accepted that acute pancreatitis arises as a result of activation of pancreatic enzymes within the gland. Three main types of pancreatic inflammation have been described in association with acute pancreatitis:

1. *Acute oedematous pancreatitis* is characterised by peripancreatic fat necrosis, interstitial oedema and inflammatory cell infiltration, with some necrosis of acinar cells at the periphery of pancreatic lobules. These pathological changes generally occur with mild clinical disease.

2. *Necrotising pancreatitis* is characterised by more widespread necrosis of glandular tissue and surrounding fat necrosis. A swollen, necrotic pancreatic mass is often referred to as a pancreatic phlegmon.
3. *Haemorrhagic pancreatitis* results from rupture of blood vessels in the gland, with both intraglandular and retroperitoneal haemorrhage. Widespread pancreatic necrosis is present.

With more severe degrees of pancreatic inflammation, a *pseudocyst* may develop. This is a collection of enzyme-rich pancreatic fluid containing variable amounts of tissue, debris and blood occurring within the pancreas, lesser sac or elsewhere in the abdomen. It can cause local pressure effects, rupture into the peritoneal cavity, become infected, result in massive haemorrhage, erode into other intra-abdominal organs or rupture through the diaphragm. Areas of pancreatic necrosis may become infected, resulting in abscess formation.

Some of the systemic features of acute pancreatitis (e.g. shock, respiratory failure) may be mediated by the release of *vasoactive peptides* (bradykinin, kallikrein) from the gland into the circulation. These and similar substances may result in vasodilatation, increased vascular permeability and myocardial depression. With severe forms of pancreatitis, *hypocalcaemia* may develop; one responsible mechanism is sequestration of calcium in areas of fat necrosis. *Hyperglycaemia* may occur with acute pancreatitis. It is considered to result from damage to the islets of Langerhans, leading to an excess of glucagon and a deficiency of insulin in the circulation.

More severe forms of pancreatitis may be associated with *pulmonary insufficiency* and *hypoxaemia*. The mechanisms responsible probably include disseminated intravascular coagulation, the action of circulating vasoactive compounds, and disruption of the alveolar-capillary membrane via the action of circulating phospholipase A_2.

Clinical features

The cardinal symptom of acute pancreatitis is abdominal pain. It may vary in intensity. It is generally localised to the epigastrium and periumbilical region, and often radiates through to the back as well as to the lower abdomen, flanks and chest. The severity of the pain is often reduced with flexion of the trunk. Nausea and vomiting are frequent accompaniments. Physical examination generally reveals a distressed patient. Low-grade fever, tachycardia and hypotension may be present. Abdominal tenderness and guarding are often present, but these signs may be unimpressive when compared with the severity of the pain and the general condition of the patient. Bowel sounds may be diminished or absent. Bluish discolouration around the umbilicus (Cullen's sign) or in the flanks (Grey Turner's sign) are rarely seen, but signify severe haemorrhagic pancreatitis.

Approximately 10–20% of patients with acute pancreatitis develop pulmonary complications. Clinically, basal crackles or evidence of a pleural effusion are the most common signs. With severe pancreatitis, patients may develop hypoxaemia and the adult respiratory distress syndrome (ARDS).

Erythematous skin nodules may be observed. These lesions result from subcutaneous fat necrosis due to the action of lipase released from the pancreas into the circulation. They may mimic erythema nodosum.

Complications

Local complications of acute pancreatitis include the development of a pseudocyst, abscess formation and retroperitoneal haemorrhage. Small bowel ileus is common; it is associated with abdominal distension and diminished bowel sounds. With rupture of the pancreatic duct, pancreatic juice can accumulate in the peritoneal cavity (pancreatic ascites). Compression of the lower end of the common bile duct by a swollen head of pancreas can result in cholestatic jaundice.

Remote complications of pancreatitis include shock, ARDS, subcutaneous fat necrosis, hypocalcaemia, hyperglycaemia and renal insufficiency.

Major risk factors for fatal pancreatitis include hypotension, the need for massive fluid and colloid replacement, respiratory failure and hypocalcaemia. The identification of such risk factors helps to identify those patients who may require ventilatory and circulatory support in an intensive care unit.

Diagnosis

Acute pancreatitis may mimic almost any abdominal emergency, and it is usually impossible to make a confident diagnosis on history and examination alone. On clinical findings, the disease may be confused with biliary tract disease, perforated peptic ulcer, mesenteric ischaemia, intestinal obstruction and acute appendicitis. In most instances, acute pancreatitis is diagnosed when compatible clinical features are associated with a serum amylase level greater than 500 IU/L.

Despite its deficiencies, measurement of total serum amylase remains the most commonly used method for confirming the diagnosis. Serum amylase will be elevated in approximately 75% of patients with acute pancreatitis. The amylase levels in blood generally rise within twenty-four hours of the onset of the illness and remain high for one to three days. Values usually return to normal within three to five days, unless there is extensive pancreatic necrosis or pseudocyst formation.

It should be emphasised that normal values for serum amylase do not exclude the diagnosis of acute pancreatitis, and that hyperamylasaemia may occur in a variety of intra- and extra-abdominal conditions. Normal serum levels of this enzyme may result from a delay in obtaining blood samples or the presence of hyperlipidaemia. In addition, patients who present with recurrent 'acute' attacks of pancreatitis associated with alcohol abuse often manifest normal serum levels. Other than acute pancreatitis, cases that may be associated with a *marked* elevation of serum amylase levels include perforated peptic ulcer, mesenteric infarction, and following endoscopic pancreatography. A number of other conditions result in *minor* elevations of total serum amylase, for example, biliary tract disease (especially choledocholithiasis) and intestinal disease.

Measurement of serum pancreatic isoamylase, serum lipase and serum trypsin levels have generally been shown to have greater sensitivity and specificity in the diagnosis of acute pancreatitis. These determinations are not in general use, however, probably because of methodological difficulties with the assays.

Plain x-rays of the abdomen (supine and erect) and chest should be obtained in every suspected case of acute pancreatitis. These investigations rarely provide the diagnosis in themselves, but are important in excluding other possible diagnoses, especially a ruptured abdominal viscus. In addition, the chest x-ray may show abnormalities (basal atelectasis and pleural effusions) consistent with the diagnosis of pancreatitis. An abdominal ultrasound study should be performed. This is the most sensitive way of detecting gallstones, and it may provide information about pancreatic morphology; however, ultrasonic images of the pancreas during acute pancreatitis may be obscured by bowel gas. An abdominal CT scan is a more reliable way of obtaining information concerning pancreatic morphology, and is the preferred method for assessment of pancreatic necrosis.

Management

Patients with suspected acute pancreatitis should be admitted to hospital. The principles of management include:

1. pain relief;
2. the maintenance of intravascular volume and correction of serum electrolyte abnormalities;
3. avoidance of pancreatic stimulation ('resting' the pancreas);
4. determining the cause; and
5. detecting the presence of complications.

Pain relief usually requires the administration of narcotic analgesics, although morphine should be avoided because of its spasmogenic effect on the sphincter of Oddi. The pancreas is best 'rested' by fasting the patient and administering fluids intravenously. In the mild case, this may be all that is necessary. With more severe pancreatitis, nasogastric suction may be instituted. This will help alleviate the symptoms of nausea and vomiting and may reduce pancreatic stimulation further by aspirating gastric acid. Specific pharmacological agents such as anticholinergic drugs, aprotinin (Trasylol), antibiotics, cimetidine, glucagon, calcitonin and somatostatin have not been shown to be of value in the management of acute pancreatitis. In fact, anticholinergic drugs may exacerbate small intestinal ileus and cause tachycardia.

As gallstones and alcohol abuse are the commonest associations of 'acute' pancreatitis, the presence or absence of these factors should be confirmed in every case where the cause is not obvious (e.g. following ERCP or trauma). A detailed alcohol consumption history should be obtained from the patient and, where possible, collaborative information derived from friends and relatives. Abdominal ultrasonography is valuable in diagnosing gallstones. Once these factors have been reliably excluded, finding the cause of acute pancreatic inflammation can be quite difficult. Hyperparathyroidism and hypertriglyceridaemia should be considered. Serum calcium and triglyceride determinations should be performed during convalescence, as these parameters can be altered by acute pancreatitis per se. The diagnosis of hyperparathyroidism can be elusive, and multiple determinations of serum calcium and serum parathyroid hormone may be required. With recurrent unexplained attacks of acute pancreatitis, a renewed search for gallstones should be undertaken. Work-up of these cases should include ERCP, which may be useful in detecting gallstones, obstructive lesions of the pancreatic duct (tumours, strictures) and pancreas divisum. Some of these patients may have a motility disturbance of the sphincter of Oddi, and should be investigated in specialised centres with an interest in biliary/pancreatic disorders.

Those individuals manifesting risk factors for severe disease should be managed in an intensive care unit providing circulatory and ventilatory support. In patients with gallstone pancreatitis and prognostic criteria suggesting the development of severe disease, urgent ERCP and sphincterotomy may reduce morbidity and length of hospital stay.

A pancreatic abscess requires thorough debridement and drainage as well as antibiotic therapy. An infected pseudocyst, or one which persists for longer than six weeks, requires drainage.

Chronic pancreatitis and exocrine pancreatic insufficiency

Associations of chronic pancreatitis and exocrine pancreatic insufficiency

Table 5.4 lists the known associations of chronic pancreatitis and exocrine pancreatic insufficiency. Gallstones *never* cause chronic pancreatitis. *Alcohol abuse* is the most common cause of chronic pancreatitis in Western society. Alcoholic pancreatitis is a chronic disease with acute exacerbations. The isolated alcoholic debauch rarely, if ever, causes pancreatitis, and clinical features of the condition usually only develop after five to fifteen years of heavy drinking. Chronic changes are believed to exist in the gland at the time of the first attack of pain. Radiological evidence of pancreatic calcification has been detected at the onset of clinical disease; moreover, pancreatic fibrosis has been found at autopsy following death during an initial episode. Only a minority of alcoholics develop clinically evident pancreatic disease, but the reasons for the selectivity of alcohol in this condition are not clear. There is evidence that dietary factors (high fat and high protein intakes, as well as malnutrition) and heredity contribute to the selection of those heavy drinkers destined to develop pancreatic damage.

Chronic calcifying pancreatitis in the absence of alcoholism has been reported in parts of Africa, India and South-East Asia, where protein-calorie malnutrition is prevalent. The clinical features of this disease closely resemble that of alcoholic pancreatitis.

Table 5.4 *Associations of chronic pancreatitis and pancreatic insufficiency*

Common	*Uncommon*
Alcohol abuse	Abdominal trauma
Idiopathic factors	Unknown inherited factors
Cystic fibrosis	Schwachman's syndrome
Protein-calorie malnutrition	Hypertryglyceridaemia
	Hyperparathyroidism
	Haemochromatosis
	Prolonged parenteral hyperalimentation

Cystic fibrosis is the major cause of pancreatic insufficiency in childhood. The disease is inherited as an autosomal-recessive trait. It is a multisystem disorder characterised by an abnormality in exocrine gland function. Schwachman's syndrome is a similar paediatric disorder, comprising pancreatic insufficiency and haematological abnormalities (neutropenia, thrombocytopenia and anaemia), but with normal sweat electrolytes.

Abdominal trauma is a well-established cause of chronic pancreatitis. Such trauma may be apparently trivial—for example, a fall from a bicycle. Hyperparathyroidism and hypertriglyceridaemia are rare but definite associations of chronic pancreatitis.

Hereditary pancreatitis is a rare disease. The pathophysiology is obscure. It is inherited in an autosomal-dominant manner, and most patients present in childhood or adolescence with recurrent attacks of abdominal pain. Progression of the disease leads to pancreatic calcification and insufficiency. There appears to be an increased incidence of intra-abdominal malignancy including pancreatic carcinoma. Aminoaciduria has been reported in some patients.

Pathology and pathophysiology

The morphology of chronic pancreatitis is characterised by an irregular fibrosis and permanent loss of acinar cells that may be focal, segmental or diffuse. All types of inflammatory cells may be observed as well as oedema and focal necrosis. Cysts and pseudocysts are often present. The endocrine pancreas appears relatively well preserved. Dilatation of the main pancreatic duct and of the smaller ducts may occur together or independently. Duct dilatation is often associated with strictures of the ducts, intraductal protein plugs or calculi, but it may occur in the absence of these factors.

The pathogenesis of chronic pancreatitis is poorly understood. Because of its prevalence in Western society, alcoholic pancreatitis has received the most attention. The most widely held hypothesis concerning the development of this condition suggests that the deposition of proteinaceous plugs in small pancreatic ducts is the initial lesion. Subsequently, the acini drained by these obstructed ducts degenerate, leading to atrophy and fibrosis. The protein plugs are the likely precursors of the calcific intraductal stones which are a common pathological feature of alcoholic pancreatitis. Other hypotheses concerning the pathogenesis of alcoholic pancreatitis postulate either dysfunction of the sphincter of Oddi or a direct toxic effect of alcohol on the acinar cell.

The basic pathophysiological defect in cystic fibrosis has recently been shown to be a genetically determined abnormality in chloride transport. A mutation in the gene coding for the cystic fibrosis transmembrane conductance regulator (CFTR) results in defective ductular chloride secretion, thereby resulting in viscous pancreatic secretions which in turn cause ductal obstruction, glandular atrophy and pancreatitis.

Chronic pancreatitis can lead to maldigestion, abdominal pain and glucose intolerance. Approximately 90% of function must be lost before maldigestion (steatorrhoea) becomes clinically apparent. The pathophysiological basis for pain in chronic pancreatitis is poorly understood. It is probably multifactorial: increased pressure within the pancreatic ductular system, pseudocyst formation, damage to pancreatic nerves and narcotic addiction may all play a role.

Destruction of the islets of Langerhans leads to the onset of diabetes mellitus. Diabetes in this setting may be very sensitive to insulin therapy, and hypoglycaemia is common. This 'brittleness' may be attributable in part to a deficiency of pancreatic glucagon secretion.

Clinical features

The cardinal clinical features of chronic pancreatitis are those of pain and pancreatic insufficiency.

As noted earlier (p. 114), individuals with chronic pancreatitis may present (especially in the early stages of the disease) with symptoms and signs identical to those found with acute pancreatitis; however, with progression of the disease, patients often complain of continual or intermittent abdominal pain. This pain is generally epigastric in location and radiates to the back, but the pain may be more intense in the right or left upper quadrant, the back, or occur diffusely throughout the abdomen (p. 225). It is often severe, and is unrelieved by antacids or food ingestion. Alcohol and fatty meals may exacerbate the pain. Narcotic analgesics are often required for its relief, and narcotic addiction is common in this setting. Weight loss is a frequent feature and may be accompanied by diarrhoea and steatorrhoea. Patients may report the passage of frank oil into the toilet—a symptom pathognomonic of pancreatic exocrine insufficiency. The symptoms of diabetes may be present.

The physical findings in patients with chronic pancreatitis are generally unimpressive. Patients may appear malnourished. Jaundice may be present, and results from either obstruction of the common bile duct as it passes through the head of the pancreas or from concomitant alcoholic liver disease. Abdominal examination may reveal some tenderness, but the findings are generally not in keeping with the severity of the abdominal pain.

Diagnosis

Table 5.5 lists tests used in the investigation of chronic pancreatitis or chronic pancreatic insufficiency.

Table 5.5 *Investigations used in the diagnosis of chronic pancreatitis and pancreatic insufficiency*

1. *Estimation of exocrine secretion*
Direct tube tests
Faecal proteases
Faecal fat estimation
Bentiromide test
Pancreolauryl test
2. *Assessment of pathology or structural changes*
Abdominal x-ray
Ultrasonography
CT scan
Endoscopic retrograde cholangio-pancreatography (ERCP)
3. *Serum tests*
Pancreatic isomylase
Trypsin-like immunoreactivity

The presence of pancreatic calcification on the plain abdominal x-ray or abdominal CT scan is virtually diagnostic of chronic pancreatitis, and no other, more invasive investigations may be necessary (Fig. 5.4). This finding generally indicates damage to about 80% of the exocrine pancreas, but is detected in only 20–30% of all patients with chronic pancreatic disease. In Western society, pancreatic calcification usually indicates alcohol-induced disease. Abdominal ultrasonography is useful for detecting the presence of pancreatic pseudocysts, while CT scan is the more reliable procedure for defining the size and shape of the pancreas.

Endoscopic retrograde cholangio-pancreatography (ERCP) is probably the most commonly employed investigation in the diagnosis of chronic pancreatitis. This investigation involves placement of the tip of a side-viewing endoscope in the second part of the duodenum, cannulation of the pancreatic duct and instillation of radiographic dye. Radiographs of the pancreatic ductal system are thus obtained. Characteristic images can be obtained of early, moderate and advanced degrees of pancreatitis. In addition, information about ductal morphology is often valuable if surgical relief of pain is contemplated. Unfortunately, the test is time-consuming, invasive and expensive. It results in clinically significant acute pancreatitis in approximately 1% of examinations.

In the absence of pancreatic calcification, other investigations may be required to make the diagnosis. Duodenal intubation, followed by stimulation of pancreatic exocrine secretion and collection of pancreatic juice, is the most sensitive test of exocrine pancreatic function. An infusion of secretin and/or cholecystokinin is instituted and the aspirated duodenal secretion is analysed for bicarbonate and enzyme content. The use of this test is confined to specialist centres, however, and it is not generally used in clinical practice.

A three-day faecal fat determination may be abnormal in patients with chronic pancreatitis and suspected steatorrhoea. A very high level of faecal fat

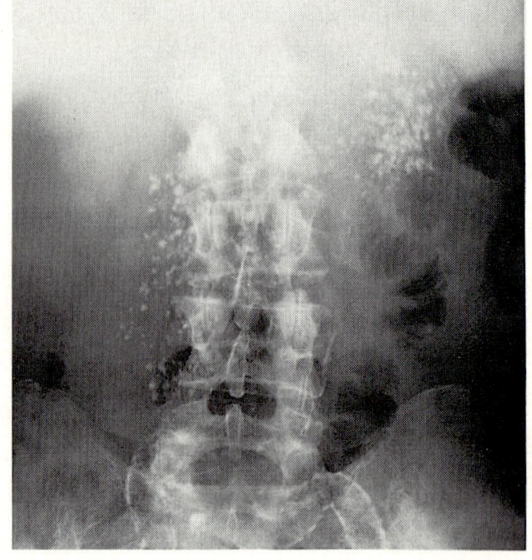

(a)

Fig. 5.4 *Chronic pancreatitis with diffuse calcification. Pancreatic calcification may be seen on plain abdominal x-ray (**a**) or CT scan (**b**) (arrows)*
DEPARTMENT OF MEDICAL ILLUSTRATION, UNIVERSITY OF NEW SOUTH WALES AND TEACHING HOSPITALS

(b)

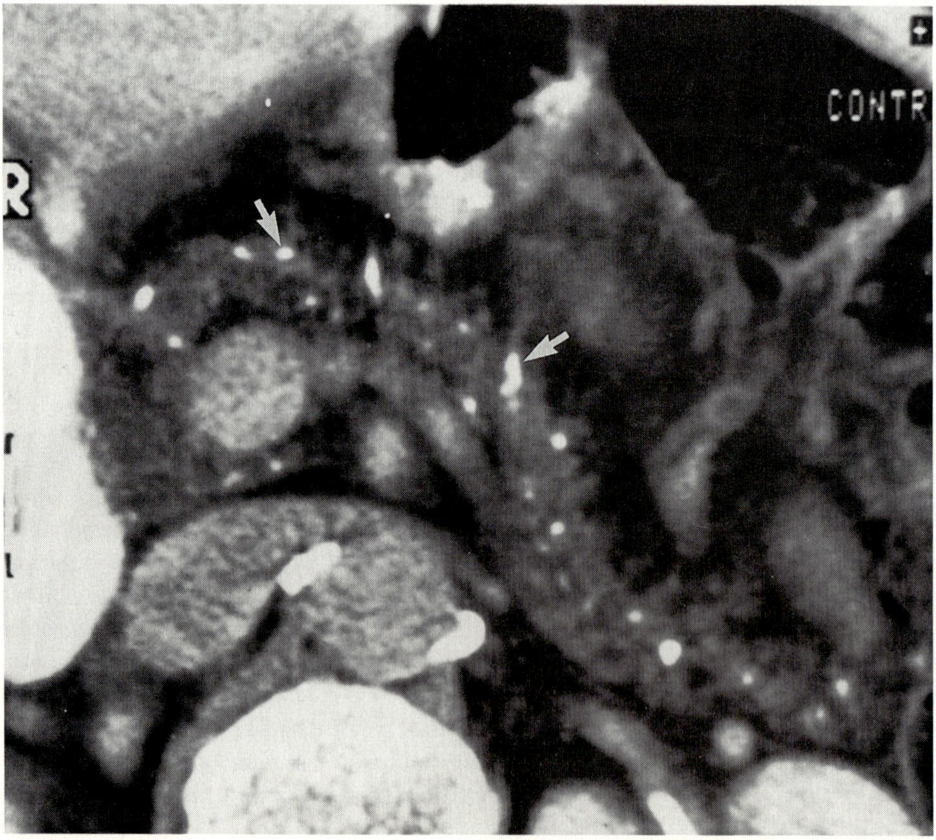

excretion (greater than 40 g per day) is virtually diagnostic of pancreatic steatorrhoea.

Because of the invasiveness of tube tests of exocrine pancreatic function and ERCP, considerable effort has been directed towards developing non-invasive tests of pancreatic function. These have included the bentiromide and pancreolauryl tests. The principles of these tests are similar: each test involves the ingestion of artificial pancreatic substrates and the subsequent measurement of metabolites in serum or urine. Compared with more invasive investigations, these tests appear to have a sensitivity and specificity of around 90%. Perhaps, as would be expected, their sensitivity appears to be better with moderate and severe pancreatic exocrine insufficiency than with slightly impaired function. False-positive results are obtained with advanced liver disease, diffuse small intestinal pathology, small intestinal bacterial overgrowth and renal failure.

The presence of low levels of circulating pancreatic isoamylase or trypsin-like immunoreactivity in the presence of steatorrhoea are highly specific for chronic pancreatitis.

Pancreatic insufficiency leads to decreased faecal excretion of proteases. Both trypsin and chymotrypsin have been measured, with chymotrypsin appearing to be the more reliable.

Once the presence of chronic pancreatitis has been established, a search should be made for the cause. If alcohol abuse has been reliably excluded, finding the cause of chronic pancreatitis may be quite difficult. Cystic fibrosis should be suspected in any child, adolescent or young adult presenting with pancreatic insufficiency. Pulmonary symptoms may not be prominent. Molecular methods now permit an accurate diagnosis. A history of abdominal trauma should be carefully sought. A family history may reveal the presence of hereditary pancreatitis (a very rare condition). As with acute pancreatitis, hyperparathyroidism and hypertriglyceridaemia should be excluded, as these are definite (although rare) causes of chronic pancreatitis.

Management

The management principles for chronic pancreatitis involve:

1. encouragement of abstinence from alcohol;
2. relief of pain; and
3. correction of pancreatic exocrine and endocrine insufficiencies.

Patients with alcoholic pancreatitis who continue to drink will do poorly. Narcotic addiction is more likely to develop in these individuals.

As the pathophysiology of pain in chronic pancreatitis is poorly understood, treatment must be empirical. In alcoholic patients, abstinence is mandatory. If the main pancreatic duct is dilated, a pancreatico-jejunostomy may be performed. Of all the surgical procedures performed for chronic pancreatitis, this operation appears to offer the best chance of success in terms of pain relief. Drainage of a pancreatic pseudocyst can often result in the dramatic relief of pain.

Ingestion of large quantities of pancreatic proteases may relieve abdominal pain in patients with mild to moderate exocrine impairment. The mechanism is believed to be via a feedback inhibition of pancreatic exocrine secretion.

Pancreatic extract therapy is the time-honoured method for the treatment of pancreatic exocrine insufficiency. An effective enzyme preparation should contain at least 600 units of lipase per tablet or capsule. In practice, six to eight tablets of a potent enzyme preparation (e.g. Viokase, Cotazym) or three capsules of enteric coated preparation (such as Pancrease), per meal, satisfactorily reduce steatorrhoea in most patients.

Carcinoma of the pancreas

Pancreatic carcinoma is an insidious and (usually) fatal disease. The factors responsible for its development are obscure, and attempts at early detection (through organ imaging or serological markers) have been disappointing.

Incidence and epidemiology

In Western society, pancreatic carcinoma is the fourth most common cause of cancer death in men and the fifth most common cause of cancer death in women. The overall prevalence of this disease is ten per 100 000 population, which rises to 100 per 100 000 population in individuals over seventy-five years of age. Men are afflicted twice as frequently as women. While factors responsible for the development of pancreatic carcinoma are largely unknown, an increased incidence has been reported in association with smoking, diabetes mellitus, chronic pancreatitis, hereditary pancreatitis, occupational exposure to certain chemicals (e.g. β-naphthylamine), and an increased dietary intake of fat, protein, and breads made from highly refined flour. Furthermore, a strong positive association between latitude and pancreatic cancer, and a strong negative association with average ambient temperature has also been reported. Although earlier epidemiological studies suggested an association between coffee consumption and pancreatic carcinoma, subsequent investigations have failed to confirm this.

Pathology and pathophysiology

Over 90% of pancreatic cancers are adenocarcinomas arising from the ductal epithelium. Approximately 5% of adenocarcinomas of the pancreas arise from islet cells. Some rarer forms of pancreatic malignancy such as cystadenocarcinomas and islet cell tumours have a considerably better prognosis. Approximately two-thirds of the tumours arise in the head of the gland. Histologically, pancreatic adenocarcinoma is characterised by dense strands of fibrous tissue in which there are scattered groups and cords of malignant cells, some forming duct-like structures. In the majority of cases, the tumour has spread to involve adjacent structures, such as the common bile duct, the duodenum, stomach and portal vein, at the time of presentation. In more advanced cases, there is extensive metastatic spread and peritoneal seeding.

Clinical features

The most frequent symptoms are:

1. persistent, central abdominal pain often with radiation through to the back;
2. progressive cholestatic jaundice; and
3. weight loss.

Vomiting usually signals gastric outlet obstruction or extensive peritoneal metastases. Infrequently, patients may present with an attack of acute pancreatitis. There is occasionally a history of recent onset of diabetes mellitus.

Physical examination may reveal:

1. no abnormality;
2. jaundice, possibly with a palpable gallbladder (Courvoisier's sign; see Fig. 5.5);
3. an abdominal mass; or
4. evidence of metastatic spread (hepatomegaly or ascites).

Diagnosis

Pancreatic carcinoma should be strongly suspected in any patient over the age of fifty years who presents with *unexplained, persistent abdominal pain* of recent onset, particularly with radiation to the back; or *painless jaundice* (even in the presence of gallstones). Other clinical features that may suggest the diagnosis include unexplained acute pancreatitis, the recent onset of pancreatic insufficiency, and the development of diabetes mellitus without predisposing factors.

To date, carcinoma of the pancreas has largely defied early diagnosis and, therefore, the prospect of curative resection. At present, diagnosis depends on:

1. imaging the tumour; and
2. obtaining tissue for histological examination (if possible).

Imaging the tumour

To image the tumour, abdominal ultrasonography and CT scanning are generally performed. The latter is the more accurate technique for defining pancreatic morphology, but the two investigations are complementary, with a combined sensitivity and specificity greater than 90%; however, the resolution of both procedures declines with pancreatic lesions of less than 2 cm in diameter. In addition to imaging the pancreas, these techniques can provide important information about other intra-abdominal structures such as the liver, biliary tree and portal vein.

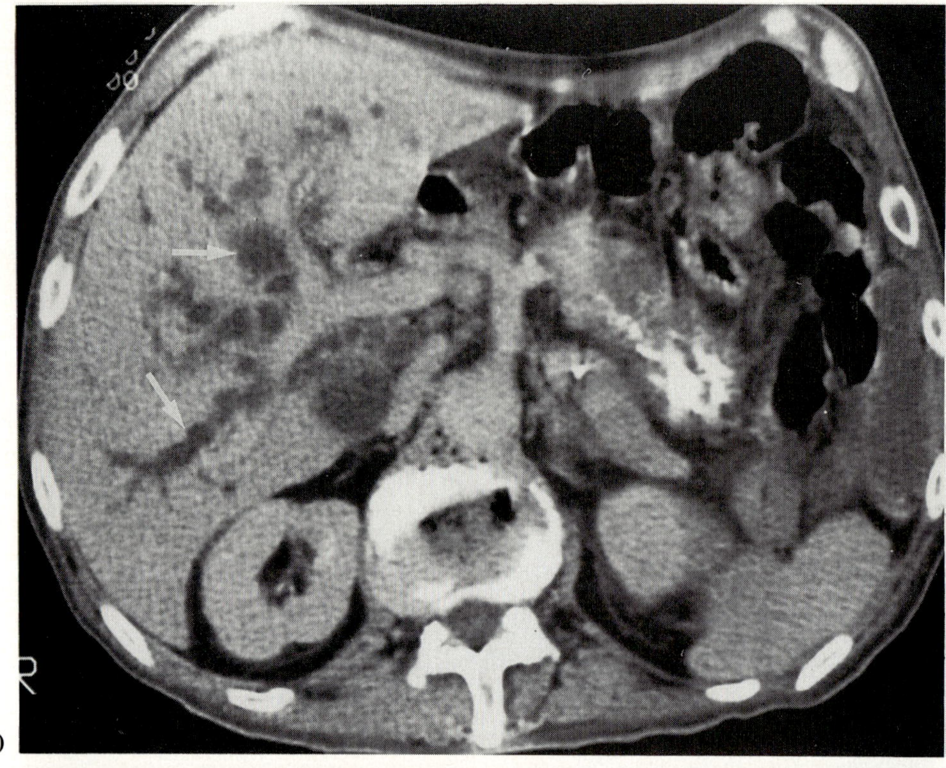

(a)

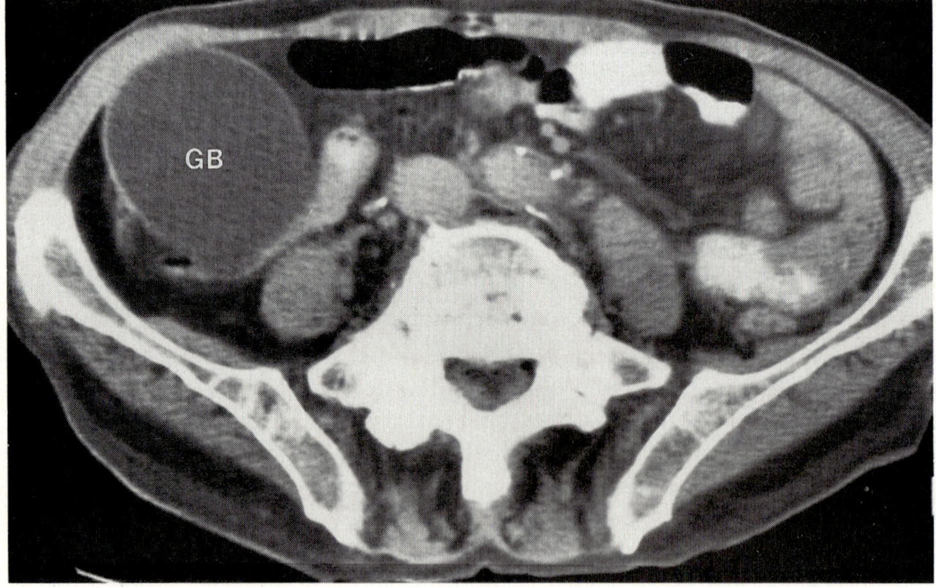

(b)

Fig. 5.5 *Abdominal CT scan of a patient who presented with progressive, painless jaundice and a palpable gallbladder (Courvoisier's sign). Dilated intrahepatic ducts are visible in (**a**) (arrows), and the distended gallbladder is seen to extend down to the pelvic brim in (**b**) (GB = gallbladder). Subsequent investigations confirmed the presence of carcinoma in the head of the pancreas* DEPARTMENT OF MEDICAL ILLUSTRATION, UNIVERSITY OF NEW SOUTH WALES AND TEACHING HOSPITALS

If pancreatic cancer is suspected, but ultrasound and CT examination yield negative or equivocal results, ERCP should be undertaken. With this procedure, infiltration of the duodenum, ampullary tumours and malignant strictures of biliary and pancreatic ducts may be observed. Endoscopic retrograde cholangiopancreatography is also useful in defining precise local anatomy in cases where surgery is contemplated. In some cases, surgery may be necessary to define fully the extent of a pancreatic mass and, hence, resectability.

Obtaining tissue

Once a pancreatic mass has been identified, histological confirmation should be sought because:

1. chronic pancreatitis may mimic pancreatic malignancy; and
2. some forms of pancreatic carcinoma (islet cell tumours, cystadenocarcinomas) have a better prognosis.

Tissue can be obtained by:

1. fine-needle aspiration under ultrasound or CT guidance;
2. ERCP; or
3. surgical biopsy.

If a pancreatic tumour is visualised by ultrasonography or CT scan, fine-needle aspiration should be undertaken. With an experienced cytologist and radiologist, this technique has a sensitivity greater than 80% and a specificity of 100% in the diagnosis of pancreatic cancer. Occasionally, the diagnosis remains unconfirmed even after surgical biopsy. Measurements of various circulating hormones (e.g. gastrin, VIP, insulin) may aid in the diagnosis of an islet cell tumour.

Management

Overall management of pancreatic cancer will depend upon the age and general condition of the patient.

Surgery

Surgery may be performed for attempted cure or for palliation. Only a minority of patients (10%) will be suitable for a curative resection. These are generally individuals with small lesions in the head of the pancreas who have presented with obstructive jaundice. The Whipple resection remains the surgical procedure of choice for such patients. This involves an en-bloc resection of the distal stomach, duodenum, common bile duct and head of the pancreas, with gastrointestinal continuity being restored by performing separate anastomoses between the pancreas and jejunum, stomach and jejunum, and common bile duct and jejunum. If a curative resection is not possible, surgery may be undertaken to relieve intestinal and biliary obstruction.

Biliary stenting

In those patients with obstructive jaundice who are unsuitable for curative resection, a biliary stenting procedure may provide an alternative to surgery. A plastic tube is placed through the ampulla of Vater and across the malignant stricture so that bile can drain freely into the duodenum. The stent is best positioned using an endoscopic approach, but a percutaneous transhepatic or combined approach may be employed. Endoscopic stenting is as effective as biliary bypass surgery in relieving unresectable malignant biliary obstruction, and may involve fewer complications.

Radiotherapy and chemotherapy

Megavoltage irradiation, either alone or in combination with chemotherapy, may limit progression of this disease; however, morbidity may be considerable, and further information is required before these palliative approaches can be recommended as a matter of routine.

Islet cell tumours of the pancreas

These are rare tumours with an annual incidence of three to five per million. They are commonly called neuroendocrine tumours because they are thought to derive from common neuroectodermal cells with the potential to differentiate into a variety of endocrine tumours. The pancreas is the most common site for the occurrence of neuroendocrine tumours of the gastrointestinal tract.

Typically, the tumours are characterised by the hormones they secrete, with the subsequent development of definable syndromes (see Table 5.6). The tumours may be benign or malignant and they often secrete multiple hormones; however, up to 50% of endocrine tumours of the pancreas may be non-functional.

Table 5.6 *Neuroendocrine tumours of the pancreas*[(a)]

Tumour	*Hormone*	*Clinical features*
Carcinoid	Serotonin	Flushing, wheezing, diarrhoea
Gastrinoma	Gastrin	Multiple peptic ulcers, peptic ulcers in unusual sites, intractable ulcers, diarrhoea, steatorrhoea
Insulinoma	Insulin	Hypoglycaemia
VIPoma	*V*asoactive *I*ntestinal *P*eptide	Watery diarrhoea, hypokalaemia, alkalosis
Glucagonoma	Glucagon	Diabetes, stomatitis, glossitis, anaemia, skin rash

[(a)] Only the more common tumours are listed in this table.

Pancreatic endocrine tumours are associated with the autosomal dominant, multiple endocrine neoplasia type 1 (MEN 1) syndrome in approximately 25% of cases. Commonly, this syndrome is also associated with parathyroid hyperplasia or adenomata and pituitary adenomata.

Gastrinoma (Zollinger-Ellison syndrome)

This syndrome is caused by secretion of large amounts of gastrin by gastrin-secreting cells in the tumour, leading to hypertrophy and hyperplasia of gastric parietal cells with increased gastric acid secretion. This tumour has an incidence in the general population of about one to three per million. Approximately 85% of gastrinomas occur in the pancreas and 10–15% in the duodenal wall or rarer sites. About two-thirds of the tumours are malignant.

Clinical features

The usual mode of presentation is recurrent or intractable peptic ulceration, with complications such as haemorrhage or perforation (see p. 25). The diagnosis should be suspected with intractable ulcers, multiple ulcers, ulcers in unusual positions (second part of the duodenum, jejunum), hypertrophy of gastric folds on endoscopy or barium meal, or unexplained diarrhoea due to acid inactivation of pancreatic lipase (causing steatorrhoea), and acid-induced damage of the small bowel mucosa.

Diagnosis

The diagnosis is made by demonstrating an elevated fasting serum gastrin (usually about 300 fmol/mL) in the presence of an increased basal acid output. Confirmation of the diagnosis can be made by intravenous injection of secretin which will increase serum gastrin concentration.

It must be remembered that hypergastrinaemia per se is not necessarily indicative of the Zollinger-Ellison syndrome. Any cause of hypochlorhydria or achlorhydria will elevate serum gastrin levels, because acid in the lumen of the gastric antrum normally inhibits secretion of gastrin by antral G cells in a negative feedback fashion. Common causes of hypochlorhydria or achlorhydria include pernicious anaemia, renal failure, vagotomy and treatment with acid suppressive therapy. These latter conditions are usually not associated with a compatible clinical syndrome and will not manifest a positive secretin test.

Tumour localisation

This can be difficult. Imaging modalities such as ultrasonography, CT scanning and angiography are only successful in about 30% of patients. The technique of portal vein sampling (via a transhepatic route) for a peak in gastrin levels has been used, but results have been generally disappointing. Endoscopic ultrasonography and scintigraphy with radio-labelled octreotide (octreotide is a somatostatin analogue and many neuroendocrine tumours possess a high density of somatostatin receptors) are two new imaging techniques which have shown initial promise.

Management

If feasible, resection of the tumour is the treatment of choice. Unfortunately, this is possible in only 20% of patients. Most patients can be successfully managed with the potent acid-suppressive agent omeprazole. The dose must be titrated against gastric acid output. If medical therapy fails, total gastrectomy is required. Chemotherapy may help with malignant gastrinomas.

VIPoma

These islet cell tumours secrete the gut hormone vasoactive intestinal peptide (VIP) and result in a syndrome of watery diarrhoea, hypokalaemia and gastric achlorhydria (sometimes called the WDHA syndrome or pancreatic cholera). About 50% are malignant at diagnosis.

Clinical features

The disorder is characterised by profuse secretory diarrhoea, hypokalaemia, acidosis and low gastric acid secretion. Vasomotor symptoms are present in about 20% of patients and manifest as flushing and hypotension.

Diagnosis

The diagnosis is made by demonstrating elevated serum VIP levels in the presence of secretory diarrhoea.

Management

Surgical removal of the tumour is the definitive therapy but is often not feasible as the tumours are often difficult to find. The long-acting somatostatin analogue octreotide can often successfully control symptoms by suppressing both secretion from the tumour and target organ (i.e. gut) responsiveness.

SUGGESTED FURTHER READING

Glazer, G. and Ranson, J. H. C. (eds), *Acute Pancreatitis: Experimental and Clinical Aspects of Pathogenesis and Management*, Bailliere-Tindall, Philadelphia, 1988.

Go, V. L. W. et al. (eds), *The Pancreas: Biology, Pathobiology, and Diseases*, Raven Press, New York, 1993.

Lankisch, P. G., Exocrine pancreatic function tests, *Gut*, 1982; 23:777–98.

Niederau, C. and Grendell, J. H., Diagnosis of chronic pancreatitis, *Gastroenterology*, 1985; 88:1973–85.

Sleisenger, M. H. and Fordtran, J. S. (eds), *Gastrointestinal Disease: Pathophysiology, Diagnosis and Management*, 5th edn, W. B. Saunders, Philadelphia, 1993.

Toskes, P. P. and Greenberger, N. J., Acute and chronic pancreatitis, in Disease-a-Month, Cotsonas, N. J. (ed.), *Year Book Medical*, New York, 1983.

Walsh, J. H., Gastrointestinal peptide hormones, in Sleisenger, M. H. and Fordtran, J. S. (eds), *Gastrointestinal Diseases*, Vol. 1, 4th edn, W. B. Saunders, London, 1988; 78–107.

CHAPTER 6

Liver and biliary tract

L. W. Powell and E. E. Powell

Relevant anatomy

The usual description of the anatomy of the liver has been modified by the description of functional internal architecture stemming from the recent French literature. Classically, the liver was described as being divided into right and left lobes at the falciform fissure. Here, the ligamentum teres is a remnant of the umbilical vein of the foetus and runs into the left branch of the portal vein. Functionally, however, the liver is divided into right and left lobes at a line which runs from the gallbladder bed anteriorly to the angle between the right and left hepatic veins posteriorly as they enter the inferior vena cava.

Internally, the liver is divided into eight segments, each of which has its own blood supply from the portal vein and the hepatic artery, and each of which is drained by a segmental bile duct which, in turn, drains into the right and left hepatic ducts. These combine to form the common hepatic duct at the hilum of the liver (porta hepatis), which then runs down to be joined by the cystic duct from the gallbladder to form the common bile duct; this then may be joined by the pancreatic duct at a common hepato-pancreatic ampulla of Vater, just prior to its opening into the duodenum (duodenal papilla).

There are three hepatic veins—right, middle and left—which run between the segments and receive branches from them before draining into the inferior vena cava just below the diaphragm (Fig. 6.1). This drainage may be individual, but more usually the middle hepatic vein joins the left and, thus, two veins run into the inferior vena cava. This description of the internal anatomy of the liver has several practical consequences.

1. Resections of the liver through the line between the gallbladder and the junction of the hepatic veins are possible, and are termed right and left hepatic lobectomy, respectively.

2. It is possible to resect the liver through the line of the falciform fissure with preservation of the left hepatic duct (extended right lobectomy, trisegmentectomy).
3. Removal of the individual segments of the liver is possible, making use of knowledge of the internal anatomy not apparent from external examination of the organ.
4. The use of ultrasound at operation is very helpful in identifying where the individual segmental ducts and vessels are located, providing a scientific basis for segmental resection.
5. The left hepatic duct remains extrahepatic and deep to the liver capsule for some 2–3 cm before its entry into the liver substance. It is, therefore, surgically accessible, and both lobes of the liver can be drained from the extrahepatic part of the left duct. This is important in resectional surgery for common hepatic duct stricture and malignancy, and also for palliative drainage where the hepatic duct malignancy cannot be removed because it has involved the portal vein and hepatic artery.

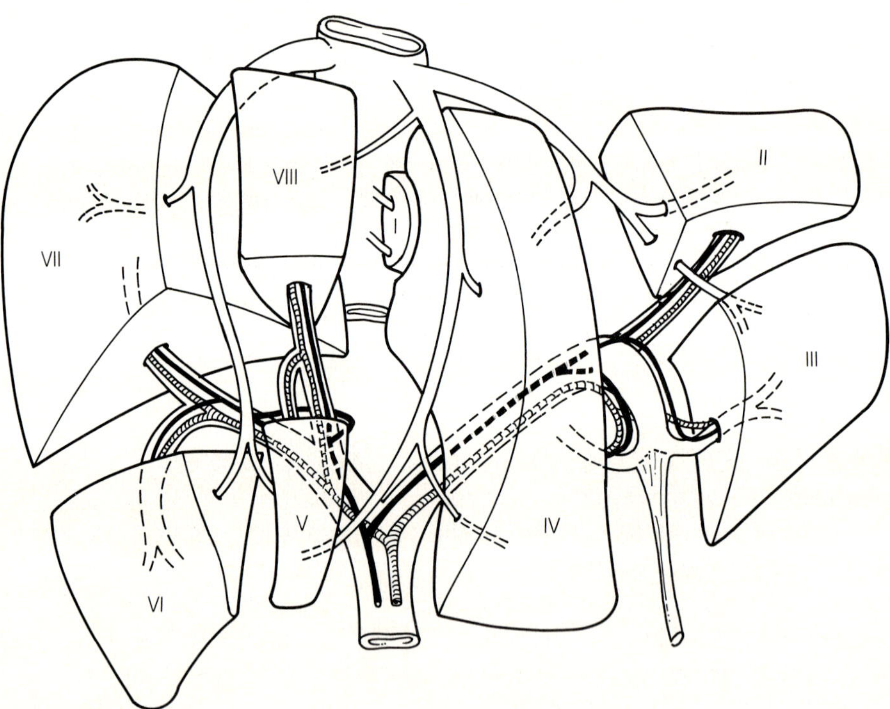

Fig. 6.1 *Segmental anatomy of liver. Three main hepatic veins divide the liver into four sectors, each of them receiving a portal pedicle (see text)* FROM BOURGEON, R. AND GUNTZ, M., *NOUVEAU TRAITÉ DE TECHNIQUE CHIRURGICALE,* MASSON S.A., PARIS, 1975, WITH PERMISSION

The portal vein drains blood from the gut and the spleen and pancreas towards the liver, and is formed behind the neck of the pancreas at the junction of the splenic and superior mesenteric veins (Fig. 6.2). It then runs upward in the posterior aspect of the free edge of the lesser omentum, behind the hepatic artery and the bile duct, to enter the liver at the porta hepatis. The arterial blood supply to the liver is from the hepatic artery, which continues upwards to the liver after giving off the gastroduodenal artery behind the first 2 cm of the duodenum. Malignancies of the bile duct grow slowly, and often involve both hepatic artery and portal vein before they obstruct the bile duct.

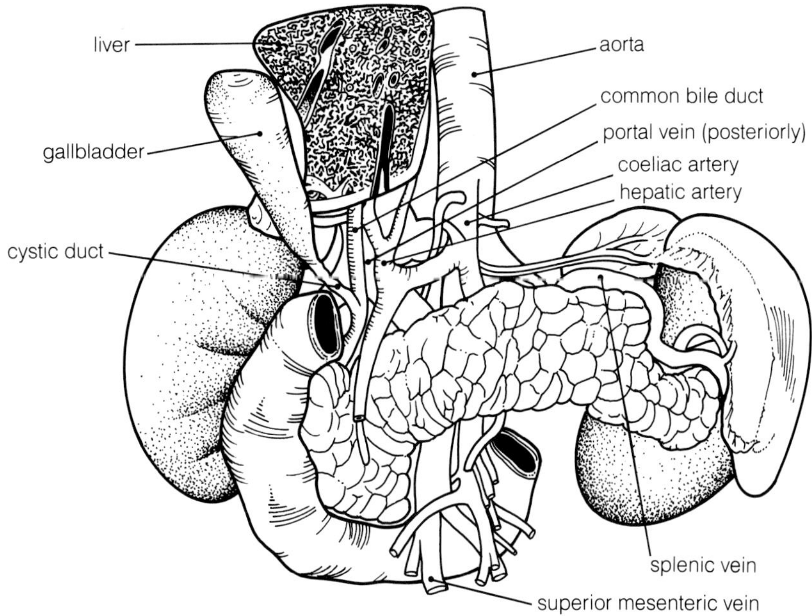

Fig. 6.2 *Anatomy of porta hepatis and biliary tract* FROM *CA—A CANCER JOURNAL FOR CLINICIANS,* AMERICAN CANCER SOCIETY, NOV./DEC. 1981, VOL. 31, NO. 6, WITH PERMISSION

The lower part of the bile duct below the duodenum runs downwards in a groove behind the head of the pancreas, and enters the duodenum about two-thirds of the way down its second part. This is usually by way of a common ampulla with the pancreatic duct, thus providing an anatomical basis for involvement of the pancreatic duct in the passage of gallstones to the duodenum and in the causation of gallstone pancreatitis (see p. 109).

At its lower end, just before entry into the duodenum, the bile duct (and, if present, the common hepato-pancreatic ampulla) is surrounded by circular and longitudinal muscle fibres derived from the duodenum. This is called the sphincter of Oddi, and may be the anatomical basis for biliary pain where a pathological abnormality (such as gallstones or stricture) is not demonstrable (biliary dyskinesia).

The gallbladder is a diverticulum of the bile duct that stores and concentrates bile prior to its release during digestion, especially after ingestion of fatty foods. Its blood supply is from the cystic artery, which usually crosses behind the bile duct from the hepatic artery. There are, however, a number of small arteries which enter the gallbladder wall directly from the liver substance, and this is why the gallbladder, when inflamed, rarely necroses and perforates (as does the appendix). Venous and lymphatic drainage of the gallbladder is to nodes in the porta hepatis and lesser omentum. Variations in the anatomy and disposition of the biliary ducts and vessels are very common.

The lymph vessels from the liver drain to nodes in the porta hepatis and thus downwards in the lesser omentum to the supraduodenal and coeliac lymph nodes. Afferent nerves from the liver and biliary tract run in the sympathetic and parasympathetic fibres originating from spinal cord segments T6–T10. Liver and biliary pain is therefore usually felt in the epigastrium or may be referred to the inferior angle of the scapula. When the liver and gallbladder are acutely inflamed, the process involves somatic nerves supplying the parietal peritoneum and the pain is, therefore, localised to the right upper quadrant of the abdomen.

Microscopic anatomy

The liver is a huge vascular sponge, into which the blood from the hepatic artery and portal vein drains to sinusoids lined by endothelial and phagocytic cells of the reticuloendothelial (RE) system. The branches of the hepatic artery and portal vein, before entering the sinusoids, run in portal triads with biliary radicles which will eventually coalesce to form the bile ducts. Within this sponge, the liver cells (or hepatocytes) are arranged in three zones (Rappaport) around the portal triad. According to this concept, zone 3 of the hepatocytes (that furthest from the portal triad) will suffer most from noxious stimuli (whether viral, toxic or anoxic), and there is a zonal heterogeneity of liver cell function (see below).

Between the hepatocytes and the sinusoidal lining cells is the space of Disse. The hepatocytes comprise about 60% of the liver, and their life span is about 150 days. They are bipolar cells, one pole facing the sinusoid and the space of Disse and the other facing their excretory system—the biliary canaliculus—which is sealed from the rest of the intercellular space by a number of junctional complexes, including tight junctions, gap junctions and desmosomes. The canalicular intralobular network drains into thick-walled terminal bile ducts (cholangioles, canals of Hering), which terminate in the interlobular bile ducts in the portal triads.

Ultrastructurally, microvilli project into the lumen of the biliary canaliculus and, along the sinusoidal border of the hepatocytes, microvilli project into the perisinusoidal tissue space. The organelles within the hepatocyte are functionally similar to those in other parenchymal cells, but with some specialisation. The rough endoplasmic reticulum (RER) synthesises proteins, particularly albumin and blood coagulation factors, and the smooth endoplasmic reticulum (SER) is the site of bilirubin conjugation and the metabolism of many drugs and other foreign compounds. The lysosomes are dense bodies adjacent to the biliary canaliculi. They contain many hydrolytic enzymes and are the site of deposition of ferritin, lipofuscin, bile pigment and copper.

The Golgi apparatus is a 'packaging' site for excretion into the bile.

Microtubules and microfilaments provide a supporting cytoskeleton. They are contractile, the microtubule containing tubulin and the microfilament, actin. They control subcellular motility, vesicle movements and cell shape.

The sinusoidal cells (endothelial, Kupffer, fat-storing and pit cells) each have important functions. The *Kupffer cells* are highly mobile macrophages attached to the endothelium. They are derived from circulating monocytes and, when activated in infections, Kupffer cells endocytose endotoxin and secrete specific factors such as interleukins and tumour necrosis factor (TNF). These secreted products mediate the toxicity of endotoxin. The Kupffer cell has specific membrane receptors for ligands including the Fc portion of immunoglobulin and C3b component of complement, which are important for antigen presentation.

Endothelial cells are sessile cells which form a continuous wall to the lumen of the sinusoid. Their fenestrae (0.1 μm in diameter) determine the exchange of fluid and the size of particulate matter passing to and fro between the sinusoid and the space of Disse and the hepatocyte. They are active in clearing macromolecules and small particles from the circulation by receptor-mediated endocytosis. They also have receptors for the Fc fragment of IgG and act as scavenger cells, removing harmful enzymes or pathogens.

Fat-storing (ITO) cells or lipocytes are stellate, sessile cells lying within the space of Disse. They store excess vitamin A, retinoids and other fat-soluble vitamins. With hepatocyte injury, they migrate to zone 3 and transform to myofibroblasts which secrete collagen. Hence, they may be important in the pathogenesis of cirrhosis.

Pit cells are highly mobile, natural killer lymphocytes attached to the endothelium, with spontaneous cytotoxicity against tumour cells and virus-infected hepatocytes.

Physiology

Bilirubin is the bile pigment resulting from the degradation of haem. Of the daily production of between 250 and 350 mg (4–6 mmol), 80% is derived from destruction of senescent red cells in the RE system and the remainder is formed from the haem proteins (e.g. cytochromes) and from ineffective erythropoiesis (defective red cells percursors). The unconjugated, water-insoluble bilirubin is transported in the plasma bound to albumin, which dissociates from bilirubin at the hepatocyte plasma membrane. Uptake of bilirubin at the hepatocyte is shared by other organic anions (e.g. indocyanine green, but not bile acids) and involves the specific cytosolic proteins, ligandin and Z protein. Conjugation of bilirubin takes place with glucuronic acid by the microsomal enzyme, uridine diphosphate glucuronyl-transferase (UDPGT). This renders the pigment water-soluble and thus able to be transported and excreted in bile. Canalicular excretion of conjugated bilirubin is also shared by other organic anions but not bile acids. Once it reaches the intestine via the biliary tree, bilirubin is metabolised by bacteria to urobilinogen. A small amount (20%) of urobilinogen is reabsorbed (enterohepatic circulation) and re-excreted into the bile. The renal handling of bile pigments should be readily deduced from the above, that is:

1. unconjugated bilirubin cannot be filtered because it is bound to the albumin (hence 'acholuric' jaundice in haemolytic states);
2. the water-soluble conjugated bilirubin is excreted, but only in detectable amounts if the plasma level is elevated or rising (e.g. in early acute hepatitis). In the later stages of cholestatic or hepato-cellular jaundice, despite high serum bilirubin levels, none can be detected in the urine. This is apparently due to the production of a bilirubin mono-conjugate which is covalently bound to albumin. This would not be filtered by the glomerulus and therefore would not reach the urine;
3. urinary urobilinogen is increased with conjugated hyperbilirubinaemia, but absent with complete extrahepatic bile duct obstruction.

Bile acids (strictly, bile salts at physiological pH) are formed in hepatocytes by the metabolism of cholesterol. They form micelles with cholesterol and phospholipids in bile to aid in the absorption of dietary fats. They are absorbed specifically in the terminal ileum and undergo enterohepatic circulation. Serum levels are elevated in liver disease but are of limited clinical value.

Functional heterogeneity of the liver

There is increasing evidence that the relative functions of hepatocytes in the periphery of the acinus (zone 3, adjacent to the central or terminal hepatic veins) are different from those in the circulatory area, or zone 1 (adjacent to the portal triads). The major differences described relate to oxygen supply, Krebs cycle enzymes and bile secretion (zone 1), and drug-metabolising P-450 enzymes (which predominate in zone 3).

Acute viral hepatitis

This is a systemic infection which predominantly affects the liver. The term 'viral hepatitis' is generally used to describe either hepatitis A, B, C, D or E infections, although an illness with similar clinical features may result from other less common viral infections. These include the Epstein-Barr virus (infectious mononucleosis), cytomegalovirus, Coxsackie and herpes simplex viruses. Hepatitis is rarely the predominant feature of these illnesses, however.

Nomenclature and features of the hepatitis antigens and antibodies

Hepatitis A

This is due to a 27 nm non-cytopathic RNA virus belonging to the picornavirus family. It is present in the stools of patients during the early prodrome of hepatitis A infection and for about one week after the onset of jaundice. Sensitive assays are now available for the detection of the hepatitis A antigen and corresponding antibody (anti-HAV). Recent (as opposed to past) infection can be determined by the demonstration of a rising titre of anti-HAV in the IgM fraction of serum.

Hepatitis B

Hepatitis B is a major cause of morbidity and mortality worldwide, with over two million deaths per annum from hepatitis B-related cirrhosis, liver failure and hepatocellular carcinoma.

Spectacular advances in knowledge of the molecular biology of this virus (HBV) followed the demonstration by Blumberg in 1965 of a new antigen in serum from an Aboriginal Australian (first called 'Australia antigen'). Three different particles are present in the serum of patients with hepatitis B, the largest of which is the intact virus, a double-shelled particle known as the Dane particle (Fig. 6.3). This particle comprises a central core containing the genome of the hepatitis B virus, a single molecule of DNA and a specific DNA polymerase. Hepatitis B is one of the hepadnaviruses which have partially double-stranded and partially single-stranded DNA. Replication involves reverse transcriptase, as with retroviruses. The core particle is generally found in the nuclei of hepatocytes, while the outer (surface) lipid-rich proteins are acquired in the cytoplasm of the hepatocyte. The core of the virus (HBcAg) is antigenically distinct from the 'surface' antigen (HBsAg), and the corresponding antibodies can be detected by sensitive radioimmunoassay.

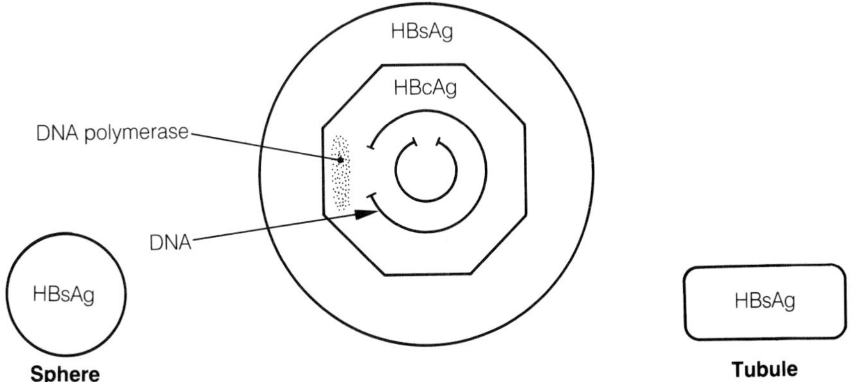

Fig. 6.3 *Diagram of the structure of the hepatitis B virus (Dane particle) and related structures found in serum. For nomenclature refer to Table 6.1. HBeAg represents a component of HBcAg. The spherical and tubular particles represent excess HBsAg. The first hepatitis B vaccine was produced from these non-infectious particles*

The other particles detected in serum are spherical and tubular forms of incomplete virus consisting entirely of HBsAg (Fig. 6.3). A further antigen—labelled HBeAg—is a protein sub-unit of HBcAg, and appears transiently in serum in every episode of acute hepatitis B, together with viral DNA polymerase (see Fig. 6.4). Its presence indicates viral replication and as such this antigen is a good marker of infectivity; however, HBV DNA is the most sensitive index of viral replication and, when present even in anti-HBe positive serum, it indicates a severe ongoing disease, possibly due to a mutant virus unable to produce HBeAg. The typical time course of appearance of the various antigens is shown in Figure 6.4 and their significance for diagnosis is summarised in Table 6.1.

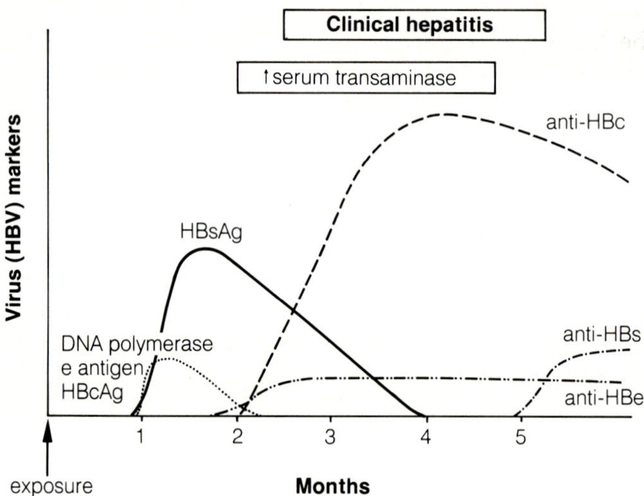

Fig. 6.4 *Time course of the appearance of the various viral markers in acute hepatitis B*

Table 6.1 *Commonly encountered serological patterns of HBV infection*

HBsAg[(a)]	*HBeAg*[(b)]	*Anti-HBs*[(c)]	*Anti-HBc*[(d)]	*Significance*
+	–	–	–	Early acute infection or chronic carrier
+	+	–	–	Early infection; high infectivity
–	–	+	–	Past infection with HBV, or vaccination
–	–	+	+	Recovery from HBV infection
—	—	—	+	Recovery from HBV infection

[(a)] HBsAg appears in the blood about six weeks after infection and disappears by three months; persistence for more than six months implies a carrier state.

[(b)] HBeAg appears early in illness and disappears within two weeks; persistence implies ongoing disease. Anti-HBe follows disappearance of HBeAg and is present for many months.

[(c)] Anti-HBs appears late (three to four months) after onset of illness and in comparatively low titre.

[(d)] Anti-HBc appears early in illness in high titre and persists indefinitely.

Hepatitis C

Hepatitis C was formerly known as posttransfusion Non-A, Non-B (NANB) hepatitis. The responsible agent has now been identified as a 10 kilobase, single-stranded RNA virus with properties similar to the flaviviruses (Group B arboviruses, including yellow fever and dengue fever). The genome of the virus has been fully sequenced and sensitive assays for the antibody (anti-HCV) and for HCV RNA are now available. Serological evidence for HCV infection can be detected in 60–90% of cases of transfusion-associated hepatitis, 70–90% of intravenous drug users and haemophiliacs, 50% of cases of sporadic NANB hepatitis and a variable percentage of patients with chronic liver diseases (see below).

Hepatitis D (delta)

Hepatitis D is a small single-stranded circular RNA virus of 1.7 kilobases, which depends on the DNA genome of HBV for its maturation, although its RNA shares no homology with HBV DNA. The core of HDV bears the antigenic protein (HDVAg) and the envelope incorporates HBsAg. Thus, HDV occurs only in HBsAg-positive individuals.

Hepatitis E

Formerly known as enteric NANB hepatitis, this agent has been isolated as a 32–34 nm non-enveloped RNA virus. It is thought to be a member of the calcivirus group (such as the Norwalk virus), which is usually associated with severe diarrhoea. The genome has recently been cloned and this should allow the development of new serological assays for HEV infection to facilitate clinical diagnosis.

Epidemiology

The major characteristics of the different types of viral hepatitis are summarised in Table 6.2.

Hepatitis A

Hepatitis A is usually transmitted by faecal-oral spread, most often by faecal contamination of food or water, but parenteral transmission is also possible. The disease occurs in sporadic cases or in epidemic form. Epidemics have been caused by faecal pollution of city water supplies and by contamination of food.

Infection with the hepatitis A virus can occur at any age, but it is most common in young children in whom it usually causes only a mild gastroenteritis. The incubation period is about three weeks (fifteen to fifty days). The high incidence of anicteric or subclinical infection makes effective control difficult. In adults, the illness tends to be more severe, particularly in white races and the higher socioeconomic groups. This is possibly because they escape childhood infection and consequent immunity, a phenomenon recognised with some other viral infections such as poliomyelitis.

Table 6.2 *Characteristics of the different types of viral hepatitis*

	Hepatitis type				
Feature	*A*	*B*	*C*	*D*	*E*
Agent	27 nm RNA virus (HAV)	42 nm DNA virus (HBV)	10kb RNA flavivirus (HCV)	1.7 kb RNA virus (HDV)	27–39 nm virus-like particle (HEV)
Antigens	HAAg	HBsAg, HBcAg, HBeAg	HCAg	HDAg	HEAg
Epidemiology	Faecal-oral	Mainly parenteral	Mainly parenteral	Parenteral (endemic in Italy)	Faecal-oral
Venereal transmission	No	Yes	Uncertain	Yes	No
Incubation period	15–50 days	50–150 days	50–150 days	60–150 days (?)	30–55 days
Age preference	Any age, but common under 20 years	Any age	Any age	Any age	Any age
Carrier state	No	Yes	Yes	Yes	No
Icteric:anicteric ratio	1:10	1:2	1:4	?	1:20
Mortality rate	0.1%	1.3%	1.2%	?	low[a]
Fulminant hepatitis	Yes	Yes	Yes	Yes	[a]
Chronicity	No	Yes (approx. 10%)	Yes (20%–50%)	Yes	No
Nasopharyngeal secretions infective	Rare	Rare	?	?	No
Protection by normal immune serum globulin	Good	Poor	?	Poor	Partial
Protection by hyperimmune globulin	Not necessary	Yes	?	?	?
Diagnostic serological markers	Anti-HAV (IgM)	HBsAg, anti-HBc (IgM)	Anti-HCV	Anti-HDV	Crude
Risk of HCC	Nil	++	+++	?	Nil

[a] High fatality rate among women in their third trimester of pregnancy.

Hepatitis B

This produces an identical clinical picture after a longer incubation period of fifty to 150 days. This virus is usually transmitted parenterally through a break in the skin or mucous membranes, through the therapeutic administration of blood and blood products or by a contaminated needle. Accidental inoculation of medical, nursing and laboratory personnel from careless handling of infected blood or needles has occurred. Venereal transmission of hepatitis B is well recognised, as is vertical transmission to infants whose mothers have the HBsAg or especially HBeAg in serum. It is also frequently spread among inmates of institutions. The latter suggests that transmission can occur via non-parenteral routes.

Hepatitis C

Screening of healthy blood donors in Australia has yielded anti-HCV positivity rates of 0.2 to 0.4%, that is, some five times more common than the HBV carrier rate.

Hepatitis C is spread primarily by blood, in a similar fashion to HBV. The risk for 'ever-users' of intravenous drugs is 70% and for those using IV drugs for more than two years over 90%. The incidence of sexual transmission from a patient with chronic HCV infection appears to be low and much rarer than for HBV and HIV. Perinatal and vertical transmission from mother to infant may occur when the mother has high circulating titres of HCV RNA, but overall it is much less common than for HBV.

Chronic HCV infection is an important cause of chronic hepatitis, cirrhosis and hepatocellular cancer (HCC). At least 50% of individuals exposed to the HCV virus become chronic HCV carriers and at least 25% of these will develop cirrhosis, although this often takes up to twenty years or more. Thus the progression of HCV-induced liver disease is usually slow, with chronic hepatitis developing over ten years, cirrhosis over twenty years and HCC over thirty years. Where the relevant studies have been performed—for example, Japan, China and Spain—the majority of HBV-marker negative patients who develop HCC are anti-HCV positive. A synergistic role for HCV and alcohol, and for HCV and iron, has been suggested.

Hepatitis D

Hepatitis D occurs in endemic form in Italy, in other Mediterranean countries and in the Third World. In addition, it is increasingly common in intravenous drug abusers, haemophiliacs and male homosexuals. The clinical picture depends on whether there is simultaneous co-infection with HBV or subsequent superinfection of chronic HBV carrier with HDV. The latter event is a well-recognised cause of 'relapse' of acute hepatitis in an HBV carrier, and the resultant liver disease is usually accelerated. Such subjects may be at increased risk for malignant hepatoma (HCC).

Hepatitis E

This RNA virus (HEV) is responsible for most epidemics of enteric non-A, non-B and non-C (NANBNC) hepatitis in developing countries. It should be considered in the differential diagnosis of acute hepatitis in the traveller. The incubation period is short, as with hepatitis A (fifteen to fifty days), and the prognosis is favourable except in pregnancy when the risk of fulminant hepatitis is up to 20%. Whether immune serum globulin produced in countries in which HEV is endemic can prevent the disease remains to be determined.

Other viral causes of hepatitis

These include the Epstein-Barr virus, cytomegalovirus (CMV), Coxsackie B virus, adenovirus, herpes simplex virus and, increasingly importantly, the human immunodeficiency virus (HIV). Diagnosis of the underlying disease is usually not difficult because of other clinical manifestations; for example, lymphadenopathy from CMV and HIV infections is more common in immunosuppressed patients. Multiple infections are common and should always be considered in drug addicts and homosexuals.

Pathology

The infection is a systemic one with inflammation of the gastrointestinal tract, pancreas, bone marrow and other organs. The essential lesion, however, is an acute inflammation of the entire liver with centrilobular necrosis and diffuse cellular infiltration most marked around the portal tracts. The reticulin framework is usually preserved and this allows complete restoration of hepatic architecture when the liver cells regenerate. Other characteristic features include prominent Kupffer cells lining the hepatic sinusoids and apoptotic (Councilman) bodies, and evidence of recent cell death. In hepatitis C, spotty lobular hepatitis and lymphoid follicles are commonly seen. More extensive disease with bridging necrosis between central veins and portal tracts tends to carry a worse prognosis.

Clinical features

These are very similar, whatever the viral aetiology. The prodromal symptoms are those of any viral infection including malaise, headache, fever, lassitude, etc. Characteristic symptoms are severe anorexia and a marked distaste for smoking. During the prodromal phase of hepatitis B, 5–10% of patients develop a serum sickness-like syndrome with arthralgia or arthritis and rash. Abdominal pain is absent. The icteric phase of hepatitis is often heralded by loss of colour of the stools, due to decreased secretion of bile pigments, and by dark urine due to bilirubinuria. With the onset of clinically evident jaundice the symptoms and fever often subside quickly. Physical examination usually reveals icterus, an enlarged tender liver and splenomegaly in 25% of cases. The convalescent stage usually begins seven to ten days from the onset of the jaundice, the stools regain their colour and the jaundice gradually clears. The illness usually lasts from two to six weeks in the adult although complete recovery, as evidenced by clinical, biochemical and histologic examination, may take up to six months.

Diagnosis

Diagnosis involves awareness of the characteristic symptomatology of acute hepatitis, especially the absence of pain and a careful history from the patient and relatives to exclude the possibility of a drug cause (see below). It is also important to ask about recent injections, inoculations and contact with jaundiced patients. The laboratory tests which are of value include:

1. serum bilirubin (total and conjugated levels), which gives an indication of the severity of the illness and it is helpful in differential diagnosis (see below);
2. serum transaminase level, which is greatly elevated in the first week or so, levels greater than 1000 IU being common;
3. serum alkaline phosphatase level, which is usually only moderately raised to less than 200 IU/L;
4. HBsAg and other hepatitis antigens (Table 6.2);
5. coagulation studies, especially the prothrombin time which is probably the most valuable prognostic factor in the acute stage;
6. ultrasonography to exclude extrahepatic obstruction if the diagnosis is not certain.

Differential diagnosis

This includes other viral illnesses such as infectious mononucleosis, drug hepatitis, chronic active hepatitis and acute cholecystitis and cholangitis if abdominal pain, nausea, vomiting and fever are marked. Gilbert's syndrome (benign familial unconjugated hyperbilirubinaemia) is sometimes misdiagnosed as viral hepatitis—hence the importance of measuring conjugated levels of serum bilirubin.

Complications

It should be emphasised that the majority of patients with viral hepatitis recover completely; however, certain sequelae are well recognised and they tend to occur more commonly with hepatitis B, C and D. They are summarised below.

Relapsing hepatitis

Some 5–10% of cases relapse in late convalescence. The reason for this is uncertain. In these patients the symptoms and signs return, and hepatic histology is similar to that seen in the original attack. Recovery is almost always complete.

Cholestasis

Some degree of biliary stasis is common in viral hepatitis, resulting in mild generalised pruritus and some elevation in levels of serum alkaline phosphatase; however, in some outbreaks intrahepatic cholestasis is moderately severe, giving rise to possible diagnostic confusion. Complete recovery is the rule.

Immune complex disease

There is increasing evidence that the clinical manifestations of acute hepatitis are determined by the immunologic responses of the host. In addition, a number of important extrahepatic manifestations of hepatitis B are due to immune complex-mediated tissue injury. During the preicteric phase a serum sickness-like syndrome occurs in about 5–10% of cases, characterised by skin rash, angio-oedema and arthritis. The syndrome is due to circulating immune complexes and activation of the complement system. Immune complexes of HBsAg and anti-HBs, HBcAg and anti-HBc or HBeAg and anti-HBe may be found, which disappear from the serum after recovery.

In patients who become chronic carriers of HBsAg after acute hepatitis B, other types of immune complex diseases are seen. The major ones are proliferative glomerulonephritis with the nephrotic syndrome and polyarteritis nodosa. In the former, immune complexes are found on the glomerular basement membrane and in the latter in the affected small and medium sized arteries. It is noteworthy that 20–30% of patients with polyarteritis nodosa have HBsAg in the serum.

Hepatitis B, C or D carrier state

In a minority of patients with these forms of hepatitis the antigens may persist in the blood. This is often indicative of chronic liver disease, although the existence of apparently healthy asymptomatic carriers is well recognised. The infectivity of these individuals is an important public health problem. For example, it has been estimated that there are as many as 300 million HBV carriers.

Fulminant hepatitis

The disease suddenly worsens, the patient becoming deeply jaundiced, confused and drowsy; the disease often progresses to coma within forty-eight to seventy-two hours. Spontaneous bleeding is common because of deficiency of prothrombin and factors V, VII and X. Once coma develops the outlook is usually grave. Histologically, massive hepatic necrosis is present with few remaining hepatocytes; however, the reticulin framework is intact and patients who survive may have complete histological recovery. This complication is common with HEV (enteric NANB) infection in pregnancy (see also p. 137).

Chronic persistent hepatitis

The term is often used to describe a benign non-progressive inflammation of the liver without distortion of architecture, which persists for six months or more after the onset of the illness (see p. 142).

Chronic active hepatitis

This is an important complication of hepatitis types B, C and D occurring in up to 10% of cases. It does not follow infection with HAV or HEV. The features which suggest progression of acute hepatitis to CAH include:

1. lack of resolution of clinical symptoms and signs;
2. failure of the serum transaminase and other biochemical test levels to return to normal within six to twelve months;

3. perilobular hepatitis with piecemeal necrosis and apoptosis histologically (see p. 144);
4. the persistence of HBsAg or HCV RNA in serum after six months.

Cirrhosis of the liver

Cirrhosis may follow bridging necrosis or chronic active hepatitis (see p. 147) in HBV, HCV or HDV infection.

Hepatocellular carcinoma (HCC)

This may follow HBV and HCV infection, and commonly develops on the basis of chronic hepatitis or a long-standing carrier state (see p. 172).

Other complications

Rare complications of viral hepatitis include pancreatitis, myocarditis, aplastic anaemia and peripheral neuropathy.

Prophylaxis

Despite the advent of active immunisation for hepatitis A and B, the control of viral hepatitis still lies in large part in good sanitation and hygiene, particularly at a personal level, together with adequate screening of blood and blood products before their administration. All excreta of patients with hepatitis A must be considered infectious, at least in the early stages of the disease.

Potential parenteral sources of hepatitis B infection include:

1. any parenteral inoculation procedure or transfusion;
2. medical and paramedical work, especially where associated closely with blood, for example, laboratories;
3. sharing of razors, toothbrushes and syringes, for example, illicit drug use;
4. ear piercing, tattooing and tribal scarification;
5. sexual intercourse, especially involving male homosexuality.

Screening of blood for anti-HCV and the 'surrogate' markers, ALT and anti-HBc, will substantially reduce the incidence of posttransfusion hepatitis.

Passive immunisation

An attack of viral hepatitis confers lifelong immunity, but only to infection with the same virus. Immune serum globulin given prophylactically is of value in preventing or attenuating type A, but not type B hepatitis unless a specific hepatitis B immune globulin (HBIG) preparation is used containing a very high concentration of antibody to HBsAg. The effect of immune serum globulin and HBIG on C and E hepatitis is uncertain.

Immune serum globulin should be given to all household contacts of hepatitis A patients as soon as the index case is diagnosed. Hepatitis B immune globulin is indicated after non-immune subjects have a definite parenteral exposure to hepatitis B, that is, after percutaneous or 'needle stick' exposure, for sex partners of patients with acute hepatitis B infection and for infants of HBsAg-positive mothers.

Active immunisation

Hepatitis A vaccines prepared from inactivated cultured virus have recently become available and will replace immune globulin for travellers and for military personnel travelling overseas. Results in more than 25 000 volunteers have shown an immune response in 95% and 99% of recipients after one or two doses, respectively, but the duration of protection is uncertain.

Active immunisation with a hepatitis B vaccine prepared by recombinant DNA technology is also possible. Ideally, universal vaccination against HBV should be introduced but the cost remains relatively high. Thus, the most cost-effective policy is to vaccinate populations at increased risk, that is, health care workers and laboratory personnel in contact with hepatitis patients and blood, male homosexuals, sex industry workers, babies born to HBsAg mothers, and patients and staff of mental hospitals. Natural or vaccine-induced immunity to HBV, that is, circulating anti-HBs, will protect against HBV infection.

Treatment of acute hepatitis

There is no specific treatment for acute viral hepatitis. Most patients prefer bed rest in the early stage and a high caloric diet is desirable. It is wise to regard all cases as potentially fatal until progressive clinical and biochemical improvement is obvious. Hospitalisation may be required for correct diagnosis, for clinically severe or worsening illness, or for socioeconomic reasons. Hospitalised patients are usually nursed in open wards, provided the principles of good personal hygiene are followed by both patients and staff, and special care is taken with bed linen and eating utensils. Cholestyramine may reduce pruritus but potentially hepatotoxic drugs should be avoided. Corticosteroids do not alter the degree of necrosis or the rate of healing and should not be used.

Patients may resume normal activity when they feel well; the serum bilirubin level should not be regarded as a contraindication to mobilisation.

Chronic hepatitis

This is generally defined as a chronic inflammatory reaction in the liver continuing without improvement for at least six months. Whatever the aetiology, the same basic underlying liver histology is seen. Chronic hepatitis has traditionally been classified into chronic persistent, chronic lobular and chronic active hepatitis (mild and severe). While there is some overlap, this classification is helpful for prognosis and treatment. Chronic persistent hepatitis does not usually progress. In contrast chronic lobular hepatitis and mild chronic active hepatitis often develop slowly towards cirrhosis. Severe chronic active hepatitis often progresses rapidly and cirrhosis may already co-exist.

The major causes of chronic hepatitis are listed in Table 6.3 but in many instances the specific aetiology is unknown.

Table 6.3 *Comparison of chronic persistent and chronic active hepatitis*

Causes	*Chronic persistent hepatitis (CPH)*	*Chronic active hepatitis (CAH)*
Viral		
Hepatitis B	+	+
Hepatitis C	+	+
Drugs		
Methyldopa, isoniazid, paracetamol, nitrofurantoin, aspirin	+	+
Alcohol		
Especially recurrent acute alcoholic hepatitis	+	+
Other		
Wilson's disease	—	+
Alpha$_1$-antitrypsin deficiency	—	+
Liver histology		
Site of inflammation	Portal	Portal, extending into lobules
Piecemeal necrosis/apoptosis	Inconstant or absent	Characteristic
Lobular architecture	Preserved	Distorted
Bridging necrosis	Absent	Common
Fibrosis	Slight or absent	Common
Progression to cirrhosis	Rare	Common
Clinical features		
Onset	Commonly acute	Commonly insidious
Recurrent episodes	Infrequent	Common
Extrahepatic features (e.g. arthritis)	Rare	Common
Signs of chronic liver disease	Rare	Common
Laboratory features		
Raised serum transaminase	Common	Common
Raised serum immunoglobulin	Rare	Common
Circulating autoantibodies	Rare	Common
Prognosis	Excellent	Variable, often poor

Chronic persistent hepatitis

This is characterised by a non-specific chronic inflammation of the portal zones of the liver and some fibrosis; however, the hepatic parenchymal cells are normal and the limiting plate between liver cells and portal zones is intact (Fig. 6.5).

Clinical features

These are usually mild, consisting of fatigue, anorexia and discomfort over the liver. The patient may be asymptomatic and diagnosed during routine blood screening at the time of blood donation or medical examination. Usually the only abnormal physical sign is a slightly enlarged liver.

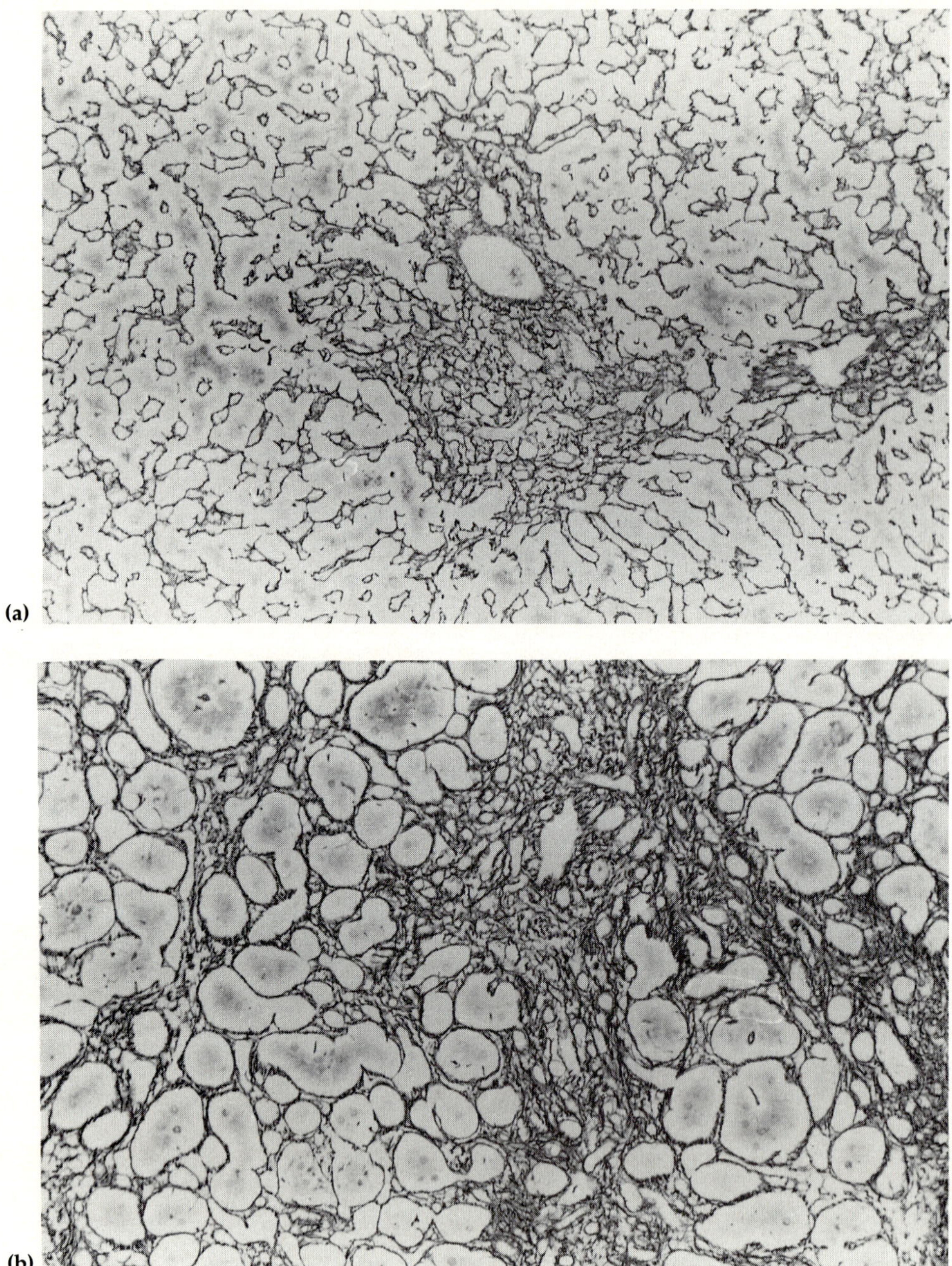

(a)

(b)

Fig. 6.5 **(a)** *Chronic persistent hepatitis. The portal tract is expanded by fibrous tissue, but the margin of the portal tract is regular and there is no penetration of the limiting plate. H-E stain, original magnification × 40.* **(b)** *Chronic active hepatitis. The portal tract is expanded by fibrous tissue, but the margin of the portal tract is irregular, with penetration of the limiting plate by the fibrous tissue. This often progresses to cirrhosis. H-E stain, original magnification × 40*

Biochemical tests

The results of these are normal except for a raised serum transaminase value up to ten times normal that usually fluctuates over months or years. A normal serum gamma globulin concentration is helpful in distinguishing CPH from CAH.

Treatment and prognosis

The outlook is usually excellent and the patient should be firmly reassured after thorough investigation which includes needle liver biopsy. No further treatment is required although an annual reassessment may be necessary if the diagnosis is uncertain. Alcohol and oral contraceptives are best avoided but the patient may eat normally and lead a normal life.

Chronic lobular hepatitis

This may be regarded as a variant of CPH in which the portal tract inflammation extends into the hepatitic lobules, but without piecemeal necrosis or disturbance of architecture. It usually has a good prognosis unless it is associated with the more sinister changes of chronic active hepatitis.

Chronic active hepatitis

This form of chronic hepatitis is characterised by an active continuing inflammation of the liver, which persists for more than six months and is associated with histologic evidence of perilobular hepatitis with conspicuous lymphocytes and plasma cell infiltration and fibrosis. The inflammatory infiltrate extends into the liver lobule causing erosions of the limiting plate, apoptosis and piecemeal necrosis (Fig. 6.5). Confluent necrosis between portal zones and central veins or from one portal zone to another ('bridging necrosis') occurs, often with fibrosis. The disorder commonly progresses to cirrhosis. The diverse aetiologies are summarised in Table 6.3.

Two main types of CAH are currently recognised (Table 6.4):

1. autoimmune CAH (usually now referred to simply as autoimmune hepatitis). In this type, viral antigens cannot be detected and the disease is believed to result from continuing host responses to unknown antigens, possibly from the liver. A variety of non-specific autoantibodies to tissue antigens are present in serum (see below), reflecting an underlying immunological disorder;
2. hepatitis B- and C-induced CAH, which are associated with the persistence of HBV and HCV, respectively.

There are several other important but less common causes of CAH. These include chronic ingestion of certain drugs, Wilson's disease and alpha$_1$-antitrypsin deficiency (see Tables 6.3 and 6.9).

Table 6.4 *Comparison of major types of chronic hepatitis*

	Autoimmune	*Type B (HBsAg-positive)*
Sex predominance	Female	Male
Age	Puberty, menopause	Neonates, older adults
Associated autoimmune diseases	Common	Rare
Serum immunoglobulins	High	Slight increase
Smooth muscle antibodies, Antinuclear antibodies	High titre (60% of patients)	Absent or low titre
LE cells	15% of patients	Absent
Risk of primary liver cancer	Low	High
Response to corticosteroids	Good	Usually poor

Clinical features

These may be minimal, the condition being diagnosed incidentally. Alternatively, the patient may present with the symptoms and signs of active hepatocellular disease of either insidious or sudden onset. Associated diseases include diabetes mellitus, inflammatory bowel disease and thyroiditis. Autoimmune CAH classically presents in women at the time of puberty or the menopause; amenorrhoea and Cushingoid features are common. In contrast, hepatitis B CAH largely affects males in the twenty-five to fifty year age group although HCV-induced CAH occurs at all ages. Physical examination may reveal no abnormality or evidence of hepatocellular failure (jaundice, splenomegaly, ascites, hepatic encephalopathy).

Biochemical tests

These reveal evidence of active hepatocellular disease with elevated serum transaminase and immunoglobulin (IgG). In the 'autoimmune' form non-specific tissue antibodies are often demonstrable in serum, including antinuclear antibody in high titre, and smooth muscle antibody. In hepatitis B CAH these tissue antibodies are absent or present in low titre, but the hepatitis B-associated antigens HBsAg, HBeAg and anti-HBc are usually detectable in serum, implying continued replication of the hepatitis B virus. HBV DNA in serum is more specific for viral replication. In hepatitis C-induced CAH, anti-HCV is usually found in the serum but circulating HCV RNA is more specifically indicative of viral replication and infectivity.

Treatment and prognosis

Corticosteroid therapy, with or without azathioprine, has been shown to induce remission and prolong life in 'autoimmune' CAH. Liver histology then shows less inflammatory activity although the progression from chronic hepatitis to cirrhosis may not be prevented. The treatment usually has to be continued for two years or more. It is difficult to decide when to stop therapy as premature withdrawal leads to relapse. Long-term, low-dose prednisone maintenance is often required.

Treatment of chronic hepatitis B is aimed at controlling infectivity, eradicating the virus and preventing the development of cirrhosis and hepatocellular carcinoma. Antiviral therapy with alpha interferon, a genetically engineered cytokine, in the replicative stage of disease (HBeAg and HBV DNA positive) may result in reduction or cessation of necro-inflammatory changes. In controlled trials 30–40% response rates have been achieved with loss of HBeAg in serum, but only 10% will clear the circulating HBsAg as well. Although the optimal dose and duration of therapy remain uncertain, usually 5–10 million units of interferon are given subcutaneously three times a week for twelve to twenty-four weeks. The most likely patients to respond to interferon therapy have recently acquired disease, high serum transaminase levels, a low serum HBV DNA titre and an active hepatitis on liver biopsy. Corticosteroids alone are contraindicated in patients with hepatitis B CAH, as such treatment perpetuates viral replication.

Chronic hepatitis following hepatitis C infection tends to be low grade with less markedly elevated serum transaminase and immunoglobin levels and absent autoantibodies. The course is usually mild although cirrhosis develops in some 20% of chronic HCV infections.

The precise role of alpha-interferon in the treatment of chronic hepatitis C is currently being more clearly defined, especially as it is expensive. At present, anti-HCV positive patients with significant symptoms, elevated ALT levels and chronic persistent hepatitis, as well as all those with chronic active hepatitis on biopsy (irrespective of symptoms) should at least be considered for such therapy. Currently, a six-month course of three million units thrice weekly costs approximately $3000 for the drug. Side effects (fevers, chills, malaise) are common but reversible.

Randomised controlled trials have already demonstrated that apparent control of hepatic necroinflammatory activity (histologically, biochemically and symptomatically) occurs in about 60% of patients treated for six months with relatively low doses of interferon. About half of those who respond to interferon (30% overall) maintain that response after treatment is discontinued. Recent viral studies indicate that most (but not all) of these long-term responses are complete cures, with clearance of HCV-RNA from serum. The remaining patients relapse within weeks of stopping interferon, although they usually respond to its re-introduction. Patients with cirrhosis are less likely to respond to interferon.

The other causes of CAH—for example, Wilson's disease—carry the prognosis of the underlying disease. The prognosis of all drug-induced CAH is usually good, provided the drug is stopped.

Fulminant hepatic failure (FHF)

This is a syndrome of massive hepatic necrosis defined as acute liver failure occurring in a previously normal liver and progressing rapidly to coma. The mortality is high (70–80%), especially with grade 4 coma. Causes include all forms of viral hepatitis, drugs and toxins, especially paracetamol (acetaminophen), Wilson's disease, fatty liver of pregnancy and Reye's syndrome (see Fig. 6.6). In the latter two conditions, microvesicular fat is a characteristic histological feature.

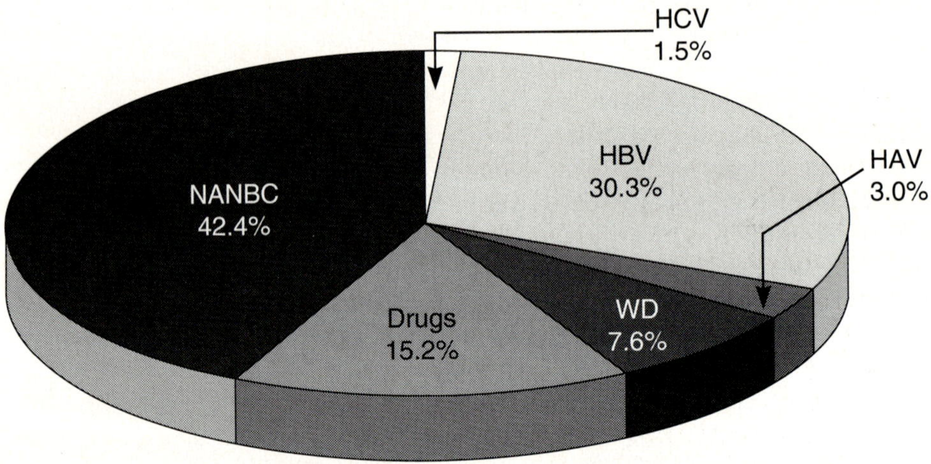

Fig. 6.6 *Causes of fulminant hepatic failure in Australia (series of 68 cases to 1994)* COURTESY DR GEOFFREY McCAUGHAN, ROYAL PRINCE ALFRED HOSPITAL, SYDNEY

Clinically, FHF presents as acute liver disease progressing rapidly to deep jaundice, coagulopathy and coma. Death results from infection, bleeding or hepatic coma with cerebral oedema.

Medical therapy is largely supportive in correcting the above complications, since the liver can regenerate in time. When FHF is due to paracetamol poisoning, N-acetyl cysteine should be given to replenish hepatic stores of glutathione which are depleted when the electrophilic metabolite of paracetamol conjugates with hepatic glutathione. In other forms of FHF no specific therapy has been shown to affect mortality, except liver transplantation which should be considered with worsening encephalopathy and coagulopathy. Such patients should be referred early to a liver transplant unit. Patients who survive FHF have a normal (regenerated) liver and do not manifest chronic hepatitis.

Cirrhosis of the liver

Definition

This is a chronic diffuse liver disease characterised by hepatic fibrosis with nodule formation. Fibrosis is not synonymous with cirrhosis, nodule formation with disturbed architecture being essential features of cirrhosis.

The condition results from liver cell necrosis, collapse of the reticulin framework with approximation of portal and central zones, and the formation of diffuse fibrous septa forming nodules of various sizes. This pattern occurs irrespective of the type of injury, since the possible responses of the liver to injury are limited.

It is important to distinguish between chronic hepatitis with some fibrosis present and established cirrhosis with nodule formation which is irreversible.

Aetiology

Up to 20% of patients with cirrhosis of the liver have no known cause for the disease (so-called 'cryptogenic cirrhosis'). Of the others, alcoholism, chronic active hepatitis and viral hepatitis account for the majority of patients, the precise incidence varying from one country to another depending on the frequency of chronic alcoholism and the hepatitis B and C viruses in the community. Less common causes are listed in Table 6.5.

Table 6.5 *Causes of cirrhosis of the liver*

1. *Alcohol*[(a)]	4. *Autoimmune*
2. *Viral hepatitis*[(a)] Hepatitis B ± delta hepatitis Hepatitis C	Chronic active hepatitis[(a)] Primary biliary cirrhosis
3. *Hereditary and metabolic* Haemochromatosis[(a)] Wilson's disease Alpha$_1$-antitrypsin deficiency Non-alcoholic steatohepatitis Cystic fibrosis Galactosaemia Type IV glycogen storage disease Tyrosinosis	5. *Drugs, e.g. methotrexate, isoniazid* 6. *Biliary obstruction (secondary biliary cirrhosis)* 7. *Neonatal hepatitis*

[(a)] These causes together account for about 75% of cases and 'cryptogenic cirrhosis' (unknown cause) for a further 20%.

Pathology

As emphasised above, the aetiology of cirrhosis cannot usually be determined from the pathological appearances. The size of the nodules in cirrhosis is related more to the persistence (or not) of the causal factor and not to any particular aetiology. Therefore, morphologic terms such as portal cirrhosis or postnecrotic cirrhosis, which implied aetiology, have been superseded by a simplified descriptive terminology which recognises three anatomical types:

1. micronodular cirrhosis characterised by uniformly small nodules (also called 'portal', 'septal' or Laennec's cirrhosis);
2. macronodular cirrhosis characterised by nodules of variable size, some containing large areas of intact or regenerating parenchyma within each large nodule (also called postnecrotic);
3. mixed micronodular and macronodular type.

The size of the liver may be small if there has been much destruction of tissue, or quite large, for example, if there has been considerable regeneration of liver tissue or associated fatty change as in alcoholic liver disease.

Symptoms and signs

These will depend on the degree to which the surviving liver cells can compensate for the disease. In the fully compensated state there may be no symptoms whatever, the disease being suspected at a routine medical examination by the finding of an enlarged liver or spleen. As the disease progresses, signs of *chronic hepatocellular failure* or *portal hypertension* appear. The clinical features, prognosis and treatment depend on the magnitude of these two major complications.

Hepatocellular failure

This leads to symptoms of fatigue, loss of weight, fluid retention and a general deterioration in health. Physical signs include:

1. spider angiomata on the skin of the upper trunk, face and forearms;
2. palmar erythema;
3. decreased body hair;
4. ascites;
5. testicular atrophy and gynaecomastia in male patients;
6. leuconychia (hypoalbuminaemia);
7. Dupuytren's contracture of the palmar fascia, parotid enlargement and peripheral neuropathy, which are pointers to alcoholism as a cause of cirrhosis;
8. a hyperdynamic circulation with flow murmurs over the precordium and the development of abdominal wall collateral veins.

In addition, jaundice, low-grade fever, the characteristic musty odour or fetor hepaticus, and increasing drowsiness are common. The precise mechanisms underlying these changes are complex and ill-understood. Impaired protein synthesis by the liver leads to hypoalbuminaemia, oedema and disordered blood coagulation.

Hepatic encephalopathy or coma and other neurological abnormalities

The clinical manifestations include personality changes, slurred speech, a characteristic 'flapping' tremor of the outstretched hands (asterixis) and a constructional apraxia (inability to write clearly or draw figures such as stars or houses). These are a consequence of an extensive portasystemic collateral circulation and consequent failure of the liver to remove ammonia and other products of protein metabolism. Neurotransmitter synthesis is controlled by the brain concentration of precursor amino acids. The aromatic amino acids are increased in liver disease and may result in increased production of the inhibitory neurotransmitter serotonin. The principal inhibitory neurotransmitter of the brain is gamma-aminobutyric acid (GABA), which can be synthesised by gut bacteria and may bypass the liver in portasystemic shunting. Recently, a GABA receptor has been demonstrated which binds not only GABA but also barbiturates and benzodiazepines. This receptor promotes chloride conductance across the postsynaptic neuromembrane, resulting in increased membrane polarisation and inhibition of postsynaptic potential. Increased sensitivity to benzodiazepine agonists leads to increased GABA-ergic tone. Flumazenil, a benzodiazepine antagonist, has been used to treat hepatic encephalopathy. It can induce variable and distinct transient improvement in about 70% of patients with hepatic encephalopathy, but these results need to be confirmed by controlled trials.

Coma may be precipitated by the administration of nitrogenous compounds, a high-protein diet or by the digestion of blood in the gut after an intestinal haemorrhage. Other precipitating factors include constipation, infection (especially spontaneous bacterial peritonitis), electrolyte imbalance (often due to diuretic therapy) and the administration of sedatives. Hepatic encephalopathy is also common after shunt surgery (see p. 158). Clinically its severity is graded as follows:

- *grade 1 (mild)*: tremor, impaired handwriting;
- *grade 2 (moderate)*: impaired intellectual function, lethargy, asterixis, constructional apraxia;
- *grade 3 (severe)*: confusion, somnolence;
- *grade 4 (coma)*: responsiveness to painful stimuli impaired or lost.

Portal hypertension

See page 154 for details of symptoms for portal hypertension.

Ascites

This develops from the combined effect of portal hypertension and hypoalbuminaemia (see p. 159).

Diagnosis

In the compensated phase this requires a high index of suspicion on the part of the clinician and confirmation by liver biopsy. History and clinical examination of the patient may reveal evidence of alcoholism or other causative factors. In the decompensated state, diagnosis is usually easy, especially in the presence of ascites, oedema, jaundice and other signs of chronic hepatocellular disease as described above.

Laboratory tests in the compensated stage of the disease may give quite normal results or show a slight to moderate increase in serum gammaglobulin, transaminase and alkaline phosphatase levels.

Organ-imaging procedures such as ultrasonography and CT scanning may also detect abnormal and uneven texture with excess fibrous tissue; however, none of the above tests is diagnostic and liver biopsy is required to confirm the diagnosis (see p. 182).

Prognosis

This varies considerably according to aetiology, to whether causative agents can be removed and to the stage of the disease. Thus the outcome for alcoholic patients is much improved if they abstain, as is that for patients with haemochromatosis if iron is removed by venesection therapy, and patients with Wilson's disease if they are treated with a chelating agent such as penicillamine to remove excess copper. In addition, early vigorous and meticulous medical care probably prolongs life and delays or prevents the onset of complications such as ascites or gastrointestinal bleeding. This is particularly important in alcoholic patients. Patients who abstain from alcohol have a five-year survival rate of about 60%, compared with 40% for those who continue to drink. Mortality figures are much higher when complications such as ascites and variceal bleeding are present. As a clinical guide to severity and prognosis, a classification was introduced in 1964 by Child and Turcotte (Table 6.6). Until more suitable quantitative tests of liver function are available this classification is of value.

Table 6.6 *Pugh modification of Child-Turcotte criteria*[a]

	Points scored for increasing abnormality[b]		
Clinical and biochemical measurements	*1*	*2*	*3*
Encephalopathy (grade)	None	1 & 2	3 & 4
Ascites	Absent	Slight	Moderate
Bilirubin (mg/100 mL)	<1–2	2–3	>3
Albumin (g/100 mL)	>3.5	2.8–3.5	<2.8
Prothrombin time (sec. prolonged)	<1–4	4–6	>6
Primary biliary cirrhosis			
Bilirubin (mg/100 mL)	<1–4	4–10	>10

[a] Table adapted from Pugh, R. N. H., Murray-Lyon, I. M., Dawson, J. L., Pietroni, M. C. and Williams, R., Transection of the oesophagus for bleeding oesophageal varices, *British Journal of Surgery*, 1973; 60:646–9.
[b] Points: grade A, 5–6; grade B, 7–9; grade C, 10–15.

Treatment

Compensated cirrhosis

All patients should be advised to take an adequate diet, preferably with evening snacks, to abstain from alcohol and to be reviewed regularly for signs of hepatocellular failure. Long-term care includes control of ascites, avoidance of drugs that may induce hepatic coma, and prompt treatment of infections and variceal bleeding.

Decompensated cirrhosis

Oedema and ascites require appropriate treatment (see p. 160).

Haematemesis and/or melaena

See page 157 for details.

Hepatic coma

Neuropsychiatric symptoms in a cirrhotic patient are usually an indication of incipient coma and require protein restriction. An additional effect can be achieved by sterilising the gut using oral neomycin or by lactulose which alters the pH in the colon. Precipitating factors should be searched for and treated appropriately. In established coma, intravenous glucose is given in addition to the above measures, to provide calories and so minimise endogenous protein catabolism and prevent hypoglycaemia. As stated above, flumazenil is promising but requires further evaluation.

Liver transplantation

Orthotopic liver transplantation (OLT)—the removal of the patient's liver and replacement by a normal donor liver—represents a major and spectacular advance in therapy for end-stage irreversible chronic liver disease, and in some circumstances for acute hepatic failure. With improved surgical techniques and immunosuppression, the one-year survival rate has risen to over 90%, with excellent prospects for good quality of life thereafter. Timing of the procedure is all important and should not be deferred until the patient is too ill to withstand the procedure.

The indications by disease category are shown in Table 6.7. Primary biliary cirrhosis is the most common indication in adults and biliary atresia is the most common in children. Age is not a major prognostic factor.

Table 6.7 *Indications for liver transplantation*

Adults	
Chronic liver disease	
• Primary biliary cirrhosis	35%
• Primary sclerosing cholangitis	8%
• Chronic active hepatitis	4%
• Cryptogenic cirrhosis	6%
• Alcoholic cirrhosis	1%
Acute liver failure	15%
Malignancy	9%
• Primary HCC (if less than 3.0 cm diameter)	
• Secondary (e.g. carcinoid syndrome)	
Other	10%
Children	
Inborn errors of metabolism	4%
• With intrinsic liver disease (e.g. α_1-antitrypsin deficiency)	
• Without intrinsic liver disease (e.g. Crigler-Najjar syndrome)	
Cholestatic liver disease	
• Biliary atresia	8%

The contraindications are listed in Table 6.8. Absolute contraindications are those which render a successful outcome impossible. The risk of recurrent disease is very high in patients with hepatocellular carcinoma greater than 3 cm diameter and in patients with HBV infection with active viral replication (serological positivity for HBeAg and/or HBV DNA). The risk is lower with acute fulminant hepatitis where the virus is not replicating. Attempts to prevent reinfection with vaccines or antiviral drugs are currently being evaluated.

Table 6.8 *Absolute and relative contraindications to liver transplantation*

Absolute	*Relative*
Active sepsis outside the liver and biliary tree	Impaired renal function
HIV positivity	Hepatitis B or D
Metastatic or hepatobiliary malignancy	Pulmonary hypertension
	Previous upper abdominal surgery
	Active post-sclerotherapy ulceration
	Bacteraemia
	Spontaneous bacterial peritonitis

HCV infection is not a contraindication to OLT because, although reinfection is common, the resulting hepatitis is usually mild.

Alcoholic liver disease poses special challenges since the survival rate and subsequent return to good health does not differ from those transplanted for other causes. The decision is often a difficult one because of social and behavioural problems (including poor compliance with medical advice, which is important following OLT), the presence of alcohol-related organic disorders such as nutritional deficiencies and cardiomyopathy, and the fear of a return to alcohol (recidivism). In patients with severe acute alcoholic hepatitis, who may die within six to eight weeks of their initial hospital admission, transplantation may be performed successfully but the risk of recidivism is high.

For further details of patient selection, timing of transplantation, operative and postoperative care, immunosuppressive therapy and complications, see the references at the end of this chapter.

Portal hypertension

The portal system includes all veins that carry blood from the abdominal part of the alimentary tract, the spleen, pancreas and gallbladder (see p. 127).

At rest portal blood flow averages 800 mL/min and portal pressure is 0.67–1.33 kPa (5–10 mm Hg), some 0.4–0.67 kPa (3–5 mm Hg) higher than the pressure in the inferior vena cava. Portal hypertension is only clinically important when the pressure is 2 kPa (15 mm Hg) or higher. A collateral circulation then develops between the tributaries of the portal circulation and the systemic circulation. The main sites for this anastomosis are the submucosa of the oesophagus (oesophageal varices) and the stomach, the submucosa of the rectum, the anterior abdominal wall, the left renal vein, lumbar veins, and the ovarian and testicular veins (Fig. 6.7).

A convenient classification of the causes of portal hypertension is according to whether the obstruction is above, within or below the sinusoidal circulation in the liver.

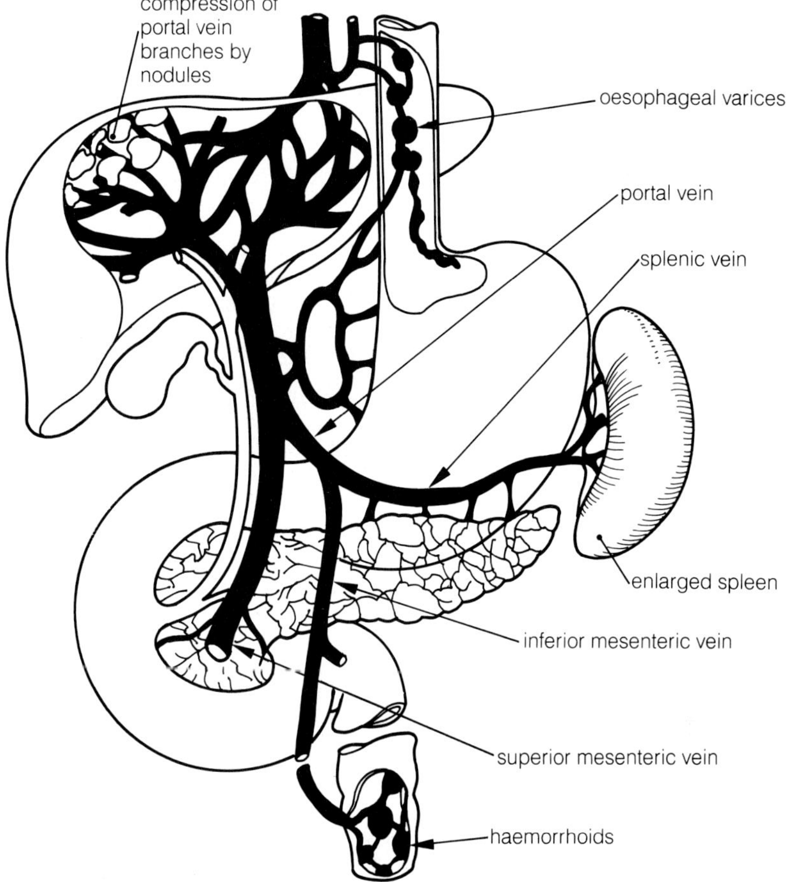

Fig. 6.7 *Diagrammatic representation of portal hypertension due to cirrhosis* FROM PIPER, D. W. (ED.), *MEDICINE FOR STUDENTS AND NURSES,* 2ND EDN, McGRAW-HILL, SYDNEY, 1980, WITH PERMISSION

Causes of portal hypertension

1. Extrahepatic
   - (a) blocked portal vein
   - (b) increased splenic flow
2. Intrahepatic
   - (a) presinusoidal
     - (i) granulomata, e.g. sarcoidosis
   - (b) sinusoidal
     - (i) cirrhosis
     - (ii) nodular transformation of the liver
   - (c) postsinusoidal
     - (i) blocked hepatic vein (e.g. Budd Chiari syndrome)
     - (ii) veno-occlusive disease

Clinical features

Those due to collateral circulations

The extensive collateral circulation that develops is clinically important because there may be gastrointestinal haemorrhage (usually from oesophageal varices) and the development of portasystemic encephalopathy. The latter is more likely to develop when large spontaneous or surgically created portasystemic shunts exist. Abdominal wall collateral veins and a venous hum may be noted. The spread of the veins around the umbilicus has been called the 'caput medusae'.

Splenomegaly

An enlarged spleen is the single most important diagnostic sign of portal hypertension. The size of the spleen bears little relationship to the portal venous pressure. With splenomegaly, thrombocytopoenia and, less commonly, leucopenia and anaemia may occur (secondary 'hypersplenism'). The thrombocytopoenia is seldom of clinical importance and its significance is best assessed by the bleeding time. It represents a pooling of normal platelets within the spleen, but the platelets usually continue to contribute to haemostasis.

Ascites

Portal hypertension alone seldom causes ascites; its presence in cirrhosis usually indicates liver cell failure with impaired albumin synthesis (less than 30 g/L) in addition to the portal hypertension.

Investigations

Biochemical studies

Liver function tests help determine the aetiology and activity of any associated liver disease.

Radiology

The demonstration of the splanchnic venous anatomy is necessary before surgery to confirm the patency of the portal vein and the extent of any collateral circulation, and to determine the feasibility of various shunt procedures. The simplest initial investigation is ultrasound (especially Doppler) examination and CT scanning. This can be followed by venography or indirect angiography for more definitive vascular imaging.

Measurement of portal pressure

A balloon catheter wedged into a hepatic venous radicle via the femoral vein measures 'wedged' hepatic venous pressure. Measurements taken with the balloon deflated reflect the 'free' hepatic venous pressure. The difference between 'wedged' and 'free' pressure is the portal venous pressure.

Liver biopsy

This is essential in determining the nature and activity of any underlying liver disease.

Medical management

Variceal bleeding

A patient bleeding from oesophageal varices requires intensive care facilities. The mortality rate from bleeding oesophageal varices is 25–50% and, of those surviving the initial bleeding, 60% will bleed again within a year. Management involves resuscitation, confirmation of the site of bleeding, control of bleeding and prophylaxis against encephalopathy and ascites.

Resuscitation

Peripheral and central venous lines should be inserted, and plasma expanders and fresh whole blood given to maintain blood volume. Platelets, clotting factors and vitamin K may all be needed in the presence of coagulopathy. During resuscitation the patient's bladder should be catheterised and all vital signs of fluid balance monitored closely.

Confirmation of bleeding site

It is important to confirm varices as the source of bleeding. Bleeding is from a non-variceal site in up to 30% of cirrhotic patients with portal hypertension, especially in patients with alcoholic liver disease. Diagnosis of the site of bleeding is dependent on fibreoptic upper gastrointestinal tract endoscopy. An experienced endoscopist is essential if reliable results are to be obtained.

Control of bleeding

Non-surgical therapy is aimed at controlling portal pressure, correcting haemostatic defects and variceal compression or obliteration.

Vasopressin produces splanchnic vasoconstriction by its actions on both the mesenteric and coeliac arterial beds, thus reducing portal blood flow and decreasing portal venous pressure. If used, vasopressin is given intravenously as a bolus of 20 units in 100 mL 5% dextrose over twenty minutes. Unfortunately, rebleeding may occur following cessation of the infusion. Somatostatin has similar haemodynamic effects to vasopressin but with fewer complications, and is now the preferred drug in this situation. It is given as a bolus followed by IV infusion.

Variceal compression

A modification of the Sengstaken-Blakemore tube (Fig. 6.8) is an effective short-term measure for the control of variceal haemorrhage, if the patient continues to bleed despite vasopressin.

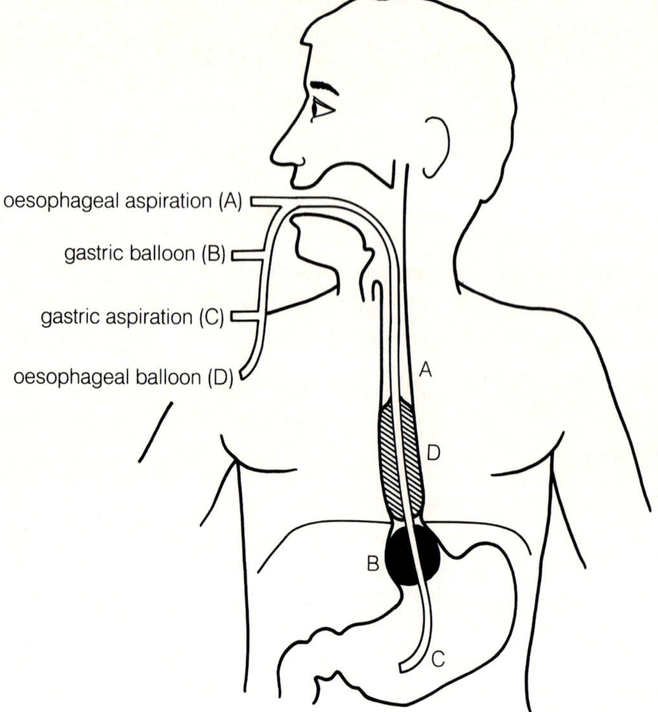

Fig. 6.8 *Sengstaken-Blakemore tube in situ*

Obliteration of oesophageal varices can be achieved by endoscopic sclerotherapy or by banding the varices. This can be used in either the acute or elective situation, and the procedure can be repeated until the varices are completely ablated.

Encephalopathy and ascites

Both lactulose and neomycin can be given to minimise encephalopathy. Electrolyte homeostasis, the early detection of infection and the maintenance of renal function are also important.

Long-term medical management to prevent recurrent bleeding

The optimal medical control of portal hypertension and the prevention of variceal bleeding has received much recent attention and evaluation by controlled clinical trials. Propranolol has been shown to decrease portal venous pressure, probably by decreasing cardiac output and blood flow to the splanchnic circulation. In some controlled trials propranolol has been as successful as sclerotherapy, especially in good risk patients. It is also of therapeutic value in patients with bleeding from portal hypertensive gastropathy and in primary prevention of bleeding where large varices have been demonstrated. A dose sufficient to reduce resting pulse rate by 25% should be given.

Prognosis

The above procedures arrest bleeding, but the ultimate survival depends on liver function. Hence patients with portal vein thrombosis and normal liver function have an excellent prognosis if the variceal bleeding can be controlled. Total abstinence from alcohol is essential for a good prognosis in alcoholic patients. Once bleeding has been controlled, consideration should be given to hepatic transplantation.

Surgical management

Portasystemic shunting (either porta-caval or distal spleno-renal) must be considered when sclerotherapy and somatostatin have failed to control variceal bleeding. Although recurrent haemorrhage from varices is eliminated, the mortality is high and postoperative encephalopathy is a major problem. Subsequent surgery for hepatic transplantation is also more difficult.

Transjugular intrahepatic portasystemic shunt (TIPSS) may be performed under local anaesthesia with ultrasound guidance, but this requires considerable technical skill. Although it avoids abdominal surgery it does appear to be complicated by hepatic encephalopathy. It can be particularly helpful in patients with portal hypertension and bleeding who subsequently proceed to liver transplantation.

Ascites

This is due to the combination of sodium retention and portal hypertension. The mechanism responsible for the development of the inappropriate renal sodium retention in cirrhosis is ill-understood and controversial. The traditional concept is that the kidney is thought to be responding to a contraction of the effective circulating plasma volume, which stimulates the renin-aldosterone system. The kidneys therefore retain sodium and water as a homeostatic mechanism to restore the blood volume. Thus, urinary sodium secretion is low (less than 5 mmol/d) and serum sodium levels are normal or low, reflecting the expanded extracellular space. Another view (the 'overfill theory') suggests that renal retention of sodium is primary, with expansion of the plasma volume and overflow into the extravascular space.

Clinical features

The patient usually has few complaints other than the cosmetic effect of a distended abdomen, but excessive ascitic fluid is uncomfortable and may contribute to the development of bleeding varices or renal failure. Some patients with ascites also develop large pleural effusions, particularly in the right hemithorax. Less than 1 or 2 L of fluid in the peritoneal cavity cannot be detected by the usual clinical signs. Larger amounts of fluid produce generalised abdominal distension extending into the flanks, marked impairment of percussion note in the flanks, shifting dullness and a fluid thrill.

Differential diagnosis

Consideration must be given to all the causes of generalised abdominal distension: fluid, flatus, fetus, faeces and fat.

In addition to liver disease, malignancy with peritoneal seeding is a common cause of ascites. Less common causes are the nephrotic syndrome, cardiac failure, myxoedema, constrictive pericarditis, pancreatic disease and tuberculous peritonitis.

Investigation

An abdominal x-ray may show a generalised loss of detail and disappearance of the outline of the lower edge of the liver; however, more sensitive techniques such as ultrasound and CT scanning can detect as little as a few hundred millilitres of intraperitoneal fluid and provide other information relevant to the cause. Diagnostic paracentesis (of about 50 mL) should always be performed to measure the protein concentration and white cell count. Aerobic and anaerobic cultures and cytological examination of the ascitic fluid should also be performed. Infection of the ascitic fluid is very common and should be suspected if a patient with cirrhosis deteriorates, particularly with encephalopathy. The ascitic fluid polymorphonuclear leukocyte cell count exceeds 250 cells per mm^3 and cultures are usually positive: the ascitic fluid should be inoculated directly into blood culture bottles.

Treatment

This is a difficult therapeutic problem. The principles are:

1. admission to hospital and careful recording of daily weight and fluid balance, including urinary sodium levels;
2. a restricted sodium diet (less than 22 mEq/d);
3. diuretics;
4. paracentesis if required.

When added to a low-salt diet, a potassium-sparing diuretic alone will elicit a response from some patients. Spironolactone up to 500 mg/d or more or amiloride 10 mg/d are the drugs of choice; however, a combination of a potassium-losing diuretic, such as frusemide 40 mg/d, and a potassium-sparing diuretic may be used with careful surveillance for electrolyte disturbances. The goal is weight loss of 0.5 kg/d, although more may be mobilised if peripheral oedema is present.

Large-volume paracentesis (4–6 L) has been shown to be cost-effective and safe, although care must be taken to avoid renal failure. Thus, if peripheral oedema is absent, salt-poor albumin should be infused intravenously at the same time.

Various manoeuvres have been introduced for the management of resistant ascites. Reinfusion of a protein-rich ultrafiltrate of ascitic fluid into the venous system or a LeVeen (peritoneo-venous) shunt may be considered for more permanent control of the resistant ascites. With this method the ascites is directly connected to the venous system by a tube containing a pressure-sensitive valve. This can be very successful but its use is restricted somewhat by complications, notably disseminated intravascular coagulation due to collagen in the ascitic fluid.

Functional renal failure in cirrhosis ('hepatorenal syndrome')

This is defined as renal failure (oliguria of less than 600 mL/d with a rising plasma creatinine level) in a patient who has no prior history of renal disease and who is volume replete (to exclude prerenal azotaemia). The urinary sodium is usually less than 10 mmol/d. This may be spontaneous or due to compartmental fluid shifts. It may be precipitated by diuretic therapy or by nonsteroidal anti-inflammatory agents. Diuresis is accompanied by a fall in plasma volume which may lead to decreased renal blood flow and a rise in plasma urea and creatinine. This is usually reversed when the diuretics are stopped. The mechanism for the functional renal failure is not understood but a major factor is probably reduction in renal blood flow. Factors contributing to this include splanchnic pooling of blood, neurogenic vaso-constriction, diuretic therapy and endotoxaemia. Treatment is unsatisfactory. Obvious precipitating factors should be reversed and the patient is managed in the traditional conservative scheme of fluid, sodium, potassium and protein restriction. The syndrome is common in patients with end-stage alcoholic cirrhosis. The prognosis is poor.

Renal tubular necrosis may complicate toxic liver injury and may also occur as a complication in patients who have marked hypotension after severe gastrointestinal bleeding.

Special types of cirrhosis

Haemochromatosis

This is a common disorder of iron metabolism in which there is inappropriately high iron absorption and progressive deposition of iron in parenchymal cells of the liver, pancreas, pituitary and other organs with eventual fibrosis and organ failure.

In its fully developed form, the disease presents as cirrhosis associated with gross increase in total body iron stores. Most cases are due to an inherited metabolic defect which has been shown to be linked to the HLA A3 locus on chromosome 6 and which results in excessive iron absorption (primary, idiopathic or genetic haemochromatosis), but the same clinical and pathological picture may also result secondarily from the accumulation of excess iron over many years due to chronic anaemia, haemolysis or other causes of increased iron absorption (e.g. mostly sideroblastic anaemia and thalassaemia major). Recent studies have shown that the disease susceptibility trait is inherited as autosomal recessive with a gene frequency in Europeans of 1:10 to 1:20 and a homozygous frequency of 1:300 to 1:400 of the population.

The deposition of iron in the tissues appears to be responsible for most of the manifestations of the condition. These are classically hepatic fibrosis or cirrhosis with gross hepatomegaly, pancreatic damage with diabetes mellitus, cardiomyopathy, skin pigmentation, gonadal atrophy and an arthropathy resembling osteoarthritis. This is due to the deposition of calcium pyrophosphate in the synovium (chondrocalcinosis). The relationship of the arthropathy to the basic abnormality in iron metabolism is unclear. Death usually results from hepatocellular failure, from cardiac failure due to cardiomyopathy resulting from iron deposition in the myocardium or in the conducting fibres, or from primary liver cell carcinoma. The symptomatic disease is more common in men and symptoms usually begin in the fifth or sixth decades; however, asymptomatic precirrhotic iron overload is diagnosed in about 25% of siblings when they are screened for the disease. The diagnosis is confirmed by a high level of saturation of the serum transferrin, an elevated serum ferritin level and needle biopsy of the liver, which demonstrates gross deposition of iron with or without fibrosis or cirrhosis and increased hepatic iron concentration. Relatives should be screened for the disease by estimating the transferrin saturation and serum ferritin level and, where these are abnormal, liver biopsy is performed. HLA typing of siblings can help define heterozygosity and homozygosity and therefore relative risk.

Treatment by regular venesection therapy, removing 500 mL once or twice per week, allows mobilisation of the iron stores and improvement in the manifestations of the disease. The prognosis in treated cases is excellent, although the risk of primary liver cell cancer remains if cirrhosis is present. Precirrhotic patients, if treated, have a life-expectancy that does not differ from the normal population.

Wilson's disease (hepatolenticular degeneration)

This is a metabolic disease inherited as an autosomal recessive trait and characterised by excess deposition of copper in the liver (leading to chronic hepatitis or cirrhosis) and in the cerebrum (resulting in tremor, rigidity, dysarthria and other extrapyramidal manifestations). The responsible aberrant gene has recently been cloned on chromosome 13 and this is responsible for an intra-hepatocyte defect in copper transport, leading to diminished biliary copper excretion. The carrier rate varies in different population groups, but in Europeans it is approximately 1:100 with a homozygous rate of about 1:30 000. Diagnosis is made from the familial nature of the disease, the presence of characteristic copper deposition at the margin of the cornea (Kayser-Fleischer rings) and by the demonstration of increased urinary copper excretion, low serum caeruloplasmin and copper levels, and an increased concentration of copper in the liver. Treatment consists of chelating the excess copper with penicillamine and this usually results in striking clinical improvement but must be continued for life. The disease is cured by hepatic transplantation.

Alpha$_1$-antitrypsin deficiency

This is a rare cause of cirrhosis in children and occasionally in adults. The protease inhibitor (Pi) system has a number of variants under the control of a single autosomal co-dominant gene with seventy-five different alleles, distinguished by isoelectric focusing or PCR analysis. The single gene locus coding for alpha$_1$-antitrypsin is on the long arm of chromosome 14. About 80% of the population are PiMM and have normal alpha$_1$-antitrypsin levels. The genotype PiZZ (homozygous alpha$_1$-antitrypsin deficiency) and the heterozygote PiZ are associated with liver disease in about 20% of patients. About 50–60% of patients with severe deficiency may develop emphysema in early adult life.

Patients with alpha$_1$-antitrypsin deficiency have an accumulation of periodic acid-Schiff positive inclusion bodies in hepatocytes. This material is an alpha$_1$-antitrypsin which is deficient in sialic acid and other carbohydrate residues; but the precise mechanism of the liver damage remains unexplained.

The disease usually presents as a neonatal hepatitis within the first few months of life and the child may die at this stage. Those who survive develop cirrhosis of the liver which becomes overt in late childhood or early adult life, with hepatomegaly and portal hypertension. The liver biopsy shows necrosis, cholestasis, inflammatory cell infiltration and a periportal fibrous reaction, together with the characteristic periodic acid-Schiff positive inclusion bodies. Replacement therapy with synthetic alpha$_1$-antitrypsin is under development to treat the pulmonary disease. Liver transplantation (for end-stage disease) corrects the basic defect. The recipient's phenotype rapidly changes to that of the donor.

Primary biliary cirrhosis (chronic nonsuppurative destructive cholangitis)

Primary biliary cirrhosis (PBC) is an uncommon disease of unknown origin characterised by a progressive nonsuppurative intrahepatic cholangitis which eventually leads to cirrhosis. Most patients are females aged thirty-five to seventy years and the disease usually begins with pruritus of insidious onset. The clinical features are those of chronic cholestasis including hepatosplenomegaly, a rising serum alkaline phosphatase level, hypercholesterolaemia, skin pigmentation and xanthomata. Thus, the clinical picture resembles that produced by unrelieved obstruction of the extrahepatic bile ducts. The prognosis of the disease is very variable, but most symptomatic patients develop complications of cirrhosis within ten years of onset of symptoms.

The disease is associated with considerable immunologic disturbance, including high titres of non-specific antibodies in serum against tissue antigens (especially mitochondria) and increased levels of IgM in serum. These observations suggest that disordered immune responses play a role in the initiation or progression of the disease, although the mechanism is unclear. The mitochondrial antibody is helpful diagnostically, since it is present in over 95% of cases and is absent from the serum in cases of obstruction of the extrahepatic bile ducts. Moreover, virtually 100% of patients have serological antibodies against M2, a specific antigen on the inner mitochondrial membrane. This antigen is a component of the pyruvate dehydrogenase complex of mitochondrial enzymes. The relationship of mitochondrial antigens and antibodies to the pathogenesis of this disease remains unclear.

Several diseases with presumptive immunological pathogenesis may occur in assocation with PBC, including Sjogren's syndrome, scleroderma, rheumatoid arthritis, thyroiditis and the CREST syndrome (calcinosis, Raynaud's phenomenon, oesophageal dysmotility, sclerodactyly, and telangiectasia).

Although ursodeoxycholic acid has shown promise in clinical trials, there is still no satisfactory specific therapy. Pruritus is relieved by cholestyramine. Liver transplantation is recommended when the disease interferes significantly with quality of life and usually when the serum bilirubin level reaches five times normal. If not delayed to the late stages this can be spectacularly successful.

Primary sclerosing cholangitis (PSC)

This is a chronic, progressive, fibrosing inflammatory process involving parts or all of the biliary tree, ultimately leading to biliary cirrhosis. About half the patients suffer from ulcerative colitis or Crohn's colitis. The clinical features are those of progressive cholestasis, particularly with pruritus and elevated serum alkaline phosphatase levels. Diagnosis rests on the demonstration of beading and stenosis of the biliary tree, usually by ERCP (see p. 117). Cholangiocarcinoma may be associated and should be suspected if localised dilatation of ducts occurs, especially at the hilum. Medical treatment is unsatisfactory and PSC, when advanced, is one of the most common indications for liver transplantation.

Secondary biliary cirrhosis (SBC)

Complete or partial obstruction of the extrahepatic biliary tree as occurs with gallstones and bile duct stricture will, if unrelieved, lead to diffuse hepatic fibrosis, cholangitis and eventually cirrhosis. The clinical picture and complications are similar to those described for PBC, except for the immunologic disturbances which are not present.

Patients with long-standing cholestasis (e.g. primary and secondary biliary cirrhosis) have elevated hepatic copper levels, and sometimes elevated serum and urinary copper levels. The relation of this disturbance in copper metabolism to the pathogenesis of the liver disease is unclear. Long-standing cholestasis also impairs the absorption of fat-soluble vitamins (A, D, E and K) with resultant side-effects, especially osteomalacia and osteoporosis.

Non-alcoholic steatosis and steatophepatitis

Fat may also accumulate in the liver in obesity, diabetes mellitus, hypertriglyceridaemia, corticosteroid therapy, protein malnutrition, fatty liver of pregnancy, Reye's syndrome, following jejunoileal bypass, parenteral hyperalimentation and drugs (valproic acid and IV tetracycline). With the exception of Reye's syndrome and fatty liver of pregnancy, which both lead to fulminant hepatic failure, fatty liver is usually benign and non-progressive; however, inflammation can occur, with a histological picture mimicking acute alcoholic hepatitis (including cirrhosis), especially after jejunoileal bypass or rapid weight reduction. Treatment consists of gradual weight reduction and good control of diabetes.

Alcoholic liver disease

Prevalence and pathogenesis

Alcohol ingestion is an important cause of acute and chronic liver disease in affluent societies. In general, the development of alcoholic liver damage is dependent on the duration and dose of alcohol ingested, severe chronic alcoholic liver damage resulting after approximately ten years of heavy drinking, or sooner in women, in amounts in excess of 100 g/d (approximately equivalent to eight to ten standard drinks). It is emphasised that only about 20% of alcoholics develop cirrhosis and the reason for this is unknown. On the other hand, less severe forms of alcoholic liver damage are more common.

There are three major types of hepatic change seen in alcoholic liver disease: fatty liver, acute alcoholic hepatitis and cirrhosis. It is emphasised that the processes of fatty change, hepatitis and cirrhosis commonly coexist in the same patient.

Fatty liver

The precise reason for the accumulation of triglyceride in the liver is uncertain. It may result from increased hepatic synthesis of triglyceride, from mobilisation of free fatty acids from peripheral stores, or from increased intestinal absorption or synthesis of triglycerides. It is believed, however, that fatty liver in the alcoholic is reversible and is probably not a precursor of alcoholic cirrhosis.

Acute alcoholic hepatitis

This is a more severe hepatic reaction characterised by focal hepatocellular necrosis, intracellular hyaline deposits (Mallory bodies) and polymorphonuclear neutrophil infiltration, particularly around necrotic cells. A characteristic lesion is fibrosis around terminal hepatic venules (central hyaline sclerosis). The pathogenesis of alcoholic hepatitis is uncertain, but it is probably a forerunner of cirrhosis.

Cirrhosis

Cirrhosis in the alcoholic often results from repeated episodes of acute alcoholic hepatitis, with recurrent necrosis and the development of fibrosis, resulting in micronodular cirrhosis.

Clinical features

Fatty liver is not usually associated with symptoms or signs other than a large liver. Alcoholic hepatitis, on the other hand, may produce severe hepatic decompensation, with vomiting, diarrhoea, fever, polymorphonuclear neutrophil leucocytosis in the peripheral blood and an enlarged tender liver. Biochemical tests reveal hepatocellular insufficiency, sometimes with intrahepatic cholestasis. The picture may closely resemble that of viral hepatitis, and so a history of a recent alcoholic bout and the leucocytosis are useful diagnostic clues. In addition, in acute alcoholic hepatitis, the serum transaminase level is rarely above 300 U/L as compared to viral hepatitis where it is commonly very high. In addition the AST/ALT ratio is often reversed and greater than 2.

Cirrhosis in the alcoholic does not differ in its manifestations from other types of cirrhosis, except that the symptoms and signs of hepatic decompensation often respond quite dramatically to alcohol withdrawal. Associated clinical features due to alcoholism may also be present, for example, parotid gland enlargement, peripheral neuropathy, cerebellar signs and Dupuytren's contractures of the palmar fascia.

Treatment

Treatment of alcoholic liver disease consists of convincing the patient of the importance of complete abstinence, and the usual measures for hepatocellular failure and portal hypertension. Psychiatric assessment may be helpful. Corticosteroids have been shown to increase the survival of very ill patients. The role of hepatic transplantation has been discussed previously (see p. 153).

Cholestasis

This is a syndrome associated with failure of bile to reach the duodenum. The abnormality may lie anywhere from the fine biliary canaliculi to the ampulla of Vater, and the clinical, biochemical and histological complications are very similar irrespective of the cause.

Aetiology

The causes of cholestasis are summarised in Table 6.9. The most common causes are drug jaundice, gallstones and carcinoma of the pancreas.

Table 6.9 *Causes of cholestasis*

1. **Intrahepatic cholestasis**
   (a) *Lesions known or presumed to be at the level of the parenchymal cell*
   Cirrhosis
   Cholestatic viral hepatitis
   Alcoholic hepatitis
   Chronic non-haemolytic jaundice (Dubin-Johnson and Rotor syndromes)
   Postoperative cholestasis
   (b) *Lesions known or presumed to be distal to the parenchymal cell (canaliculi, cholangioles or intrahepatic bile ducts)*
   Drugs (e.g. chlorpromazine and C-17 alkylated anabolic steroids)
   Cholestasis of pregnancy
   Benign recurrent cholestasis (familial or idiopathic)
   Pericholangitis of ulcerative colitis
   Sclerosing cholangitis
   Cholangiocarcinoma of hepatic ducts
   Parasitic infestation (e.g. *Clonorchis sinensis*)
2. **Extrahepatic bile duct obstruction (e.g. gallstones, carcinoma, bile duct stricture)**

Pathology

With the light microscope, bile pigment is seen to accumulate in the liver cells, particularly in the centrizonal areas, the Kupffer cells and the biliary canaliculi, and this is sometimes associated with mononuclear cellular infiltrate. When large duct obstruction is present, oedema of portal tracts and proliferation of small bile ducts are prominent features.

Clinical features

In contrast to patients with hepatocellular jaundice, patients with cholestasis are often asymptomatic and show little evidence of physical deterioration. Their major symptom is pruritus, which has previously been attributed to retained bile acids; however, it has not been possible to correlate pruritus with the concentration of any naturally occurring bile acid in serum or in skin. With prolonged cholestasis there may be deposition of lipids in the skin (xanthomata) and generalised skin pigmentation. Steatorrhoea is usually present and results from deficiency of bile salts in the intestine. The impaired absorption of fat-soluble vitamins D and K leads respectively to osteomalacia and spontaneous bleeding.

With mechanical obstruction to the large bile ducts ('surgical' cholestasis) the liver becomes enlarged and the gallbladder may be palpable and tender. Additional features sometimes present are pain (due to stretching of the liver capsule, to gallbladder disease, or to a primary tumour) and fever (due to ascending cholangitis).

Laboratory tests

The findings characteristic of cholestasis include elevations of serum bilirubin, alkaline phosphatase, gamma glutamyl transpeptidase and 5 nucleotidase. The aminotransferase levels are usually normal or only slightly elevated. Very high levels of serum alkaline phosphatase (>500 IU/L) are seen with prolonged intrahepatic obstruction (e.g. bile duct carcinoma).

Diagnosis

Identifying a responsible drug may be very difficult, requiring repeated questioning of the patient and close relatives. The differentiation of intrahepatic cholestasis from obstruction to the main bile ducts can usually (but not always) be made on the basis of history, physical signs, laboratory tests and ultrasonography. The distinction between the two is obviously important. High resolution ultrasonography has greatly simplified this distinction between intrahepatic cholestasis and extrahepatic obstruction. In the latter instance the dilated bile ducts can usually be delineated together with any gallstones present (Fig. 6.9). Endoscopic retrograde cholangiopancreatography (ERCP) or transhepatic cholangiography is often necessary to localise or exclude a large duct obstruction.

Treatment

This obviously depends on the cause, which should be identified and removed if possible. Replacement therapy with parenteral fat-soluble vitamins and clotting factors may be necessary with prolonged cholestasis.

Drug-induced liver damage

Because of the liver's central role in drug metabolism it is particularly susceptible to injury. Drugs are responsible for about 2% of all cases of jaundice in hospitalised patients and about 25% of cases of fulminant hepatic failure. Drug reactions can mimic virtually every known liver disease; hence in every patient with liver disease it is mandatory to record all medications taken over the previous six months.

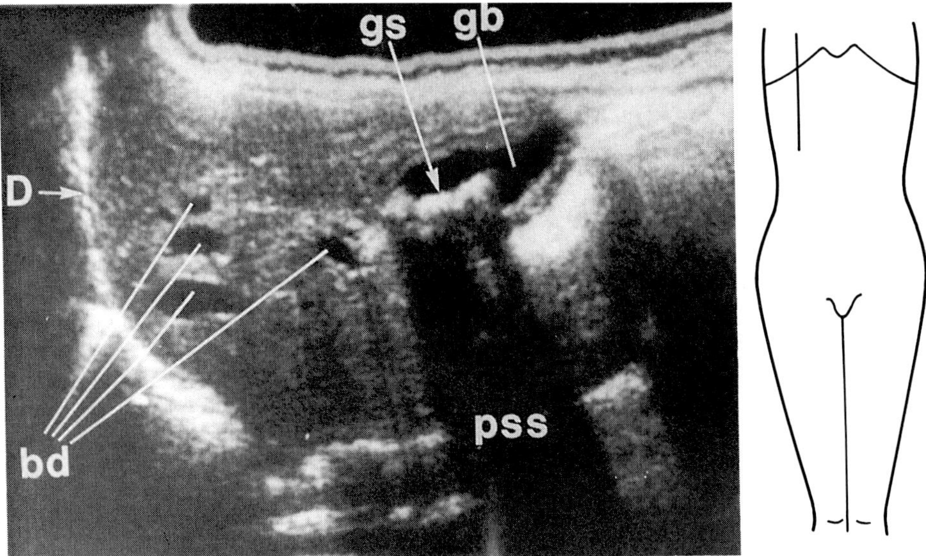

Fig. 6.9 *Ultrasonography of liver and gallbladder in a patient with extrahepatic bile duct obstruction due to gallstones. The site of the examination is indicated in the accompanying figure. gb = gallbladder; gs = gallstone; pss posterior sonic shadowing; bd = bile ducts (dilated); D = diaphragm*

Hepatic injury due to drugs can be classified according to the type of liver disease produced (Tables 6.10 and 6.11) and broadly as predictable or unpredictable, depending on the mechanism by which they cause liver injury.

Predictable drug-induced liver injury

The main features that distinguish predictable hepatotoxins are:

1. All individuals develop hepatic injury if a sufficient quantity of drug is given.
2. The severity of the liver injury is dose-dependent.
3. The injury is usually reproducible in laboratory animals.
4. The hepatic lesion that results is usually distinctive and consistent.

Some of the more common types of predictable liver injury and their causative agents are listed in Table 6.10.

Table 6.10 *Some types of predictable liver injuries and their causative agents*

Reaction	*Cause*
Fatty change	Tetracycline, corticosteroids
Centrizonal necrosis	Carbon tetrachloride, paracetamol (acetaminophen)
Hepatitis	Acetaminophen, salicylates
Cholestasis	Anabolic steroids
Fibrosis (±cirrhosis)	Methotrexate, vitamin A
Hepatic angiosarcoma	Polyvinylchloride

Many of the toxic drug reactions occur because of the hepatic conversion of drugs to chemically reactive (electrophilic) metabolites which covalently bind macromolecules in the hepatocyte, causing hepatic necrosis. This occurs, for example, with paracetamol (acetaminophen). The toxicity of this agent is augmented by phenobarbitone, which enhances its cytochrome oxidation and conversion to reactive and toxic metabolites.

Unpredictable drug-induced liver injury

Many drug-induced hepatic lesions are rare and idiosyncratic. Sometimes these appear to be due to hypersensitivity reactions and are accompanied by fever, skin rash and eosinophilia. Examples of drugs causing this type of reaction are phenytoin, sulphonamides and penicillin.

Other drugs produce liver disease only in subjects with genetically determined abnormalities of hepatic drug metabolism. An example of such a mechanism is isoniazid, which produces liver damage principally in subjects who are 'fast acetylators' and metabolise isoniazid rapidly to its toxic metabolite, acetylhydrazine.

Other examples of inherent predisposition to drug-induced liver disease are the cholestasis produced by oestrogens (also seen in pregnancy) and halothane hepatitis which occurs in approximately one in 10 000. In such subjects an alternative (reductive) pathway of drug biotransformation occurs with the formation of electrophilic metabolites. The reaction is much more common after multiple exposures and in obese older females. Chlorpromazine induces a cholestatic hepatitis with features of hypersensitivity in 0.5% of subjects, but it has been suggested that the liver injury is produced by a toxic effect rather than hypersensitivity. Features which suggest hypersensitivity to toxic metabolites include:

1. a very low incidence (<1%) in exposed individuals;
2. the injury is not dose-related;
3. the lesion cannot usually be reproduced in animals;
4. children are usually unaffected;
5. there are often systemic manifestations of hypersensitivity, for example, fever, rash, arthralgia, eosinophilia.

Because the lesion is not commonly reproducible in laboratory animals, the reactions are often not detected in toxicological studies and in initial clinical trials. Some of the more common types of unpredictable liver injury and the causative agents are listed in Table 6.11.

The prognosis of drug-induced liver injury is variable, although in general most lesions improve once the offending agent is removed. An important exception is the acute hepatic reaction associated with halothane and monoamine oxidase inhibitors; this carries a mortality rate of approximately 25%.

Although important, hepatic injury induced by adverse reactions to drugs is relatively uncommon. In particular, reactions to contraceptive steroids and to

Table 6.11 *Some types of unpredictable liver injuries and their causative agents*

Reaction	*Cause*
Viral hepatitis-like[(a)]	Halothane, monoamine oxidase inhibitors (e.g. iproniazid), isoniazid, methyldopa, ketoconazole
Cholestatic hepatitis[(b)]	Phenothiazines (e.g. chlorpromazine), erythromycin estolate, azathioprine, flucloxacillin
Pseudoalcoholic hepatitis[(c)]	Amiodarone, perhexilene maleate
Cholestasis	Contraceptive steroids, chlorpropamide
Chronic active hepatitis ($\pm$cirrhosis)	Methyldopa, isoniazid, nitrofurantoin
Granulomata	Sulphonamide, phenylbutazone, allpurinol, carbamazepine
Neoplasms (adenoma, malignant hepatoma)	Anabolic and contraceptive steroids
Microvesicular fat	Sodium valproate, i.v. tetracyline

[(a)] This type of reaction closely resembles acute viral hepatitis.
[(b)] This type of reaction has the clinical, biochemical and histological features of both hepatitis and cholestasis.
[(c)] This type of reaction resembles acute alcoholic hepatitis histologically.

halothane are rare in relation to the large number of persons exposed to these agents.

Benign hepatic neoplasms

Benign neoplasms include adenomas, haemoangiomas, cysts and focal nodular hyperplasia.

Hepatic adenomas

These are benign tumours consisting of plates of hepatocytes more than one cell thick with absent Kupffer cells (hence no uptake of technetium on liver scan). They are seen most often in women taking oral contraceptives or men using anabolic steroids. They present with right upper quadrant discomfort, pain or mass, or occasionally as haemoperitoneum after rupture. Although they may regress on stopping the drugs, surgery is usually required for large lesions.

Haemangiomas

Haemangiomas are the most common benign hepatic lesions, and are often discovered incidentally during ultrasound or CT examination. The nature of the lesion is resolved by organ imaging and, if necessary, by angiography. Therapy is rarely indicated.

Cysts

These may be simple or multiple, small or large. They are usually asymptomatic unless multiple and associated with renal cysts as part of the fibropolycystic disease syndrome, which includes polycystic disease, microhamartoma, congenital hepatic fibrosis, congenital intrahepatic dilatation (Caroli's disease) and choledochal cyst. Complications depend on the extent of the lesion, but include portal hypertension and cholangitis.

Focal nodular hyperplasia

This is a well circumscribed lesion which presents as a nodular mass in an otherwise normal liver. It characteristically has a stellate, central scar containing an artery from which septa radiate, simulating cirrhosis. The lesion is more common in women, and oral contraceptives cause it to enlarge and occasionally bleed. Most cases are asymptomatic and treatment is conservative.

Malignant hepatic neoplasms

Malignant tumours of the liver include mainly primary hepatocellular carcinoma and cholangiocarcinoma.

Primary hepatocellular carcinoma (malignant hepatoma)

Although this is relatively uncommon in Western countries, it is probably the most common internal malignancy on a world-wide basis. In Africa and Asia it accounts for up to 30% of all malignancies. The major aetiological factors are viral hepatitis B and C.

In Western countries liver cancer is seen more often as a complication of cirrhosis due to hepatitis B infection, haemochromatosis, alcohol or alpha$_1$-antitrypsin deficiency. Symptoms and signs include vague gastrointestinal complaints, weakness, lassitude, right upper quadrant pain, ascites and loss of weight. Hepatomegaly is common, and there is often a friction rub or bruit over the liver. Diagnosis has been considerably aided by the use of ultrasonography, hepatic scintiscanning, selective coeliac angiography and by the demonstration of a foetal protein, alpha-foetoprotein, in the plasma of a high proportion of patients with primary liver cancer. Levels over 500 ng/mL occur in over 75% of patients in Africa and Asia. In Western countries the figure is around 45%. This probably reflects the degree of anaplasia of the tumour.

Cholangiocarcinoma

Cholangiocarcinoma or primary bile duct cancer is less common and more benign and insidious in onset (usually with cholestatic jaundice). It is a recognised association with ulcerative colitis, sclerosing cholangitis and some forms of fibropolycystic disease. Treatment is largely palliative via insertion of drainage tubes or surgical decompression.

Congenital hyperbilirubinaemia

Idiopathic unconjugated hyperbilirubinaemia (Gilbert's syndrome)

This relatively common syndrome is characterised by chronic mild unconjugated hyperbilirubinaemia without evidence of overt haemolysis. Some patients have a deficiency of the microsomal enzyme bilirubin uridine diphosphoglucuronyl transferase, while in others the uptake and transport of unconjugated bilirubin by the liver cell may be at fault. In addition, many patients have a slightly reduced red cell survival. The syndrome is inherited as an autosomal dominant trait; males are more frequently affected. It has been suggested that the condition represents, simply, the upper end of the normal range of serum bilirubin concentration, particularly in subjects whose conjugating enzymes and red cell survival are at the lower end of the normal range. The condition is compatible with normal life expectancy. Its importance lies in accurate diagnosis and distinction from more serious causes of jaundice.

Clinical features

This disorder is usually detected incidentally. Vague symptoms such as abdominal pain and discomfort, nausea and malaise are frequent. Physical examination reveals a healthy person who may be slightly jaundiced.

Investigations

The serum bilirubin is elevated, usually between 25 and 40 μmol/L and it is mostly unconjugated. The levels fluctuate and at times fall within the normal range. Bilirubin levels increase when the patient fasts and this relationship between serum bilirubin values and caloric intake may explain some of the fluctuations in bilirubin levels. Hepatic histology is normal.

Gilbert's syndrome must be distinguished from other causes of unconjugated hyperbilirubinaemia. Tests to exclude haemolysis and liver biopsy are normal.

Management

There is no specific therapy. The patient should be reassured firmly.

A rare, more severe form of unconjugated nonhaemolytic hyperbilirubinaemia is the Crigler-Najjar syndrome. This usually develops shortly after birth when the infant becomes deeply jaundiced, the serum bilirubin concentrations varying between 250 and 400 μmol/L. Kernicterus occurs in 85% of the affected infants.

Conjugated hyperbilirubinaemia

There are two main types of congenital hyperbilirubinaemia with predominantly conjugated bilirubin in plasma. The prognosis of both conditions is good and their importance lies in accurate diagnosis.

Dubin-Johnson syndrome

In this syndrome there is dark pigment in the liver cells. The patients often complain of right upper quadrant pain and discomfort, and are mildly jaundiced. There is an excretory defect of the liver cells and serum bilirubin levels rise to 30 to 100 μmol/L because of failure to excrete conjugated bilirubin. Bile salt transport is normal, as are the results of conventional tests of liver function. The syndrome is familial and the mode of inheritance is autosomal recessive. Some patients also demonstrate abnormal excretion of the isomers of urinary coproporphyrin and a deficiency of factor VII. Liver biopsy appearances are characteristic and show normal cells containing dark melanin-like pigment.

Rotor syndrome

In this syndrome the excretory defect is present but the liver cells do not contain any abnormal pigment and the oral cholecystogram appears normal.

Diseases of the gallbladder and bile ducts

Gallstones (cholelithiasis)

Gallstones in the gallbladder are found in more than 25% of autopsies done in the Western world on people over the age of sixty years. They are formed by precipitation of biliary constituents. The major component is cholesterol, with calcium salts of bilirubin and small amounts of calcium carbonate, phosphate and palmitate. Pigment stones in the gallbladder occur in states of chronic haemolysis and consist mainly of calcium bilirubinate. Primary bile duct stones may also occur with chronic partial biliary obstruction and infection.

Aetiology

Supersaturation of gallbladder bile with cholesterol results in its precipitation and the production of gallstones. The cholesterol to bile salt ratio is an important factor. 'Lithogenic bile' occurs when the biliary secretion of cholesterol is increased or the bile salt component is low, either as a result of a reduced bile salt pool or from reduced synthesis in the liver.

Recognised risk factors include age, female sex, pregnancy, obesity (all associated with increased biliary cholesterol) and ileal disease or resection (associated with decreased bile salt pool).

Once the conditions for gallstone formation are in place, the concentration of the bile and infection in the gallbladder are important factors in inducing the precipitation of cholesterol from solution and allowing the growth of stones.

There may be one large stone or a number of small ones. Most have a nucleus of cholesterol or bile pigment, and further layers of these substances, together with bile salts and calcium salts, are deposited on this nucleus, often in concentric layers. Once gallstones have formed, further stone formation is very common. This has proved to be a significant limiting factor for methods of treatment not involving cholecystectomy.

Symptoms

Gallstones may exist in the gallbladder for many years without producing symptoms. Prospective studies have shown that, over the first five years after diagnosis, about 2% per year of previously asymptomatic patients develop symptoms. Migration of a gallstone to the neck of the gallbladder or the bile duct will produce biliary pain, which is usually felt in the epigastrium and may be referred to the inferior angle of the scapula. Although it is often referred to as 'colic', it is an intense, constant pain which may last for many hours. Inflammation of the gallbladder as a result of obstruction of the cystic duct and secondary bacterial infection will involve the somatic nerves of the parietal peritoneum, and cause pain and tenderness under the right costal margin. The most common organisms in gallbladder bile are of enteric origin—coliforms, streptococci and anaerobes and, occasionally, staphylococci and salmonella. The antibiotic treatment indicated is therefore a combination of gentamycin and amoxycillin, or a later-generation cephalosporin. Occasionally, stones may pass down the cystic duct to the bile duct without causing pain, but they usually result in partial obstruction of the common bile duct with intermittent jaundice with or without cholangitis. 'Painless jaundice' is much more frequently caused by malignancy than by gallstones.

Complications

Acute cholecystitis

The gallbladder is distended and the mucosal lining acutely inflamed, usually following an attack of acute, biliary pain. There is tenderness under the right costal margin, especially on deep inspiration (Murphy's sign). There may also be fever and a palpable mass made up by the distended, inflamed gallbladder and surrounding adherent bowel and omentum.

Most attacks of acute cholecystitis will subside without operation on conservative treatment. Further attacks, however, are almost the rule, and the gallbladder wall becomes thickened and adherent to surrounding viscera (chronic cholecystitis).

Chronic cholecystitis

There is usually a history of recurrent attacks of biliary pain, perhaps associated with tenderness and fever. These may be due to acute exacerbations of cholecystitis or to cystic duct obstruction.

Jaundice

This usually means that a gallstone has passed down the cystic duct and lodged in the bile duct, obstructing flow to the duodenum. Jaundice from stones in the bile duct is a dangerous complication because it is commonly associated with bile duct infection (cholangitis), which implies infection within the intrahepatic biliary radicles from which the bacteria enter the sinusoids, and this may result in septicaemia.

Empyema of the gallbladder

If the obstruction of the cystic duct and the acute inflammatory process in the gallbladder does not resolve with antibiotic therapy, the organ may fill with pus. Perforation of the gallbladder is rare, but may cause a localised or generalised biliary peritonitis. Sometimes, partial resolution of the process may result in a distended, thick-walled, gallbladder full of mucus (mucocele of the gallbladder).

Pancreatitis

Passage of gallstones down the bile duct to the duodenum may result in acute pancreatitis. Gallstone pancreatitis is probably caused by obstruction (usually transient) of the pancreatic duct at the hepato-pancreatic ampulla.

Biliary enteric fistula

Rarely, a fistula may form between the chronically infected gallbladder and surrounding viscera, allowing passage of stones into the bowel, where they may impact and cause obstruction (gallstone 'ileus').

Carcinoma of the gallbladder

Although gallstones coexist in about 75% of cases, there is no definite evidence of a cancer relationship.

Diagnosis

This is suspected from an analysis of the symptoms and signs. Proof of the presence of gallstones may be obtained by:

1. *Plain x-ray of the abdomen*: this may show radio-opaque gallstones; however, only 10% of gallstones are radio-opaque.
2. *Abdominal ultrasound*: the investigation of choice. It has the advantage that it can be performed in pregnancy and in the presence of jaundice, and also images the gallbladder wall and the surrounding viscera. Gallstones, on ultrasound, show up as sonolucent structures in the gallbladder with a very characteristic postsonic shadowing (see Fig. 6.9). Ultrasound also will show the calibre of the bile ducts, providing vital information for diagnosis and management in the jaundiced patient.
3. *Endoscopic retrograde cholangiopancreatography (ERCP)*: this method, together with percutaneous transhepatic cholangiography (PTHC), provides accurate imaging of the bile duct. It is especially useful if a stone in the common bile duct is suspected.
4. *HIDA scan*: the gallbladder can be visualised by the use of a radioisotope excreted in the bile and concentrated in the gallbladder. This is of most use in diagnosing cystic duct obstruction; however, in most instances, clinical appraisal supplemented by ultrasound examination is sufficient for diagnosis.
5. *Oral cholecystography*: tablets of a radio-opaque contrast medium are ingested the night before the examination, are absorbed from the gut and

concentrated in the liver and gallbladder, thus outlining that organ to x-rays. This method of imaging, as well as the related intravenous cholangiography, has largely been supplanted by abdominal ultrasound.

6. *Computerised tomography (CT scanning)*: this may give accurate information on anatomy and incidental pathology, but is less accurate than ultrasound in the diagnosis of gallstones.

Management

Cholecystectomy

Once gallstones have become symptomatic, it is generally accepted that surgical treatment is indicated in order to forestall further symptoms or complications of gallstones. Operation is usually deferred until acute symptoms have subsided, but is occasionally necessary when acute disease does not settle with pain relief, antibiotics and intravenous fluids. Modern cholecystectomy is usually performed using laparoscopic surgery and is a safe operation, with minimal morbidity and mortality. It may be combined with operative cholangiography, where contrast agent is injected into the bile duct at operation to locate bile duct stones. The major advantage of laparoscopic surgery is that there is a reduction in post-operative pain, hospital stay and recovery time.

Endoscopic papillotomy

Endoscopic papillotomy (ES) and extraction of bile duct stones is the treatment of choice for residual or recurrent bile duct stones, particularly in the elderly or the unfit. Endoscopic papillotomy and leaving the gallbladder in situ is an option for bile duct stones in this group as well, but around 30% of such patients will require cholecystectomy for recurrent symptoms.

Gallstone dissolution

Dissolution using cheno- or ursodeoxycholic acid has been used where operation is not desired but, unfortunately, few patients are suitable for treatment (small numbers of stones in a functional gallbladder), the treatment takes several years, and the recurrence rate on stopping treatment is around 50%.

Extracorporeal biliary lithotripsy

The breaking up of gallstones with ultrasound waves is being actively investigated with some success. The same problems apply as with dissolution: only a minority of patients are suitable for treatment and the recurrence rate is high, probably because the diseased gallbladder is left in situ.

Diagnostic techniques in liver disease

Note: The tests most appropriate to a given clinical problem should be selected, their potential risks and cost considered, and the results interpreted in relation to the clinical findings.

Clinical tests

Serum bilirubin

Normal levels: total up to 17 μmol/L, conjugated up to 7 μmol/L. Separation into conjugated and unconjugated varieties is important in diagnosing congenital forms of jaundice (e.g. Gilbert's syndrome).

Urine bilirubin and urobilinogen

These are of limited value diagnostically; however, bilirubinuria is often present before clinical jaundice and the test is therefore useful as a screening procedure. Persistent absence of urobilinogen from the urine in a jaundiced patient is indicative of complete biliary obstruction or an unconjugated hyperbilirubinaemia.

Serum transaminases (aspartate aminotransferase or AST; and alanine aminotransferase or ALT)

Normal: up to 40 IU/L. Very high serum levels of these enzymes occur in acute diffuse hepatocellular disease; lesser degrees of elevation (up to 300 IU/L) may occur in extrahepatic or intrahepatic cholestasis or in chronic hepatocellular disease.

Serum alkaline phosphatase (SAP)

Normal: up to 80 IU/L in adults, higher in children, adolescents and in pregnancy. This liver isoenzyme is found in the biliary canalicular epithelial cells and excreted in bile. Marked elevations occur in extrahepatic and intrahepatic cholestasis and in infiltrative disease, for example, malignancy. Concomitant elevation in levels of 5-nucleotidase (derived from liver) is useful in distinguishing elevated hepatic from other isoenzymes, for example, bone. Milder elevations in SAP levels may coexist with high AST levels in hepatitis.

Gamma glutamyl transpeptidase (GGT)

Normal: up to 65 IU/L. This is a microsomal enzyme probably involved in protein synthesis. The serum level is elevated in most forms of hepatocellular and cholestatic liver disease and is a highly sensitive, but therefore nonspecific, test for the presence of liver disease. Thus, levels tend to rise earlier and be higher than those of AST, SAP and 5-nucleotidase. This sensitivity makes the serum GGT level a commonly used screening test for liver disease, (e.g. alcoholism, malignancy, etc.); however, false-positive results are common as the serum level may be elevated merely by enzyme induction (e.g. by phenytoin, alcohol).

Serum proteins

Serum albumin

Normal: >35 g/L. This protein is synthesised by the liver and has a half-life of about twenty days: thus the serum concentration is a valuable prognostic index in chronic hepatocellular disease, especially cirrhosis. With ascites, albumin may be secreted directly into the ascitic compartment and low serum albumin levels may be present in the face of increased albumin synthesis.

Serum globulin

Normal: 15 to 30 g/L. The α_1-globulins (glycoproteins and hormone-binding globulins) tend to be low in hepatocellular disease. The α_2 and β-globulins include lipoproteins and high levels may be found with biliary disease. The α-globulins rise in cirrhosis due to increased production by plasma cells in the bone marrow and liver. Serum IgG is increased in chronic active hepatitis and cryptogenic cirrhosis; IgM is increased in PBC; IgA is increased in alcoholic cirrhosis. These patterns are only suggestive and not diagnostic.

Prothrombin time (PT)

Normal: 12 to 13 s. This provides an index of the liver's ability to synthesise and release clotting factors (II, VII and X). An abnormal value may also be encountered in cholestatic jaundice due to bile salt insufficiency in the gut and malabsorption of vitamin K. In this instance the prolonged PT is correctable with parenteral vitamin K.

Lipoproteins

Cholestasis is associated with an increase in total serum cholesterol. The mechanism is uncertain but may be due to regurgitation of biliary cholesterol and lecithin into the circulation, increased hepatic synthesis of cholesterol and reduced plasma LCAT (lecithin cholesterol acyl transferase) activity. In hepatocellular disease and in cholestatic jaundice, the plasma triglycerides are often increased. The percentage of cholesterol esters is reduced due to LCAT deficiency caused by impaired formation.

Serum iron and ferritin

Normal values: iron 10 to 30 μmol/L for women, 15 to 31 μmol/L for men; ferritin 20 to 350 μg/L for men, 10 to 150 μg/L for women. Elevation of serum iron levels associated with increased percentage saturation of the serum transferrin (>55%) may reflect an increase in iron stores, for example, as seen in haemochromatosis. On the other hand raised levels are also seen in acute hepatitis, haemolysis and ineffective erythropoiesis from vitamin B12 or folic acid deficiency. Serum ferritin levels more closely reflect body iron stores, although levels also increase with inflammation and cell injury. Liver iron concentration is a more accurate indicator.

Serum copper and caeruloplasmin

Normal: 11 to 24 μmol/L and 250 to 500 mL/L, respectively. Classically, both are low in Wilson's disease. Liver copper concentrations (normal less than 25 mg/100 g dry weight) are elevated to very high levels in Wilson's disease and to a lesser extent in chronic cholestasis (e.g. primary biliary cirrhosis).

Immunologic tests

Antinuclear antibody

Antinuclear factor (sometimes associated with circulating LE cells) and smooth muscle antibody are commonly present in patients with chronic active hepatitis.

Mitochondrial antibody

These are also non-specific tissue antibodies and are present in serum in up to 90% or more of patients with primary biliary cirrhosis. The M2 antigen is more specific (see p. 163).

Hepatitis B surface antigen (HBsAg) and related antigens

See page 133 and following pages for details.

Alpha-foetoprotein

This is normally present in large amounts in foetal but not in normal adult serum. Levels greater than 500 ng/mL are highly suggestive of primary hepatocellular cancer.

Radiological studies and organ imaging

Barium swallow and meal

These may reveal evidence of oesophageal varices (confirming portal hypertension), gastric pathology or pancreatic carcinoma; however, with upper gastrointestinal endoscopy these are used less.

Oral or intravenous cholangiography

These procedures are used infrequently now, but are sometimes of value in delineating bile ducts and the presence of cholelithiasis. Concentration of the dye is poor if the serum bilirubin level exceeds 34 μmol/L.

Ultrasonography

This is a non-invasive procedure which is very useful for detecting dilated bile ducts, gallstones and focal disorders (see Fig. 6.9).

Hepatic scintiscanning

Radionuclides, which are taken up by the hepatic parenchymal or reticuloendothelial cells, are injected intravenously. The image of the liver and spleen may reveal filling defects due to tumours or cysts. Patchy uptake is seen in patients with cirrhosis and other diffuse parenchymal disease. Similarly, radionuclides that are excreted in the bile are used to outline the biliary tract (see p. 176).

Computed tomography

Although expensive, this procedure is very useful for the diagnosis of focal diseases, for example, hydatid cysts and tumours (see Fig. 6.10).

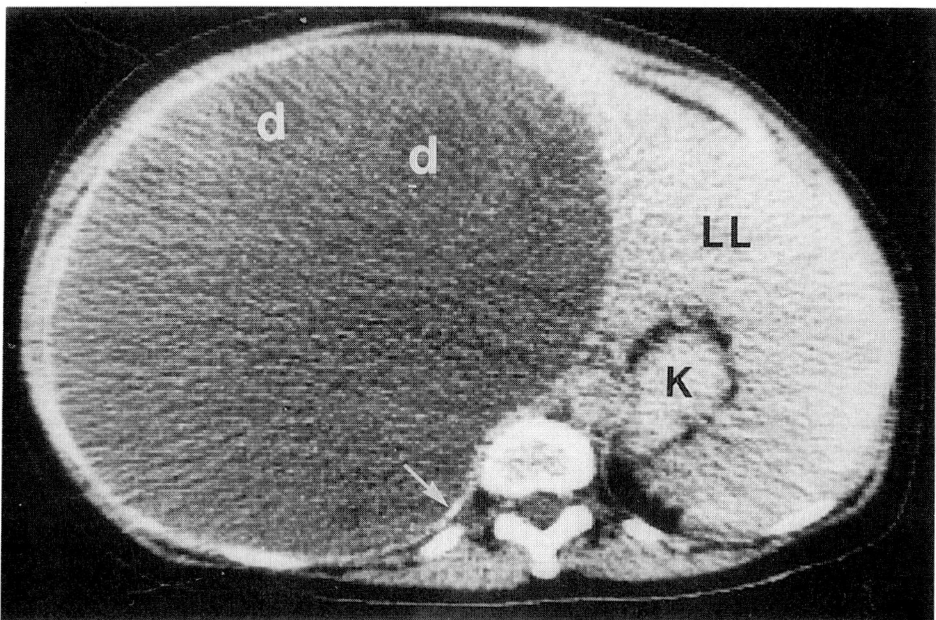

Fig. 6.10 *Computed tomography of the abdomen in a patient with a large hydatid cyst of the liver. LL = left lobe of liver; K = kidney; d = daughter cysts. The arrow points to calcification in the wall of the cyst*

Endoscopic retrograde cholangio-pancreatography (ERCP)
This procedure requires considerable expertise to perform, but it can confirm or exclude extrahepatic bile duct obstruction.

Percutaneous transhepatic cholangiography
This is particularly useful for diagnosing high bile duct obstruction.

Angiography
This includes selective coeliac, gastric or splenoportography, including measurement of portal venous pressure. In selected patients these procedures are helpful in outlining the state of the portal circulation before surgery for portal hypertension, and for demonstrating the vascular supply of hepatic tumours and cysts.

Ascitic fluid examination

This should be performed in all patients with ascites. Possible abnormalities include evidence of infection, tumour, exudate or haemorrhage. Microscopy, culture, estimation of protein content and amylase and lipase concentrations are performed.

Quantitative tests of liver function

These are more accurate in assessing the functional liver cell mass but are still cumbersome. The ones that are currently under investigation include the 14C-aminopyrine breath test, caffeine and antipyrine clearance and lignocaine metabolism. Simplified tests are awaited, especially for serial measurements of functional liver cell mass.

Percutaneous liver biopsy

This provides only a small sample of liver; it is thus of more diagnostic value in diffuse than in patchy disease. The clinical indications are:

1. to diagnose the severity and chronicity of hepatitis (especially to confirm chronic hepatitis);
2. to confirm the presence and aetiology of chronic liver disease where doubt exists (may provide specific diagnosis, e.g. alcoholic liver disease, haemochromatosis);
3. to diagnose pyrexia of uncertain origin (PUO), especially with raised SAP levels suggesting infiltrative disorders of the liver (e.g. Hodgkin's disease, sarcoidosis);
4. to diagnose systemic disorders associated with hepatomegaly;
5. to confirm suspected intrahepatic cholestasis;
6. for suspected primary or secondary malignant disease of the liver.

Clinical value

- Confirmation of clinical diagnosis: 60%
- Alter diagnosis: 20%
- Non-contributory (including inadequate specimen): 15%
- Erroneous diagnosis: 5%

Contraindications

These are bleeding disorder, unavailability of blood replacement, unco-operative patient, local sepsis, complete extrahepatic obstruction.

SUGGESTED FURTHER READING

McIntyre, N., Benhamou, J-P., Bircher, J., Rizetto, M. and Rodes, J. (eds), *Oxford Textbook of Clinical Hepatology*, Oxford University Press, Oxford, 1991.

Millward-Sadler, G. H., Wright, R. and Arthur, M. J. P. (eds), *Wright's Liver and Biliary Disease*, 3rd edn, W. B. Saunders & Co., London, 1991.

Sherlock, S. and Dooley, J., *Diseases of the Liver and Biliary System*, 9th edn, Blackwell Scientific Publications, Oxford, 1993.

Zakim, D. and Boyer, T. D., *Hepatology*, 2nd edn, W. B. Saunders & Co., Philadelphia, 1990.

CHAPTER 7

Infectious diseases of the gastrointestinal tract

T. C. Sorrell

Acute enteritis and enterocolitis

Diseases causing diarrhoea are the most common cause of morbidity and mortality, world-wide. Eighty per cent of fatal cases of infectious diarrhoea occur in infants less than one year of age, in whom the predominant pathogens are rotavirus and enteropathogenic *Escherichia coli* (EPEC). After weaning, diarrhoea may be caused by a wide range of micro-organisms, depending on environmental and host factors. The extent of morbidity is influenced by the pathogen, the age, nutritional state and enteric defences of the host, and the rapidity with which appropriate management is instituted.

Pathophysiology and clinical features

Infection is usually acquired by the oral route. Host defences in the gastrointestinal tract include gastric pH (see Chapter 2, p. 17), intestinal motility, humoral and cellular immunity, and enteric microflora. Abnormalities in any of these put the host at increased risk of symptomatic or severe disease. It has been recognised in animal models that the presence of specific receptors on mucosal cells or in intestinal mucus is necessary for pathogenicity of enterotoxigenic *Escherichia coli* (ETEC). Breast milk contains protective factors such as antibodies, lactoferrin, lysozyme, phagocytes, high lactose, low protein, low phosphate and low pH, all of which, in association with the reduced exposure to contaminated foodstuffs afforded by breast-feeding, are protective against infection.

Enteric pathogens cause symptoms via elaboration of toxins and/or through mucosal invasion. Enterotoxins elicit the production of high volume, watery diarrhoea which contains no inflammatory cells, through stimulation of adenylate cyclase (causing increased levels of cAMP) or guanylate cyclase (causing increased levels of cGMP) in small intestinal enterocytes. Elevation of cAMP in mucosal crypt cells results in secretion of chloride and bicarbonate, with associated paracellular efflux of sodium ions. Water enters the bowel lumen in response to osmotic forces generated by these ionic movements. In contrast to the secretory crypt cells, villous tip cells are the primary site of electrolyte, water and nutrient absorption. In the absence of lumenal nutrients, active reabsorption of sodium ions coupled to hydrogen ion extrusion is the principle mechanism of sodium and water absorption. This mechanism is inhibited by increases in cAMP. Enterotoxins such as *Cholera* toxin, *Clostridium perfringens* toxin and the heat-labile enterotoxin in *E. coli,* which act by stimulation of adenylate cyclase and hence cAMP, increase secretion and inhibit absorption of water and electrolytes. The net effect is the accumulation of many litres of fluid in the small intestinal lumen. Diarrhoea results because the large volumes of fluid and electrolytes, which are then presented to the colon, exceed its 2–3 L absorptive capacity. Two cAMP-independent mechanisms of sodium absorption remain intact under these circumstances—the inwardly directed hydrogen-oligopeptide cotransport system, which can stimulate sodium-hydrogen exchange and the nutrient (glucose, galactose, aminoacid)-sodium cotransport mechanism. Use is made of these in the treatment of diarrhoea with oral rehydration solutions (see below). Certain enterotoxins—such as the heat-stable enterotoxin of *Escherichia coli*—stimulate guanylate cyclase, which in the small intestine is concentrated in the villous tip cells. As a result, absorption of salt and water is inhibited, but secretion is not stimulated.

Bacterial cytotoxins, such as those produced by *Clostridium difficile,* cause direct mucosal cell damage and an inflammatory response similar to that elicited by enteroinvasive bacteria such as *Salmonella typhimurium* and *Shigella sonnei.* Mucosal secretion and absorption of fluid and electrolytes are both affected, especially absorption. Certain pathogens, such as *Shigella dysenteriae* Type I, are both toxigenic and enteroinvasive; others are enteroadherent (e.g. enteroadherent *E. coli, Cryptosporidium parvum*) or penetrate through the epithelium to elicit an inflammatory response in the lamina propria (e.g. *Salmonella typhi*). The mechanism by which enteroadherent bacteria cause diarrhoea is unknown.

Neurotoxins elaborated by bacteria cause clinical manifestations other than diarrhoea, for example, botulinum toxin (p. 189), emetic toxins of *Staphylococcus aureus* (p. 189) and *Bacillus cereus* (p. 189).

In contrast to enteroinvasive bacteria, viruses such as rotavirus and Norwalk-like agents infect and destroy mature enterocytes selectively, resulting in destruction of absorptive villous tip cells. In addition, brush border enzymes are reduced during active infection, leading to the clinical syndrome of lactose intolerance. As the inflammatory response is patchy, fever is mild and faecal leukocytes scanty. Disruption of the absorptive surface may also be involved in small intestinal infections or infestations associated with villus tip flattening or microvillus destruction (e.g. bacterial overgrowth syndromes, giardiasis, cryptosporidiosis, strongyloidiasis).

It follows from the above discussion, that the clinical concomitants of non-inflammatory diarrhoea and inflammatory syndromes can be related to the predominant site of bowel involvement and the mechanism of tissue dysfunction. Large-volume watery diarrhoea and steatorrhoea are characteristic of small intestinal involvement. Fever and faecal leukocytes are associated with mucosal inflammation and their absence, with enterotoxin-mediated viral or protozoal diarrhoea. The passage of frequent, small stools containing bright blood and/or mucus are features of colonic inflammation. Rectal involvement is manifest by faecal urgency and tenesmus. The clinical features of colonic and rectal inflammation characterise the syndrome known as dysentery.

Outbreaks or clusters of gastrointestinal illness are a feature of food-borne infection. The incubation period of the disease is shortest when caused by ingestion of preformed toxin (one to six hours) and longest in enteroinvasive disease (at least sixteen hours). In the former, nausea and vomiting often occur more frequently than diarrhoea.

Approach to the diagnosis of gastrointestinal infection

As most cases of infectious diarrhoea are mild and self-limited, identification of the pathogen is frequently not warranted. Even after full laboratory work-up, the diagnosis is made in less than 50% of patients with epidemiological features of infectious diarrhoea. A history of travel, consumption of suspect foods, presence of an epidemic or household outbreak and acuteness of onset suggest an infectious aetiology, but it should be remembered that the differential diagnosis of non-inflammatory and inflammatory diarrhoea is extensive, ranging from drug-induced causes (including laxative abuse) to ulcerative colitis, Crohn's disease and ischaemic colitis.

Laboratory investigation

Stools should be examined macroscopically for volume, consistency, blood, mucus, steatorrhoea, undigested food and helminths. Microscopic examination of fresh stool samples may reveal the presence of leukocytes. Such samples should be submitted for bacterial culture and microscopic examination for *Entamoeba histolytica*. In the absence of faecal leukocytes or blood, patients with significant dehydration or prolonged diarrhoea should have three fresh stool specimens examined for *Giardia lamblia (Giardia intestinalis)*. Bacterial cultures should also be requested, as not all enteroinvasive diarrhoeas are associated with faecal leukocytes. In diarrhoeal stools from infants, rotavirus and enteric adenovirus may be identified by rapid techniques such as latex agglutination. Depending on the clinical setting, parasites such as *Entamoeba histolytica, Cryptosporidium parvum*, microsporidia and *Strongyloides stercoralis* should be sought by microscopy of appropriately prepared and stained stool samples.

Sigmoidoscopy is essential in all cases of diarrhoea lasting more than one week, when the diarrhoeal stools contain blood or if significant diarrhoea develops while the patient is receiving antimicrobial therapy. The presence of a pseudo-membrane or discrete (e.g. amoebic) ulcers may be diagnostic. A rectal biopsy should be obtained at the time of sigmoidoscopy for histological evaluation and culture, to differentiate infection from inflammatory bowel disease. *Duodenoscopy* and small bowel biopsy may be required to diagnose some cases of giardiasis, cryptosporidiosis and microsporidiosis.

Three blood cultures should be obtained in any patient with high fever, systemic toxicity or profuse faecal leukocytes. *Serological tests* are not indicated in individual cases, except in the diagnosis of invasive amoebiasis.

Principles of management of infectious diarrhoea

Infantile gastroenteritis must be treated promptly, with particular attention to fluid and electrolyte balance. Where possible, breastfeeding should be continued, since even in the face of lactose intolerance, breast milk is better tolerated than proprietary formulae with lower lactose levels. Reintroduction of frequent, small feeds consisting of dilute formula and/or bland, low-lactose solids (e.g. cereal, potato, rice) should begin within twenty-four hours to prevent malnutrition or worsening malnutrition, which has a significant influence on morbidity and mortality. Lactose-containing feeds need be reduced again only if there is clinical evidence of lactose intolerance (marked increase in stool volume due to osmotic diarrhoea, abdominal distension, frothy stools, flatulence, acid pH, positive Clinitest for glucose). *Intravenous* fluid and electrolyte replacement is necessary in severely dehydrated or shocked infants and in the presence of continued vomiting or abdominal distension. *Oral rehydration solutions* (ORS) based on the World Health Organisation formula (Na^+, 90 mmol/L; K^+, 20 mmol/L; Cl^-, 80 mmol/L; HCO_3^-, 30 mmol/L; glucose, 110 mmol/L) are suitable for moderately dehydrated infants.

It should be noted that the use of glucose-supplemented ORS does not reduce the volume of diarrhoea. In contrast, solutions containing polysaccharides or polypeptides (e.g. mashed potato or rice, wheat, sorghum, maize or millet flour), lessen diarrhoeal loss and may be nutritive, in addition to providing rehydration fluid. In these solutions the glucose in standard ORS is replaced by 50–60 g of cereal flour or 200 g of mashed, boiled potato per litre of water. Antidiarrhoeal agents and antiemetics are to be avoided in infantile gastroenteritis. Antimicrobial agents are indicated for specific pathogens, depending on the severity of illness and/or the need to reduce the period of excretion as a public health measure (see below).

Older children and adults with gastroenteritis should be treated according to the severity of the illness. Mild cases usually respond to rest and oral fluids containing glucose and electrolytes. The use of kaolin-pectin or other adsorbents results in stool of increased form, although efficacy in reducing fluid and electrolyte loss has not been demonstrated. Antimotility drugs such as diphenoxylate, loperamide or codeine phosphate provide symptomatic relief; however, diphenoxylate and loperamide are potentially hazardous in children because of neurological toxicity, including respiratory depression.

Antimotility drugs are contraindicated in severe diarrhoea as they cause excessive fluid trapping in the bowel, and in patients with high fever, toxicity and/or dysenteric symptoms, because of the risk of precipitating toxic megacolon (see Chapter 4, p. 74). These drugs should also be avoided in infections caused by enteroinvasive bacteria, when they may result in prolongation of illness and delayed clearance of the pathogen. Mild to moderate dehydration can be corrected with ORS. In patients with severe diarrhoea, or dehydration associated with weight loss of more than 10% in twenty-four hours, initial intravenous replacement of fluid and electrolytes is indicated. Specific antimicrobial therapy is not required, except as discussed below under individual pathogens.

Causative agents of non-inflammatory infectious diarrhoea

These include viruses, protozoa and bacterial enterotoxins.

Viral diarrhoea

Rotavirus

Rotavirus is the most common cause of infantile gastroenteritis, being especially common at the time of weaning. Multiple attacks of diarrhoeal illness are possible because of the existence of at least four antigenically distinct serotypes of human rotavirus. Infection is often mild or asymptomatic, particularly in neonates, older children and adult contacts of infant cases. Symptomatic infection presents with vomiting and diarrhoea of sudden onset. Upper respiratory tract involvement, especially pharyngitis, may also be noted. Mild fever is usual and dehydration is common. Lactose intolerance is evident during the acute infection. Recovery occurs within one to two days. Morbidity and mortality are increased significantly in malnourished infants. A specific diagnosis is not usually sought because of the cost and the self-limited nature of the illness. In severe cases or in nosocomial outbreaks, rotaviruses should be looked for directly in stool by rapid techniques such as latex agglutination or ELISA. Other methods include electron microscopy and tissue culture. Serodiagnosis is reserved for epidemiological studies. Treatment is supportive.

Norwalk and related agents

These viruses typically cause winter outbreaks of nausea and vomiting in older children and adults. Abdominal pain, cramps and diarrhoea are usually mild. Outbreaks have been traced to contaminated oysters and salads, presumably via faecal contamination of the water supply, with an incubation period of twenty-four to forty-eight hours. Where required, diagnosis can be made by detection of viral particles in stool using immune electronmicroscopy, or by serology. Treatment is supportive.

Other viruses

Adenoviruses (especially the enteric, non-cultivable serotypes 40 and 41) caliciviruses, astroviruses and coronaviruses have also been implicated in diarrhoeal illness of infants and young children. Illness resembles that caused by rotavirus, except that associated upper respiratory symptoms are characteristic of certain cultivable serotypes of adenovirus. Diagnosis usually requires direct detection of viral particles in stool, as most of these agents are not cultivable. Treatment is supportive.

Common protozoal infestations

Giardiasis

Giardia lamblia (G. intestinalis) is a ubiquitous protozoan parasite, which infests the proximal small intestine. It is usually acquired by drinking water contaminated with human faeces. It has been implicated in traveller's diarrhoea. Other risk groups include children in daycare centres and patients with common variable immunodeficiency, X-linked agammaglobulinaemia and possibly, selective IgA deficiency. Asymptomatic cyst passage is reportedly frequent in homosexual men. An incubation period of seven to fourteen days is followed by the onset of watery diarrhoea and one or more of the signs of nausea, abdominal cramps, bloating, flatulence and weight loss. Lactose intolerance is usually present and may persist for several weeks. Most cases are self-limited; however, steatorrhoea may supervene and progress to a syndrome of chronic, intermittent diarrhoea interspersed with constipation and a normal bowel habit.

At least three stool samples should be examined for the presence of cysts. Trophozoites may be seen early in the illness. Without concentration techniques, the sensitivity of this method of diagnosis is only 50%. In the appropriate clinical setting, the diagnosis may be inferred by response to a therapeutic trial of tinidazole (2 g for adults; 50 mg/kg for children). If symptoms recur despite therapy and clinical suspicion is high, examination of a duodenal aspirate (using the string 'Enterotest') with or without jejunal biopsy should be considered. Specific therapy with a single dose of tinidazole is effective in 90% of cases. A second dose after seven days will improve the response rate in patients with continuing diarrhoea. Useful alternative drugs include furazolidone and quinacrine.

Cryptosporidiosis

Cryptosporidium parvum is a cosmopolitan, coccidian protozoan, which is transmitted to man by ingestion of infective oocysts of animal or human origin. Contamination of environmental waters may be responsible for outbreaks, including cases in travellers. A characteristic, severe form of disease is found in patients with AIDS.

Mature oocysts release sporozoites in the bowel lumen. These implant in epithelial lining cells and mature into trophozoites, which initiate asexual and sexual cycles of division. The asexual cycle results in the production of invasive merozoites. The sexual cycle leads to the formation of new oocysts and subsequent excretion or autoinfection. Infestation causes blunting and loss of villi with an inflammatory response in the lamina propria. The small intestine is involved most frequently, although in immunocompromised patients, cryptosporidia have been identified along the length of the gastrointestinal tract, in the gallbladder, pancreatic and bile ducts and in the lung.

In the normal host, an incubation period of two to fourteen days is followed by the explosive onset of watery diarrhoea, cramping abdominal pain, anorexia, flatulence, weight loss and malaise. As with giardiasis, malabsorption and steatorrhoea may occur, with resolution in ten to fourteen days. In the immunocompromised host, symptoms often arise insidiously, increasing in severity as immune function worsens. Symptoms are prolonged, with marked loss of fluid and electrolytes (1–25 L/d), weight loss in excess of 10% of body weight, severe abdominal pain and malabsorption. Cholecystitis and bile duct changes suggestive of sclerosing cholangitis have been reported in patients with AIDS.

The diagnosis is made readily by demonstration of oocysts in the stool using a modified acid-fast stain or fluorescent-labelled monoclonal antibodies.

There is no effective drug therapy. Symptomatic relief from antidiarrhoeal agents is variable. Careful attention to handwashing is necessary to prevent person to person spread of infection.

Enterotoxin-mediated diarrhoea

Short-incubation illness (1–6 h)

Ingestion of food contaminated with bacterial toxin(s) may cause outbreaks of nausea and vomiting within one to six hours of ingestion. The predominant pathogens are *Staphylococcus aureus* and *Bacillus cereus*.

S. aureus elaborates toxins responsible for vomiting (through a central mechanism) and diarrhoea (through stimulation of cyclic nucleotide production). The source of these toxins is usually contaminated dairy products, especially whipped cream. Illness is manifest by the abrupt onset of severe nausea, vomiting and abdominal cramps, usually without fever. Watery, non-inflammatory diarrhoea occurs in up to 75% of cases. Disease is self-limited, lasting twelve to twenty-four hours. The diagnosis is usually clinical, although large numbers of enterotoxin-producing *S. aureus* may be cultured from contaminated food. Treatment is supportive.

Bacillus cereus may also cause a self-limited, short incubation illness characterised by vomiting and abdominal cramps. Diarrhoea and fever are uncommon. The usual source of toxin is contaminated fried rice which has been allowed to stand at room temperature for some hours before ingestion. Diagnosis, which is usually clinical, may be confirmed by isolation of large numbers of *B. cereus* from the incriminated food. Treatment is supportive.

Medium-incubation illness (8–16 h)

Enterotoxin-mediated abdominal cramps and diarrhoea can occur within eight to sixteen hours of ingestion of food contaminated with *Clostridium perfringens* or *B. cereus*. Colonisation of the small intestine is followed by toxin production *in vivo*, hence the longer incubation period. Clostridial food poisoning usually follows ingestion of contaminated meat products in home preserves, stews or soups which have been kept at room temperature for several hours after cooking. *Bacillus cereus* has been isolated from meat and vegetable sources. Diagnosis is clinical, with confirmation by culture of the pathogen from suspect food. Treatment is supportive.

A severe, fatal form of clostridial infection, 'Pig Bel', characterised by haemorrhagic necrosis of the small bowel, shock, dehydration, bloody diarrhoea and death, has been reported in New Guinean natives consuming inadequately cooked pork.

Long-incubation illness (more than 24 h)

Enterotoxigenic *E. coli* (ETEC) is the most common cause of traveller's diarrhoea. It is also responsible for outbreaks of gastroenteritis in neonatal nurseries and for enteritis in infants. Plasmid-mediated enterotoxin production results in acute onset of malaise, anorexia and abdominal cramps, followed by watery diarrhoea, within two to four days of the ingestion of contaminated food or water. Salads and raw vegetables are particular risk foods for travellers to developing countries. Low-grade fever, nausea or vomiting occur in a minority of cases. Disease is self-limited, generally subsiding within one to five days. Diagnosis is usually clinical, as currently available methods of toxin detection are time consuming, costly or not readily available. Therapy is primarily supportive. In more severe cases, antimicrobial therapy with trimethoprim, trimethoprim-sulfamethoxazole or in adults, with a fluoro-quinolone such as norfloxacin, limits the duration of diarrhoea. Newer quinolones are not approved for use in children because they cause arthropathy when given to certain species of immature animals.

Most cases can be prevented by exercising care in the selection of food and drink (including the consumption of boiled water). Prophylaxis with doxycycline is effective but potentially toxic, due to photosensitivity reactions. Widespread use of antimicrobial therapy is also associated with the emergence of resistance.

Cholera is an acute enterotoxigenic disease due to *Vibrio cholerae* biotype 01. It is characterised by profuse watery diarrhoea and abdominal cramps. Initially there is a feeling of abdominal fullness associated with frequent passage of bulky stools. Vomiting may occur. The typical rice-water stool is opalescent, watery and flecked with mucus. Fluid and electrolyte loss result frequently in hypotension and muscular cramps. Hypoglycaemia may be severe. The infection is transmitted by ingestion of food or water contaminated with human faeces, with an incubation period of one to three days. Water is the main route of epidemic spread. Cholera is endemic in Asia, Africa, the Middle East and parts of Oceania.

Diagnosis is based on clinical features and stool culture. *Vibrios* may be visualised by dark field or phase contrast examination of a wet preparation of stool and immobilised with specific antisera. Therapy requires aggressive replacement of fluid and electrolytes. Antibiotics shorten the duration of diarrhoea and reduce fluid losses. Tetracycline is the treatment of choice, except in children and pregnant women in whom trimethoprim sulfamethoxazole and furazolidone, respectively, are preferable.

Prevention of cholera requires adequate attention to sanitation and hygiene. Use of boiled or treated water is preferable to bottled water as outbreaks of cholera have been reported following ingestion of the latter. The vaccine available currently for parenteral use contains two pathogenic serotypes (Ogawa and Inaba). It has provided protection from disease for three to six months in 60–70% of populations with high levels of natural immunity. Reduced efficacy and duration of effect are likely in non-immune persons such as travellers to developing countries. Cholera is an uncommon cause of diarrhoea in the latter group.

Enteropathogenic *E. coli* (EPEC) is associated with epidemic diarrhoea of the newborn in hospital nurseries, and with sporadic cases in infants and young children. Clinical features of listlessness, irritability and poor feeding develop over three to six days, with passage of watery green stool, abdominal distension and failure to gain weight. Fever and vomiting are infrequent; leucocytes are absent from the stool. Dehydration and shock are common in malnourished neonates. Symptoms may persist or relapse for several weeks. The pathogenic mechanism is unknown, but the EPEC serotypes exhibit a specific type of adherence to the intestinal epithelium, in the absence of mucosal inflammation or toxin production. Definitive diagnosis is based on clinical features and identification of virulence plasmids by DNA probing of *E. coli* isolated from stool. Mild cases respond to oral, non-absorbable antibiotics such as neomycin or gentamicin. Parenteral antibiotics should be selected according to antimicrobial sensitivity patterns and appropriate infection control measures should be instituted.

Causative agents of inflammatory diarrhoea

Virtually all bacteria that cause mucosal damage exhibit effects in the small and large intestine, but in the clinical expression of infection, features of one or the other site of involvement may predominate. In contrast, large bowel disease is characteristic of infestation with the protozoan, *Entamoeba histolytica.*

Salmonella species

Salmonellae are non-spore forming, Gram-negative bacilli of the family Enterobacteriaceae. On the basis of serotyping, they have been categorised as *Salmonella typhi* (the major cause of enteric fever), *Salmonella choleraesius* (which causes a bacteraemic syndrome often associated with metastatic infection) and a large group (1700 serotypes) of which the most common human pathogen is *Salmonella typhimurium* (the cause of up to 80% of cases of salmonella enterocolitis).

Salmonella enterocolitis

Enterocolitis is characterised by transient nausea, vomiting and headache followed by the sudden onset of colicky abdominal pain and watery diarrhoea, six to forty-eight hours after ingestion of contaminated food or water. Although fever and chills are common, bacteremia is noted in less than 5% of cases. Occasionally the clinical picture is that of cholera or of acute dysentery. Symptoms persist for two to five days. More severe disease occurs in young children, the elderly, and patients with a high gastric pH, malnutrition, leukaemia, lymphoma, AIDS and sickle cell anaemia.

The most common source of human infection is contaminated poultry and poultry products, especially eggs. The diagnosis is made by stool culture. Blood cultures should be performed in febrile or severely ill patients; they are more likely to be positive in the risk groups noted above than in normal patients. There is no evidence that antimicrobial therapy is efficacious in patients with uncomplicated enterocolitis; indeed faecal excretion of salmonellae may be prolonged. Specific therapy should, however, be considered in patients with significant systemic toxicity and in groups at increased risk of bacteremia. The choice of drug should be guided by antibiograms. Trimethoprim-sulfamethoxazole or a fluoroquinolone are the treatment of choice, although because of potential toxicity in children, quinolones should only be used for multiple drug-resistant salmonella infection.

Enteric (typhoid) fever

Enteric fever is most often due to the exclusively human pathogen *Salmonella typhi*, although other serotypes may cause the same syndrome. Illness is characterised by sustained fever, headache, relative bradycardia, abdominal tenderness, splenomegaly and a transient, rose-coloured, macular eruption on the trunk. Cough and watery diarrhoea may occur early in the illness. Constipation is a later feature. Intestinal haemorrhage or perforation may complicate hyperplasia of lymphoid tissue in the terminal ileum. The mortality of untreated infection is 10–20%. Transmission occurs via water or food contaminated with human excreta, particularly in areas where sanitation is poor. The disease is endemic in developing countries where it occurs predominantly in school-aged children. Common source outbreaks in developed countries occur when food is contaminated by chronic salmonella carriers. Blood cultures are generally positive in the first two weeks of illness, and urine and stool cultures, during the second and third weeks. Bone marrow (aspirate) cultures remain positive for longer. Specific antimicrobial therapy should be prescribed and continued until patients have been afebrile and improved clinically for at least seven days. Traditional therapy with chloramphenicol, ampicillin, amoxycillin or trimethoprim-sulfamethoxazole is effective in most cases. In certain areas, including the Indian subcontinent and South-East Asia, drug resistance is common and a fluoro-quinolone (such as ciprofloxacin) or third-generation cephalosporin (ceftriaxone or cefotaxime) should be preferred, pending the result of antimicrobial sensitivity testing.

Up to 3% of patients continue to excrete salmonellae for more than twelve months. As chronic carriers they are asymptomatic but pose a public health risk. Biliary tract disease is associated with an increased incidence of chronic enteric carriage; chronic urinary carriage may occur in patients with schistosomiasis of the urinary tract. Prolonged therapy with ampicillin, or amoxycillin plus probenecid or with ciprofloxacin may eliminate chronic carriage. Cholecystectomy is usually curative in patients with biliary disease in whom the enteric carrier state is unresponsive to antimicrobial agents.

Prevention of typhoid fever depends on appropriate public health measures. A parenteral (killed) vaccine and oral vaccines are now available for travellers to, and residents, especially children, in countries where typhoid fever is endemic. The degree of protection decreases as the inoculum of *S. typhi* increases; it is probably greater in those already partially immune from natural infection.

Shigella species

Bacteria of the genus *Shigella* are small, non-motile, Gram-negative bacilli of the family Enterobacteriaceae, and are divided into four groups. Groups B, C and D (*S. flexneri*, *S. boydii* and *S. sonnei*, respectively) generally cause less severe illness than group A (*S. dysenteriae*), the classical cause of bacillary dysentery. Within twenty-four to seventy-two hours of ingestion of an inoculum as small as 100—200 bacteria, patients present with an acute onset of abdominal cramps and large volume, watery diarrhoea due to multiplication of bacteria in the small intestine. High fever occurs in some patients. Invasion of the colonic mucosa is associated with a decrease in fever and a change to small volume stools of increased frequency. This is followed in 40% of cases by the appearance of blood and mucus in the stool, with or without faecal urgency and tenesmus. Diarrhoea remains profuse in dysentery caused by the Shiga bacillus (*S. dysenteriae* type I) because of the production of cholera-like enterotoxin. Transmission of infection occurs via contaminated water supplies or direct contact (often hand transmission) more often than via contaminated food. Flies may transmit infection. A history of intra-household or institutional spread of a febrile, diarrhoeal or dysenteric illness, with an interval of one to three days between cases, is suggestive of shigellosis. Young children are at particular risk, as are travellers to countries where infection is endemic. Diagnosis is confirmed by stool culture; bacteremia is rare.

Although mild infection responds to supportive measures, a five to ten day course of antimicrobial therapy will shorten the duration of both illness and excretion of the pathogen. *In vitro* susceptibilities should be performed because of increasing resistance to the previously effective agents, ampicillin and trimethoprim-sulfamethoxazole. Amoxycillin is not effective. Infections caused by multiple antibiotic resistant isolates generally respond to fluoro-quinolones or third-generation cephalosporins.

Campylobacter jejuni

Campylobacteriosis is a cosmopolitan zoonosis caused by motile, comma-shaped, Gram-negative bacilli of the genus *Campylobacter.* Most human cases of enterocolitis are caused by *Campylobacter jejuni.* The clinical features are those of an enteritis, with an acute onset of fever, headache, malaise and myalgia, followed by abdominal cramps and watery, large-volume diarrhoea. More than 80% of patients recover spontaneously within one week. Relapses may occur. Infection may also be manifest as an acute dysenteric syndrome or in adolescents and young adults, as pseudo-appendicitis (terminal ileitis and mesenteric adenitis). Reactive arthritis is a recognised complication. Symptomatic infection is most common in infants and young adults from developed countries and arises two to four days after consumption of contaminated food or water. Unpasteurised milk, undercooked meat (especially poultry) raw clams, salads and non-chlorinated surface water have been implicated in outbreaks. Oral transmission from infected household puppies, kittens or infants who are not toilet-trained, may also occur. *Campylobacter jejuni* is an important cause of traveller's diarrhoea.

The diagnosis can be confirmed by culture of stool samples on selective growth media; blood cultures are usually negative. Other species of *Campylobacter* such as *C. coli* or *C. fetus* can be cultured from the stool of patients with enterocolitis, but *C. fetus* is isolated more frequently from the blood of immunocompromised patients presenting with a chronic, relapsing syndrome associated with bacteremia. Specific antimicrobial therapy is not usually indicated, as in mild cases of *C. jejuni* enterocolitis the course of the illness is not influenced by antibiotics. Oral erythromycin is the treatment of choice in patients with severe, persistent diarrhoea or dysentery. Doxycycline, tetracyclines and the fluoroquinolones are also effective. Where intravenous therapy is required, gentamicin plus chloramphenicol are recommended.

Vibrio parahaemolyticus

This halophilic (salt-requiring) non-cholera *Vibrio* is a major cause of acute diarrhoea in Japan and is ubiquitous in coastal waters world-wide. Within twenty-four hours of ingestion of contaminated raw or undercooked seafood, cramping abdominal pain and profuse, self-limiting, watery diarrhoea develop acutely. Headache, fever or vomiting occur in a minority of cases. Cholera-like diarrhoea or dysentery occur rarely.

Diagnosis requires culture of stool samples on selective media. Treatment is supportive. Infection is prevented by adequate cooking and refrigeration.

Yersinia enterocolitica

Yersiniosis is caused by this motile, Gram-negative bacillus of the family Enterobacteriaceae and has been reported most frequently in Northern Europe; however, *Y. enterocolitica* has been isolated from animals, surface waters and soil in cooler climates, world-wide. Disease manifestations are age-dependent and arise one to eleven days after the ingestion of contaminated foods, especially pork and pork products, milk or untreated water. Transmission via transfused blood products has also been reported, reflecting the ability of *Y. enterocolitica* to multiply at 4°C. Young children usually manifest a self-limited syndrome of abdominal pain, watery diarrhoea, fever and an occasional erythematous rash. Pseudoappendicitis due to terminal ileitis and mesenteric adenitis is typically found in older children and young adults; this syndrome may also be caused by *Y. pseudotuberculosis*. In adults, fever, diarrhoea and/or pharyngitis may be followed within one to two weeks by the postinfectious complications of seronegative arthritis, Reiter's syndrome or erythema nodosum. Syndromes of enteric fever, bacteremia and/or metastatic infection also occur, particularly in the presence of iron-overload states, diabetes mellitus, malnutrition or immunosuppressive therapy.

The diagnosis can be made by culture of stool on standard growth media using cold enrichment, but is delayed for up to four weeks. Blood cultures are rarely positive in gastrointestinal yersiniosis. Serological diagnosis is available in some centres.

Antimicrobial therapy is required for systemic infection, focal extraintestinal infection and enterocolitis in compromised hosts. Doxycycline or trimethoprim-sulfamethoxazole are effective drugs. In bacteremic patients an aminoglycoside should be added until antimicrobial susceptibilities are available.

Aeromonas

Epidemiological evidence has implicated the motile Gram-negative aeromonads, *Aeromonas hydrophila* and *Aeromonas sobria*, in water-borne cases of enterocolitis, especially in young children during summer months. Infection presents as a febrile secretory diarrhoea associated with epigastric pain. Vomiting is common in younger patients. In a minority of cases diarrhoea persists for several weeks. Dysenteric and cholera-like forms of illness have been described. Disease appears more severe in patients with gastric hypochlorhydria, concurrent gastrointestinal or hepatic disease or in patients who have received recent antimicrobial therapy. The diagnosis is made by stool culture on selective media. Blood cultures are usually negative in *Aeromonas* enterocolitis unless the host is immunocompromised. Antimicrobial agents are indicated only in severe or bacteremic infection. Doxycycline or trimethoprim-sulfamethoxazole should be combined with an aminoglycoside if bacteremia is suspected. Third generation cephalosporins may also be effective.

Plesiomonas shigelloides

This is a motile Gram-negative bacillus which has been associated with enterocolitis occurring after ingestion of contaminated fresh water or undercooked, freshwater seafood. Several cases have been reported in Japan. The diagnosis is made by isolation of *P. shigelloides* from stool samples. Antimicrobial therapy is required only in severe cases and should be based on antibiograms.

Enteroinvasive *E. coli*

Certain serotypes of *E. coli* produce a dysenteric syndrome identical to that found with *Shigella*, two to three days after ingestion of contaminated food. Diagnosis requires specialised tests for invasive potential.

Clostridium difficile

Clostridium difficile is a spore-forming, Gram-positive, anaerobic bacillus which is the classical cause of cytotoxin-mediated colitis associated with broad-spectrum antimicrobial therapy. Most cases arise within four to nine days of commencing clindamycin, lincomycin, ampicillin, amoxycillin or a cephalosporin; however, diarrhoea may be noted as early as two days after initiation, and as late as four to six weeks after cessation, of antimicrobial therapy. Only bacitracin has been exempt from causing *C. difficile*-associated colitis. Disease is most frequent and severe in the elderly, debilitated, seriously ill patient. Abdominal surgery is a risk factor. Nosocomial outbreaks have been reported.

Lumenal production of at least two toxins by *C. difficile* (toxins A and B) is followed by the development of a diffuse superficial colitis which, when severe, is associated with pseudomembrane formation. Toxin A appears to act primarily as an enterotoxin, with minor cytotoxic activity, whereas toxin B is a potent cytotoxin and stimulant of peristalsis. Colitis is manifest by the acute onset of watery or green, mucoid, foul-smelling diarrhoea, with fever, abdominal cramps and tenderness. Progression to bloody diarrhoea may occur but is uncommon. Pseudomembranous colitis (PMC) should be suspected in patients with high fever, marked abdominal tenderness and peripheral blood leukocytosis. Toxic megacolon is a potentially fatal complication of PMC.

The diagnosis of *C. difficile*-associated colitis may be suspected from the history and the presence of a pseudomembrane at sigmoidoscopy or in rectal biopsy specimens; confirmation requires the demonstration of *C. difficile* cytotoxin in the stool and takes up to forty-eight hours using standard tissue culture assays. Rapid diagnostic tests are available but may lack sensitivity and/or specificity.

Mild cases of colitis will respond to appropriate fluid and electrolyte replacement, plus withdrawal of the offending antimicrobial agent. Symptomatic therapy with cholestyramine has been used to bind *C. difficile* toxin, but this therapy does not eliminate organism. Specific antimicrobial therapy is required in persistent or severe illness. A seven-day course of oral vancomycin, metronidazole or bacitracin is usually effective, although relapse may occur. Pseudomembranous colitis complicated by toxic megacolon is associated with bacteremia arising from normal bowel flora and requires additional antimicrobial therapy, effective against aerobic and anaerobic pathogens of bowel origin. Because of the risk of nosocomial transmission of *C. difficile*, patients should be nursed in isolation.

It should be noted that although more than 96% of cases of PMC are caused by *C. difficile* cytotoxin, most patients with mild diarrhoea associated with antimicrobial therapy have neither colitis nor *C. difficile* cytotoxin demonstrable in their stool. Occasional cases of PMC associated with antibiotic use are caused by *Staphylococcus aureus*; large numbers of staphylococci are present in the stool in such patients.

Entamoeba histolytica

Infestation with the protozoan parasite, *Entamoeba histolytica*, is estimated to affect more than 10% of the world's population, being especially prevalent under conditions of poor sanitation and/or overcrowding. *Entamoeba histolytica* is an important cause of traveller's diarrhoea and has been implicated in bowel syndromes described in homosexual males.

Transmission of infection occurs when the cyst form of the parasite, which can survive for long periods in moist environments, is ingested in water or foodstuffs (e.g. salads or uncooked vegetables) contaminated with infected human excreta. Trophozoites, which are released after dissolution of the cyst capsule in the small intestine, invade the colonic mucosa, resulting in shallow, flask-like ulcers. Amoebae seed the liver from the colon via the portal vein and thence the diaphragm, lung, pericardium and/or skin. Further encystment occurs in the bowel lumen, thus maintaining the human faecal reservoir of *E. histolytica*.

Intestinal amoebiasis

Asymptomatic passage of cysts is the commonest form of amoebiasis. Symptomatic disease usually presents with colicky, lower abdominal pain and altered bowel habit. The stool may be loose; mucus and/or blood may be present. The severity of these features varies and symptoms may be intermittent or persistent. Lower quadrant tenderness is often present. Extensive colonic involvement is associated with fever and dysentery. The rare complications of secondary peritonitis and toxic megacolon present as an acute abdomen. Tender hepatomegaly has been noted, even in the absence of an amoebic liver abscess. Other intestinal sequelae include haemorrhage, stricture formation, amoeboma, postdysenteric colitis and a chronic, non-dysenteric syndrome of intermittent diarrhoea, abdominal pain, flatulence, weight loss and the passage of mucus in the stool. The latter two syndromes must be differentiated from Crohn's disease and ulcerative colitis.

Extra-intestinal amoebiasis

The liver is the most common site of involvement. Hepatic abscesses usually involve the right lobe and present acutely or subacutely with right upper quadrant abdominal pain or pain referred to the tip of the right shoulder. Fever, cough, weight loss and hepatomegaly are common, and intercostal point tenderness or pleural effusions may be noted. Concurrent intestinal symptoms or a past history of dysentery are noted in less than 50% of cases. Large hepatic abscesses may rupture into the pleural, pericardial or peritoneal cavities, resulting in acute deterioration in the clinical state of the patient.

Diagnosis

Diagnosis of intestinal amoebiasis is made by the demonstration of trophozoites or cysts in samples of stool, rectal scrapings or rectal biopsy. Culture of fresh stool is performed in some centres. The diagnostic yield from a single stool sample may be as low as 30%, hence at least three specimens should be examined. Alternatively, the yield may be increased by collection of stool passed after a saline purge. Sigmoidoscopic examination may reveal typical punctate areas of haemorrhage or small ulcers with exudative centres and hyperaemic borders. Biopsies and scrapings should be obtained from suspicious lesions.

Serology is positive in 85% of patients with extra-intestinal or invasive intestinal amoebiasis. An indirect haemagglutination titre of more than 1:128 is commonly accepted as evidence of invasive disease, but remains positive for many years.

Amoebic liver abscesses must be distinguished from other space-occupying lesions in the liver. Basal collapse of the lung, right-sided pleural effusion and/or elevation of the right hemidiaphragm may be evident on chest x-ray. More sensitive and accurate localising techniques include ultrasonography, CT scan and radionuclide scans. Serum alkaline phosphatase is elevated in 80% of cases. Aspiration biopsy is rarely necessary, as therapy is commenced on the basis of history, identification of an hepatic lesion consistent with amoebiasis and positive amoebic serology. Stool examination is often negative in patients with amoebic liver abscesses.

Management

Management of intestinal amoebiasis varies in different countries. In highly endemic areas, therapy is usually restricted to symptomatic cases, whereas in countries such as Australia and the United States, asymptomatic infection is also treated, on public health grounds. Ninety per cent of patients with mild to moderate intestinal disease or amoeboma will be cured by tissue-active drugs (e.g. tinidazole or metronidazole). Subsequent therapy with a lumenal amoebicide (e.g. diloxanide furoate, di-iodohydroxyquinoline or paromomycin) is recommended as these drugs have proven more effective than nitromidazoles in the eradication of *E. histolytica* from bowel contents. An alternative regimen of the intestinal wall-active drug, tetracycline, followed by diloxanide furoate, is almost as effective but must be avoided in children because of tetracycline-induced staining of the teeth.

Metronidazole and tinidazole are the agents of choice for severe dysentery, where intravenous therapy, fluid, electrolyte, nutritional and blood replacement may also be necessary. Alternative regimens include tetracycline plus chloroquine followed by diloxanide furoate, or intramuscular dehydroemetine or emetine, followed by diloxanide furoate.

Asymptomatic cyst passers should receive diloxanide furoate or di-iodohydroxyquinoline.

Metronidazole is the treatment of choice for extra-intestinal amoebiasis, followed by a course of diloxanide furoate or di-iodohydroxyquinoline, to eliminate lumenal infestation. In seriously ill patients with ruptured abscesses, dehydroemetine or emetine plus chloroquine may be preferred as initial therapy. Needle aspiration of liver abscesses is indicated if the lesion is large or pointing.

Amoebic infestation is prevented by eradicating faecal contamination of food and water. In endemic areas drinking water should be boiled.

Causative agents of non-inflammatory diarrhoea containing blood

Enterohaemorrhagic *E. coli* (EHEC)

Specific serotypes of *E. coli*, including 0157:H7, produce a verotoxin responsible for the clinical syndrome of abdominal cramps and watery diarrhoea followed by the passage of bright blood per rectum, in the absence of significant fever or faecal inflammatory exudate. Barium studies are suggestive of an ischemic colitis with thumb printing. Outbreaks of haemorrhagic colitis have been traced to consumption of beef products, including hamburgers, with an incubation period of four to eight days. The same EHEC strains cause the haemolytic uremic syndrome in young children and thrombotic thrombocytopenic purpura. Diagnosis is based on clinical features and identification of the causative *E. coli* by serotyping and/or production of verocytotoxin. Specific antimicrobial therapy is indicated in severe disease.

Pathogens, sources of infection and techniques of laboratory diagnosis in enterocolitis are summarised in Table 7.1.

Chronic enteritis and enterocolitis

Non-inflammatory diarrhoeal syndromes

Syndromes of chronic, non-inflammatory diarrhoea are characterised by features of malabsorption associated with malaise, weight loss, borborygmi, abdominal cramps, abdominal distension and the passage of watery or fatty bowel motions.

Table 7.1 *Pathogens, source and diagnosis of enterocolitis*

Pathogen	*Common source(s)*	*Method of detection in stool*	*Comments*
Non-inflammatory enteritis			
Rotavirus	Human infants, children	Enzyme immunoassay Latex agglutination Electron microscopy	Winter epidemics Very common in children
Enteric adenovirus	Human	Immune electron microscopy	Common in children
Norwalk agent	Contaminated oysters, salads	Immune electron microscopy	Winter outbreaks
Giardia lamblia	Contaminated water	Light microscopy for cysts and trophozoites	Cause of traveller's diarrhoea
Cryptosporidium parvum	Contaminated water, food	Light microscopy; special stains	Zoonosis or human to human spread Association with AIDS
Staphylococcus aureus enterotoxin	Contaminated dairy products	N/A	Culture from suspect food
Bacillus cereus enterotoxin	Contaminated fried rice, meat products, vegetables	N/A	Culture from suspect food
Clostridium perfringens enterotoxin	Contaminated red meat stews, soups, preserves	N/A	Culture from suspect foods
Enterotoxigenic *E. coli*	Contaminated water, salads, raw vegetables	Toxin detection (not routine); DNA probing for virulence genes[a]	Most common cause of traveller's diarrhoea
Enteropathogenic *E. coli*	Human newborns	Culture and serotyping (not routine). DNA probes for virulence genes[a]	Cause of epidemic diarrhoea
Vibrio cholerae	Contaminated water or food	Culture (requires special media)	
Inflammatory enterocolitis			
Salmonella species (non-*S. typhi*)	Contaminated poultry, poultry products	Culture	Cause of traveller's diarrhoea
Shigella species	Contaminated water, food; direct contact with faeces, flies	Culture	Cause of traveller's diarrhoea
Campylobacter jejuni	Contaminated poultry, faecal–oral spread from pets, infants	Culture on selective media	Cause of traveller's diarrhoea
Vibrio parahaemolyticus	Contaminated, undercooked seafood	Culture on selective media	Common in Japan
Yersinia enterocolitica	Contaminated pork products, milk, water	Culture on selective media, cold enrichment, prolonged incubation	Common in Northern Europe
Aeromonas species, *Plesiomonas shigelloides*	Contaminated water	Culture (not routine)	More common in summer
Clostridium difficile	Broad-spectrum antibiotic therapy—humans	Toxin detection	Nosocomial spread reported

(continues)

Table 7.1 *Continued*

Pathogen	*Common source(s)*	*Method of detection in stool*	*Comments*
Entamoeba histolytica	Contaminated water, salads, raw vegetables	Light microscopy	Cause of traveller's diarrhoea; serology for invasive disease
Enterohaemorrhagic *E. coli*	Contaminated beef products	Culture and serotyping; DNA probes for virulence genes[(a)]	

NA = not applicable.
[(a)] Not yet available routinely.

The differential diagnosis of infectious causes includes giardiasis, cryptosporidiosis (see p. 188), infestation with *Isospora belli*, microsporidia (see section on diarrhoea in patients with AIDS, p. 203), capillariasis (see section on Helminths), sprue-like syndromes and bacterial overgrowth syndromes.

The aetiology of tropical sprue has not been defined although the clinical and epidemiological features are those of an infectious process. Colonisation of the jejunum with specific strains of *Klebsiella pneumoniae, E. coli* or *Enterobacter cloacae* has been implicated in the pathogenesis of disease. The diagnosis is one of exclusion, particularly of giardiasis. A six-month course of folic acid, vitamin B12 and tetracycline is usually curative.

Bacterial overgrowth syndromes occur in patients with disorders that impair the mechanical enteric defences, predisposing patients to colonisation of the jejunum with enteric bacteria, including *E. coli* and *Bacteroides fragilis.* Thus patients with achlorhydria (p. 21), blind-loop syndromes, scleroderma, diabetic neuropathy, surgical strictures, diverticulae and cholangitis are at increased risk of presenting with chronic, non-inflammatory diarrhoea. The diagnosis is based on the presence of enteric bacteria in duodenal contents (at concentrations exceeding 10^5 per mL) or on the ^{14}C glycocholic acid breath test for bacterial deconjugation of bile salts (p. 49). Symptoms may be controlled with antimicrobial therapy directed against coliform bacteria and anaerobes.

Inflammatory diarrhoeal syndromes

These syndromes present with fever, abdominal pain, diarrhoea, weight loss, or other systemic manifestations, which are often indolent, slowly progressive or relapsing. The differential diagnosis includes prolonged bacterial infection (e.g. *Campylobacter, Salmonella, Shigella,* EPEC enterocolitis), amoebiasis, gastrointestinal tuberculosis, syphilis and, rarely, systemic fungal infections.

Gastrointestinal tuberculosis

Extrapulmonary tuberculosis, including intestinal tuberculosis, occurs predominantly in developing countries in association with high rates of tuberculous infection, poor nutritional status and an increased prevalence of tuberculosis in young persons. Infection of the gastrointestinal tract is most often secondary to pulmonary disease caused by the human pathogen, *Mycobacterium tuberculosis*. Primary infection of the bowel occurs in miliary tuberculosis and following ingestion of mycobacteria. Unpasteurised milk is a potential source of infection with *Mycobacterium bovis*. Intestinal tuberculosis most often involves the terminal ileum and caecum, and is associated with involvement of other abdominal sites, for example, the peritoneum, the liver and lymph nodes.

Clinical features include abdominal pain, often relieved by defecation, anorexia and low-grade fever. Weight loss is more frequent in patients with pulmonary tuberculosis. In cases with involvement of abdominal lymph nodes, an abdominal mass may be noted. Diarrhoeal motions containing mucus and, rarely, blood occur in only one-third of patients and denote extensive disease. Tuberculous peritonitis may present with night sweats, abdominal swelling, gastrointestinal disturbance, malaise and weight loss, although symptoms are often insidious.

The diagnosis of gastrointestinal tuberculosis is often difficult on radiological investigation; the differential diagnosis includes infectious and non-infectious causes of ileocaecal abnormalities. Patients with pulmonary or miliary tuberculosis and abdominal symptoms or signs should be investigated for intestinal and intra-abdominal involvement. Stool samples are rarely positive. The best diagnostic method is direct biopsy and culture of material visualised at peritoneoscopy, or peritoneal biopsy. Ascitic fluid is typically exudative in nature; the yield of *M. tuberculosis* from culture of ascitic fluid is significantly lower than that from peritoneal biopsy. Treatment of tuberculosis requires a minimum of isoniazid and rifampicin for nine months. Most authorities prefer the addition of pyrazinamide, with or without ethambutol, for the first two months in order to hasten sterilisation of lesions and because of an increasing incidence of drug resistance in developing countries.

Traveller's diarrhoea

Traveller's diarrhoea affects 20–50% of short-term travellers from industrialised to developing countries. Persons with achlorhydria, previous gastrectomy or who are taking potent, long-acting anti-ulcer drugs such as omeprazole appear to be at increased risk (p. 27). Approximately one-third of travellers to developing countries complain of diarrhoea, often with abdominal cramps, within one week of arrival. Fever, vomiting or blood in the stool are noted in a minority of cases. Symptoms typically resolve within seven days. *Escherichia coli*, particularly ETEC, is the most common cause of traveller's diarrhoea; other pathogens show regional variation and include bacteria such as *Shigella* species, *Salmonella enteritidis*, *Campylobacter jejunii*, *Aeromonas* species (especially in Thailand), *Plesiomonas shigelloides* and non-cholera *Vibrios* (especially in coastal areas). Viral pathogens include rotavirus and Norwalk agent; these may be isolated concurrently with enteric bacterial pathogens. *Giardia lamblia* and *Cryptosporidium parvum* are common in travellers to certain areas, including parts of Russia, especially Leningrad. *Entamoeba histolytica* is a relatively uncommon cause of traveller's diarrhoea.

Prevention is best achieved by exercising care in choice of food and drink. Antimicrobial agents (e.g. trimethoprim-sulfamethoxazole and fluoroquinolones) are effective prophylactic drugs, but should be prescribed only in exceptional circumstances because of the risks of emerging drug resistance and of toxicity.

Rehydration is the basis of therapy. Antimotility agents (e.g. imodium) may be used short-term provided there is no systemic toxicity, malabsorption, or blood or mucus in the stool. Specific antimicrobial therapy is indicated in severe cases (see under individual pathogens).

Enterocolitis and proctocolitis in patients with AIDS

Enterocolitis

Enterocolitis occurs frequently in patients with AIDS; the resultant diarrhoea is generally more severe and prolonged than in the normal host. Haematogenous spread of infection is a common sequel of bacterial enterocolitis in this group. Recognised enteric pathogens are identified in up to 85% of symptomatic cases (see Table 7.2). The human immunodeficiency virus (HIV) itself causes an enteropathy, the pathogenesis of which is uncertain but may include a direct effect of the virus on mucosal cells, HIV-associated autonomic neuropathy or immune dysregulation in the bowel, lactase deficiency and bacterial overgrowth secondary to hypochlorhydria.

Table 7.2 *Aetiology of enterocolitis in patients with AIDS*

Viruses	Cytomegalovirus
	HIV
Protozoa	*Cryptosporidium parvum*
	Microsporidia (*Enterocytozoon bieneusi*)
	Isospora belli (Sarcocystis hominis)
	Cyclospora species
Bacteria	*Salmonella* (non-typhi)
	Shigella species
	Campylobacter species
	Clostridium difficile (toxin)
	Mycobacterium avium-intracellulare

Note: Other enteric pathogens may cause diarrhoea in patients with HIV infection, but the evidence that they are more common or cause more severe disease is inconclusive.

Of the pathogens listed in Table 7.2, cytomegalovirus, *Salmonella* species, *Shigella* species, *Campylobacter* species and *C. difficile* cause an inflammatory diarrhoeal syndrome, whereas non-inflammatory diarrhoea of small bowel type is typical of protozoa, *M. avium* and HIV. Diagnosis is based on light microscopy of stool (protozoa, *M. avium*), culture (*M. avium, Salmonella, Shigella, Campylobacter*), presence of toxin in the stool (*C. difficile*) or demonstration of the pathogen in biopsies of small bowel (HIV, cryptosporidia, microsporidia) or colon (cytomegalovirus). Multiple pathogens may be present concurrently.

There is no effective antimicrobial therapy for cryptosporidiosis, microsporidiosis or *Cyclospora* infestation. Control of symptoms caused by other enteric pathogens can be achieved with specific antimicrobial therapy (see under individual pathogens) although eradication of the pathogen is more difficult.

Proctocolitis

As in HIV-negative homosexual males, distal proctocolitis in patients with AIDS is caused by the sexually transmitted pathogens, Herpes simplex virus, *Neisseria gonorrhoeae* and *Chlamydia trachomatis*. Isolated ulcers may be caused by *Treponema pallidum* or *Haemophilus ducreyi* (the cause of chancroid). Diagnosis is made by microscopy and/or culture. Specific antimicrobial therapy should be curative.

Helminth infestation of the gastrointestinal tract

Gastrointestinal parasitisation with helminths (worms) is extremely common. Acquisition of infection occurs via the oral route or the skin and results in disease manifestations which are proportional to the adult worm burden. Gastrointestinal symptoms are frequently minor. Abdominal pain is more common than diarrhoea. Eosinophilia is characteristic of most helminth infestations.

Nematodes (roundworms)

Ascaris lumbricoides *(giant roundworm)*

Ascariasis is the most common helminth infestation of humans. Following ingestion of raw vegetables, fruits or soil contaminated with embryonated eggs, larvae are released in the human small intestine and transported to the lung, where they give rise to transient pulmonary symptoms associated with peripheral blood eosinophilia. Cranial migration through the tracheobronchial tree is followed by maturation of adult worms in the small intestine. Heavy infestation may cause non-specific complaints of fever, anorexia, nausea and abdominal discomfort. Vomiting and intestinal, biliary or pancreatic duct obstruction and gastrointestinal blood loss have been reported. Diagnosis is made readily by identification of eggs or adult worms in the stool. When required, mebendazole is the treatment of choice. Pyrantel pamoate and piperazine are also effective.

Capillaria philippinensis

This parasite is restricted primarily to small areas in the Philippines and Thailand. Jejunal autoinfection can lead to protracted symptoms of abdominal pain, borborygmi and large volume, watery diarrhoea, accompanied by nausea, vomiting, severe weight loss, features of malabsorption and protein-losing enteropathy. Raw or undercooked freshwater fish appear to be the vehicle of transmission. The diagnosis is made by identification of eggs in the stool. Fever and eosinophilia are uncommon. A prolonged course of mebendazole is the treatment of choice.

Enterobius vermicularis *(pinworm)*

This small, thread-like worm is common in temperate climates. Infection is transmitted from human to human by the faecal–oral route and is common in family groups. Deposition of eggs occurs at night in the perianal and perineal regions, causing the main presenting symptom of marked pruritis ani. A diagnostic yield of more than 99% is achieved by examination of three specimens obtained by pressing adhesive cellophane tape against the perineal region early in the morning. Patients and household members should be treated with a single dose of pyrantel pamoate or mebendazole or with two doses, two weeks apart. In some cases, weekly treatment for up to six weeks may be necessary because of reinfestation. Personal hygiene is important in containing the spread of infection.

Strongyloides stercoralis

Strongyloides stercoralis is distributed widely in the tropics. This nematode is unique because of its ability to cause autoinfection, and hyperinfection in the immunocompromised host. The tiny adult worms inhabit and lay eggs in the upper small intestine. Rhabditiform larvae, which are passed in the faeces, differentiate into free-living adult worms or undergo metamorphosis into filariform larvae. Humans are infected via skin contact with contaminated soil. Filariform larvae penetrate the skin, causing a local pruritic, papular, erythematous rash. Migration through the lungs to the tracheobronchial tree may result in pulmonary manifestations of cough, dyspnoea and a Löffler-like syndrome with eosinophilia. Symptoms of intestinal infestation include epigastric pain, nausea, vomiting, flatulence, weight loss and constipation or diarrhoea. Malabsorption and protein losing enteropathy occur in severe cases. Autoinfection occurs when filariform larvae develop during the passage of eggs through the bowel lumen. The hyperinfection syndrome in immunocompromised adults includes severe abdominal pain and distension, secondary Gram-negative bacterial sepsis and diffuse pulmonary involvement. Eosinopenia is a poor prognostic sign in this setting. Definitive diagnosis is dependent on identification of larvae in stool samples; eggs are found rarely. Because larvae are sparse in stool, multiple samples should be examined in wet preparations and following concentration techniques. Harada culture is available in some centres. Examination of duodenal contents for larvae and eggs should be considered if stool examination is negative. Thiabendazole is the treatment of choice but is associated with substantial toxicity.

Trichuris trichuria *(whipworm)*

Infestation with this 3–5 cm long worm is common. Humans are the principle host and excreted eggs are transmitted directly via the faecal–oral route, via fomites such as contaminated soil, fruit and vegetables or via flying insects. Larvae released from embryonated eggs penetrate intestinal villi and attach to colonic mucosa. Heavy worm burdens cause symptoms of abdominal pain, distension, bloody or mucoid diarrhoea, tenesmus and weight loss, and are noted especially in older children. Anaemia and rectal prolapse are uncommon complications. The diagnosis is made by identification of the characteristic eggs in the faeces. Treatment with mebendazole is warranted only in patients with heavy worm burdens.

Ancyclostoma duodenale *and* **Necator americanus** *(hookworm)*

These two species of hookworm are found in tropical and subtropical areas, and are estimated to infest one-quarter of the world's population. Larvae hatch from eggs excreted by the human host. Infection occurs via penetration of the skin and is associated with intense local pruritis, erythema and a papulo-vesicular rash. Migration through the lung to the tracheobronchial tree may produce a Löffler-like syndrome with eosinophilia. Transient abdominal pain, weight loss and diarrhoea may be noted when worms attach to the intestinal mucosa; however, the major manifestations of infestation are iron-deficiency anaemia and hypoalbuminaemia, secondary to intestinal blood loss. The diagnosis is made by identification of eggs in stool samples. Mebendazole is the treatment of choice.

Trichinella spiralis

Trichinosis is caused by this tissue-dwelling nematode, which is acquired by ingestion of encysted larvae in undercooked pork and pork products, and which has a world-wide distribution except for Australia and many Pacific Islands. Approximately twenty-four hours after ingestion, larvae excyst in the small intestine and develop rapidly into adult worms. Invasion of the small intestinal mucosa may be associated with transient nausea, vomiting, abdominal discomfort and diarrhoea. Larvae are produced, which then seed skeletal muscle via the blood, causing systemic features of fever, periorbital oedema, myositis and eosinophilia within two to three weeks. Laboratory investigations reveal an elevated creatine phosphokinase and lactic dehydrogenase; serology becomes positive within three weeks but is available in few centres. Biopsy of tender, swollen muscle is diagnostic but not usually necessary. Treatment of muscle infestation is unsatisfactory. Adult worms may be eradicated from the gut by treatment with thiabendazole, mebendazole or pyrantel pamoate. Corticosteroids are often necessary to control systemic toxicity.

Trematodes (flukes)

Blood flukes

Schistosomiasis is prevalent in major areas of agricultural development in tropical countries of Africa, South America and Asia. The geographical distribution of the five species of human pathogen—*Schistosoma mansoni* (Africa, Arabia, South America, the Caribbean), *Schistosoma japonicum* (Japan, China, the Philippines), *Schistosoma mekongi* (South-East Asia), *Schistosoma haematobium* (Africa, the Middle East) and *Schistosoma intercalatum* (West and Central Africa)—is determined by the habitat of the specific snail intermediate host. Adult worms of *Schistosoma haematobium* reside in the vesical venous plexus; those of all other species reside in the mesenteric veins. Eggs are excreted and undergo an aquatic life cycle in which the snail is the intermediate host. Infective cercariae penetrate intact human skin, causing a transient, papular, pruritic rash—'swimmers' itch'. Acute schistosomiasis or Katayama fever, which occurs at the time of deposition of eggs by the mature worms of *S. japonicum*, is manifest by fever, chills, headache, cough, sweats, hepatosplenomegaly, lymphadenopathy and eosinophilia. Chronic schistosomiasis results from egg deposition, granuloma formation and fibrosis. Infestation with *S. mansoni, S. japonicum* or *S. mekongi* may present with chronic abdominal pain, intermittent diarrhoea and dysentery, or as hepatosplenomegaly. Cirrhosis and liver failure are late sequelae. *Schistosoma intercalatum* may cause abdominal pain and bloody diarrheoa. *Schistosoma haematobium* involves the urinary tract causing obstruction, dysuria and terminal haematuria. The diagnosis is based on history and quantitation of eggs in urine or stool. Eggs may also be identified on biopsy of involved tissue. Praziquantel is the treatment of choice.

Liver flukes

The major species of liver fluke affecting man are *Clonorchis sinensis* (found in China, Japan, Vietnam and Korea), species of *Opisthorchis* (which are common in South-East Asia and the Commonwealth of Independent States) and *Fasciola hepatica* (found on all continents).

Opisthorcis *species and* Clonorchis sinensis

Man is an incidental host, becoming infected by ingestion of raw or pickled freshwater fish which contain encysted cercariae. Adult flukes reside in the human biliary capillaries and excrete eggs which are ultimately passed in the stool and enter the aquatic stage of their life cycle. Heavy infestation produces cystic dilatation of intrahepatic bile ducts, recurrent cholangitis, hepatitis with hepatomegaly and biliary cirrhosis. Weight loss and abdominal pain are common. Cholangiocarcinoma has been associated with long-standing infestation. The diagnosis is made by demonstration of ova in faeces or biliary aspirate. Praziquantel is the treatment of choice.

Fasciola hepatica

Fasciola hepatica most commonly infests sheep and cattle. Human infestation is acquired by ingestion of aquatic plants contaminated with encysted metacercariae. In the acute hepatic migratory phase there is liver enlargement, fever and marked eosinophilia. The fluke rarely pierces the intestinal wall, causing perforation, peritonitis and haemoperitoneum. Late sequelae of biliary obstruction and/or cirrhosis are rare. Diagnosis requires concentration of faeces or bile to demonstrate the characteristic eggs. Praziquantel is the treatment of choice.

Intestinal flukes

Fasciolopsis buski

Human infestation with this large intestinal fluke is endemic in the Far East and South-East Asia, and is acquired by ingestion of encysted cercariae on aquatic plants. Attachment of *F. buski* to the duodenal and jejunal mucosa is usually asymptomatic. Heavy infestation results in abdominal pain and a malabsorption syndrome. Detection of cysts in the stool is enhanced by the use of concentration techniques. Praziquantel is the treatment of choice.

Heterophyes heterophyes

This is a smaller fluke with a life cycle similar to that of *F. buski*, involving the snail as an intermediate host. It is common in the Nile delta, the Far East and South-East Asia. Metacercariae encyst in freshwater fish, hence infection is acquired by consumption of undercooked or salted fish. Clinical features include abdominal pain and mucous diarrhoea. The diagnosis is made by identification of eggs in the stool. Praziquantel is the treatment of choice.

Cestodes (tapeworms)

These segmented helminths cause human disease in either of two stages of their life cycle—the adult stage, which causes symptoms referable to the presence of adult worms in the gastrointestinal tract, and the larval stage, which causes signs and symptoms due to enlargement of larval cysts in various tissues or organs. The human is the definitive host for *Taenia saginata* (the beef tapeworm), *Taenia solium* (the pork tapeworm), *Diphyllobothrium* (the fish tapeworm) and *Hymenolepsis nana* (the dwarf tapeworm).

The dog is the definitive host for *Echinococcus granulosis* (the cause of hydatid disease in humans). Developing tapeworms attach to the intestinal mucosa by the scolex or head. Eggs are produced in worm segments or proglottids, which are passed in the stool and allow a specific diagnosis to be made. Eggs ingested by the intermediate host develop into larvae, which are contained within cyst-like structures. The life cycle is completed when tissue containing these cysts is ingested by the definitive host.

Taenia saginata infestation follows ingestion of poorly cooked beef and is common in areas where grazing lands can be contaminated with human faeces. Disease is prevalent in Yugoslavia, Moslem countries, Ethiopia, Kenya, Central Africa and South America. Intestinal symptoms are uncommon, and consist of mild abdominal cramps or discomfort from passage of gravid proglottids.

Taenia solium is acquired by eating poorly cooked pork and occurs most commonly in Eastern Europe, Central and South America, Spain, Portugal and parts of Africa, India and China. Intestinal infestation is usually asymptomatic. Humans can act as both the intermediate and definitive host for *T. solium*. Ingestion of *T. solium* eggs in water, food or from hands contaminated with faecal material, results in the development and dissemination of larval stages, and the syndrome of cysticercosis.

Diphyllobothrium latum is acquired by eating undercooked fish and is common in Sweden, Finland, Japan, the Baltic countries and the Eskimos of North America. Gastrointestinal symptoms are mild. Vitamin B12 deficiency occurs in chronic infestation due to competition for it by the parasite.

Hymenolepsis nana is the only tapeworm in which the life cycle can be maintained by humans acting as both the definitive and intermediate host. Mucosal irritation by adult and cysticercoid stages results in abdominal cramps and diarrhoea.

Niclosamide or praziquantel constitute effective therapy for these four species of tapeworm.

Echinococcus granulosis

Hydatid disease caused by *E. granulosis* occurs in most sheep and cattle-raising areas of the world, including Greece, Lebanon, Australia, New Zealand, Argentina, Uruguay, Chile, parts of Africa and the Middle East. The dog is the definitive host; sheep, cattle and humans are intermediate hosts. When ingested, *E. granulosis* eggs hatch, penetrate the intestinal wall and reach tissues where encystment occurs (particularly the liver and lung) via the blood. Symptoms result from enlargement of hydatid cysts and compression of surrounding structures. Spontaneous or induced leakage of hydatid fluid may cause an acute allergic reaction, including anaphylaxis. X-ray may reveal a calcified mass. Diagnosis is based on clinical suspicion and serology. The most specific test available currently is the arc 5 diffusion test. Drugs used in medical treatment include mebendazole and albendazole. If this fails, surgical treatment is indicated. Successful prevention requires interruption of the dog cycle by treatment of canine tapeworms and proper disposal of potentially infected carcasses and offal.

Neurotoxin-associated food poisoning

Botulism

Botulism is a potentially fatal paralytic syndrome produced by neurotoxins elaborated by the spore-forming, Gram-positive, anaerobic bacillus, *Clostridium botulinum*. Most cases of food poisoning are due to consumption of preformed toxin type A, B or E in home-canned or preserved foods. Symptoms are generally manifest within twelve to thirty-six hours of ingestion of contaminated food, by weakness, lassitude, dizziness and less often, nausea and vomiting. Toxin-mediated interruption of cholinergic nerve fibre transmission results in dryness of the mouth and throat, blurred vision, constipation and urinary retention. Neurological manifestations include diplopia, photophobia, dysphonia, dysarthria, dysphagia, weakness of the respiratory muscles and symmetrical, descending weakness of the limbs. Patients are afebrile. Eye signs may include fixed, dilated pupils and extra-ocular palsies. Motor weakness is accompanied by normal or diminished tendon reflexes and normal sensory examination.

Recovery is usually gradual. The diagnosis should be suspected in the appropriate clinical setting. Electromyography may be suggestive, but definitive diagnosis requires demonstration of toxin and/or *C. botulinum* in stool, gastric contents or suspect food. Toxin may also be found in blood. Specific tests are available only in special centres. Treatment includes ventilatory and other supportive measures combined with immediate intravenous and intramuscular administration of specific polyvalent antitoxin.

Ciguatera poisoning

This form of fish poisoning is responsible for outbreaks of vomiting, diarrhoea and neurological manifestations. Ciguatera toxin is produced by the dinoflagellate marine algae, *Gambierdiscus toxicus*, and is transferred up the food chain through herbivorous fish to carnivorous tropical reef fish (schnapper, Spanish mackerel, grouper, dolphin, barracuda), in which it is concentrated. The toxin is harmless to the fish and is resistant to cooking and freezing. Symptoms arise within four to thirty hours of toxin ingestion and include nausea, vomiting, diarrhoea, perioral and peripheral paraesthesiae, a metallic taste in the mouth, hot-to-cold reversal dysaesthesiae, increased salivation, pupillary dilatation, strabismus, ptosis, weakness, myalgia of the legs, inco-ordination and even paralysis. Pruritus may be severe. Treatment is symptomatic and supportive. Symptoms may persist or recur for several months and may be worsened by eating chicken.

SUGGESTED FURTHER READING

Bartlett, J. G., Belitsos, P. C. and Sears, C. L., AIDS enteropathy, *Clinical Infectious Diseases*, 1992; 15:726–35.

Ericsson, C. D. and Du Pont, H. L., Traveler's Diarrhoea. Approaches to Prevention and Treatment, *Clinical Infectious Diseases*, 1993; 16:616–26.

Mandell, G. L., Douglas, R. G. Jr and Bennett, J. E. (eds), *Principles and Practice of Infectious Diseases*, 3rd edn, John Wiles & Sons, New York, 1990.

CHAPTER 8

Motility and functional disorders of the gastrointestinal tract

J. E. Kellow

Gastrointestinal motor physiology and pathophysiology

General principles

Gastrointestinal motility encompasses two basic components: *motor* (contractile) activity, and *transit* (movement of contents) through the digestive tract. Motor activity is the main determinant of transit. Normal motility depends on appropriate interaction of the main functional elements, the gastrointestinal smooth muscle and the intrinsic and extrinsic nerves.

Continuous and spontaneous oscillations in membrane potential occur in the smooth muscle cells; the frequency of this myoelectrical *slow wave activity* determines the maximum rate of contraction in each region of the gut. The specific orientation of the circular and longitudinal smooth muscle layers provides a potentially infinite range of movements for intestinal segments. *'Pacemaker'* areas in the stomach, duodenum and colon are sites of specialised neuromuscular tissue which ensure that the trend of contraction in the gut is generally aboral.

The myenteric and submucosal plexuses, located between the muscle layers of the intestine, together with the neural connections to these plexuses, comprise the *enteric nervous system (ENS)*. Extrinsic nerves connecting the ENS to the central nervous system (CNS) include the sympathetic nerves travelling by the prevertebral ganglia, and parasympathetic nerves, travelling by the pelvic and vagus nerves. These anatomical arrangements provide multiple levels for control or modulation of gut motility, and also explain how CNS disturbances, as well as more local ENS influences, can produce motor dysfunction.

Regional gastrointestinal motility

The major motor functions of the stomach are to temporarily store ingested food during the process of breakdown of solids, to empty chyme appropriately into the small bowel, and to empty indigestable solids remaining in the stomach after a meal. Vagally-mediated *receptive relaxation* of the proximal stomach occurs in response to swallowing during ingestion of a meal. This prepares the proximal stomach to receive oesophageal contents, and is followed by *gastric accommodation,* whereby the proximal stomach progressively relaxes to accommodate increasing volumes, while maintaining a relatively constant intragastric pressure. Solid emptying is largely controlled by antral and pyloric motor activity. Phasic contractions sweep from the midstomach to the pylorus, at a frequency of 3/min, mixing and grinding the food until particles are approximately 1 mm in size. Emptying of liquids is controlled by co-ordinated motor activity in the fundus body and antrum. Proximal gastric tone appears to be of particular importance in liquid emptying. The pylorus is an important functional component of the gastro-duodenal region and also regulates solid and liquid emptying. The rate of gastric emptying is regulated by additional factors such as the osmolality and fat content of the meal, the amount of gastric acid secreted, and duodenal motility. Liquids empty more rapidly than solids; the time taken for half the gastric contents to empty after ingestion of a standard mixed meal is about ninety minutes for the solid phase, and about thirty minutes for the liquid phase (see Fig. 8.1).

In the small intestine, intermittent segmenting and propulsive contractions occur after ingestion of food, mixing it with digestive secretions and transporting the chyme aborally. Each propagated contraction is preceded by a propagated relaxation, a phenomenon termed the *peristaltic reflex.* The overall duration and intensity of postprandial motor activity depends upon the caloric content, and the proportion of fat, carbohydrate and protein, in the meal.

The jejunum acts primarily as a mixing and conduit segment, while the ileum, which has specialised absorptive properties, retains chyme until digestion and absorption are largely complete. The terminal ileum and ileo-colonic junction control the rate of emptying of ileal contents into the colon. Fat prolongs transit through the intestine, while fibre shortens it. In between meals, and particularly during sleep, motility in the stomach and small intestine undergoes regular cycles of activity every few hours, termed *migrating motor complexes.* These complexes migrate slowly along the small bowel, clearing away residual food and secretions.

In the colon, proximal colonic motor activity promotes the mixing of contents, absorption of water and electrolytes, and metabolism of colonic contents by bacteria. The recto-sigmoid region stores faeces and generates specific motor programs enabling convenient elimination. Contractions in the colon occur at irregular intervals; there are two main types—individual phasic contractions and high amplitude propagated contractions or *giant migrating contractions.* The latter are the major propulsive motor events in the colon, producing the so-called *mass*

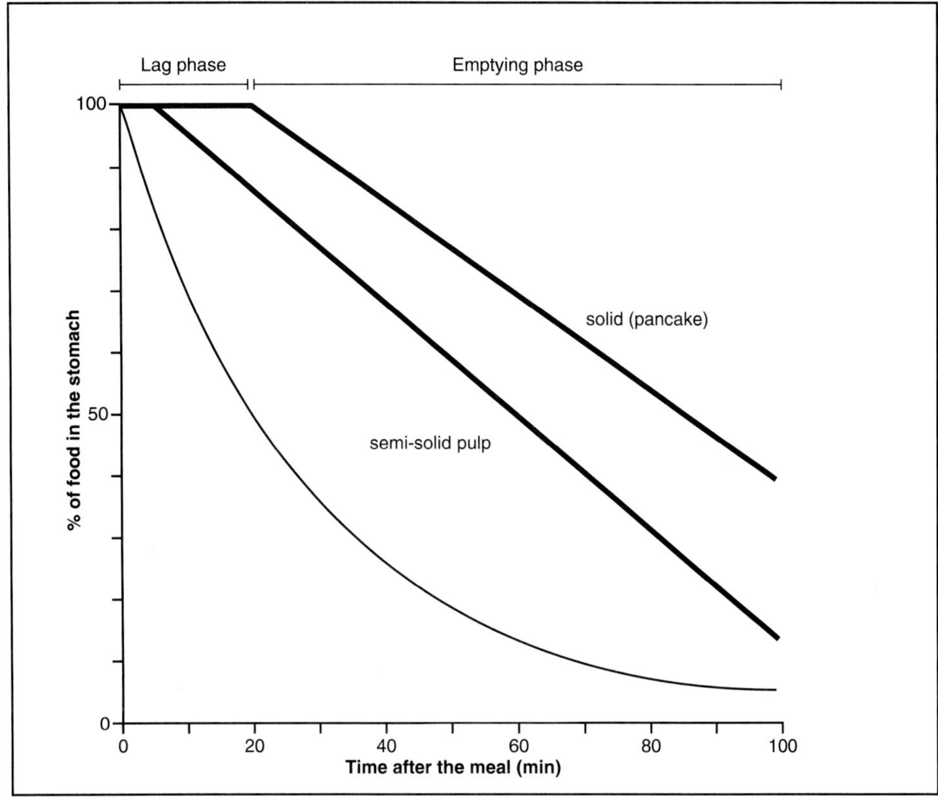

Fig. 8.1 *Gastric emptying of a liquid, semi-solid, and solid meal: normal curves. Lower curve represents liquid emptying* REPRODUCED WITH PERMISSION FROM SMOUT, AJPM AND AKKERMANNS, LMA, *NORMAL AND DISTURBED MOTILITY OF THE GASTROINTESTINAL TRACT*, WRIGHTSON BIOMEDICAL PUBLISHING LTD, PETERSFIELD, 1992, P. 96

movements. After eating, colonic motor activity and tone increases (*gastro-colic reflex*) in both the proximal and distal colon. Intestinal gas originates from three sources—the majority (about 70%) from swallowed air, a proportion from gases (carbon dioxide, hydrogen, methane, oxygen and nitrogen) produced by bacterial fermentation of incompletely absorbed food and fibre in the colon, and a very small amount by way of diffusion from the blood. On an average diet, material takes up to three days to pass through the colon, accounting for about 90% of whole gut transit time in healthy subjects.

Distension of the rectum by faeces produces relaxation of the internal anal sphincter (*recto-anal inhibitory reflex*). If defecation is to proceed, relaxation of the muscles of the pelvic floor results in perineal descent. Hip flexure, in the sitting or squatting position, produces further opening of the anorectal angle. External anal sphincter relaxation occurs voluntarily, and the rectal contents are discharged by rectal contraction and increased intra-abdominal pressure in response to a Valsalva manoeuvre. Faecal continence during micturition and the passage of flatus is maintained by contractile activity in both the anal canal and external anal sphincter.

Pathophysiology

A delay in gastric emptying of solids and/or liquids, often in association with antral hypomotility, or other regional gastric motor dysfunction, can produce symptoms of postprandial abdominal discomfort, nausea, vomiting, bloating, anorexia and early satiety; excessively rapid emptying of gastric contents, especially liquids, such as occurs after truncal vagotomy, can lead to symptoms of 'dumping'. There is not always a good correlation, however, between symptoms and altered rates of gastric emptying.

Delayed transit through the small and large intestine, and increased absorption of water can lead to symptoms of constipation and/or abdominal pain. Accelerated transit may result in diarrhoea and/or abdominal pain. Unco-ordinated or abnormally high pressure contractions may lead to distension of the intestinal lumen, or trap pockets of intestinal gas which distend the bowel and produce abdominal pain. Stools of small or 'normal' volume that are passed more frequently may result from the combined effect of rapid small bowel transit, colonic dysmotility and rectal hypersensitivity to distension.

Functional gastrointestinal disorders

Functional gastrointestinal disorders are the most common gastrointestinal disorders presenting to the practising doctor, accounting for up to 50% of consultations for digestive complaints. There are as yet no clearly defined 'organic' lesions in these disorders. In many cases, however, motor dysfunction of the stomach, small intestine, colon or anorectum appears to be crucial; it is likely that in the future the broad group of functional gastrointestinal disorders will be subdivided into more specific syndromes of motor dysfunction, possibly with specific aetiologies.

In some less common, often systemic, disorders, definite morphological abnormalities are present in the enteric nervous system or smooth muscle cells, resulting in gastrointestinal dysmotility and symptoms; however, consideration of these entities is beyond the scope of this text. A functional classification of gastrointestinal motility disorders, based on alterations in gastrointestinal transit, is shown in Table 8.1. (Oesophageal motility disorders are discussed in Chapter 1.)

Irritable bowel syndrome

Irritable bowel syndrome (IBS) is the most common of the functional gastrointestinal disorders. It is a chronic disorder characterised by disordered motor

Table 8.1 *Gastrointestinal motor disorders*

Delayed transit	*Accelerated transit*
Common	
IBS-predominant constipation	IBS-predominant diarrhoea
Aerophagy	Infectious diarrhoea
Idiopathic gastroparesis[(a)]	Duodenal ulcer disease[(a)]
Drugs, e.g. nicotine,[(a)] anticholinergics, antidepressants, iron, opiates	Drugs, e.g. laxatives (see p. 70)
Colonic diverticular disease (see p. 81)	
Pregnancy	
Diabetes mellitus[(a)]	
Uncommon or rare	
Postsurgical, e.g. adynamic ileus, vagotomy,[(a)] Roux-en-Y	Postsurgical, e.g. gastrectomy,[(a)] vagotomy, intestinal resection
'Slow transit' constipation	
Hyperthyroidism	Hyperthyroidism
Hypercalcaemia	
Scleroderma	
Anorexia nervosa/bulimia[(a)]	
Hirschsprung's disease	
Amyloidosis	
Chronic idiopathic intestinal pseudo-obstruction	

IBS = irritable bowel syndrome.
[(a)] Major motor abnormality is delayed or accelerated gastric emptying.

and/or secretory function of the gastrointestinal tract (particularly the small and large intestines), in the absence of identifiable disease. Most patients present under the age of forty years, but it can occur at any age. The ratio of women to men is more than 2:1.

Pathogenesis

The fundamental cause is unknown, but various factors have been postulated to play a role by affecting gastrointestinal sensorimotor function. Abnormalities of basal (fasting) and stimulated motility in both the large and small intestine have been reported. The primary phenomenon, however, may be sensitisation of the afferent neural pathways from the gut to the CNS, producing a heightened perception of normal gut distension and contraction. This heightened perception may then itself reflexly trigger disordered motor activity.

1. Psychological factors

Irritable bowel syndrome patients are generally more neurotic, anxious and depressed than are patients with organic gastrointestinal disorders or than the general community; whether this association is one of cause or effect remains to be determined. Acute psychological stress clearly can affect motility, but the effects of chronic stress are more difficult to assess. Psychological factors may be most important by influencing the individual's decision to seek medical attention.

2. Dietary factors

The role of diet has not yet been defined. Certain foods and/or chemicals may cause diarrhoea in some patients in an idiosyncratic, probably non-immunological fashion ('food intolerance'). Excessive ingestion of sugars, such as lactose in milk products and fructose and sorbitol in fruits and some confectionery, can provoke diarrhoea with flatulence and bloating. Low fibre intake may be important if constipation is the predominant symptom.

3. Postinfective factors

The fact that an acute attack of infectious diarrhoea can lead to symptoms of IBS well after it has subsided is well documented, and may be due to initial minor damage to the ENS. Symptoms in this type of IBS can persist for months or years.

Clinical syndromes

The cardinal symptoms are abdominal pain, diarrhoea and constipation, and these can be present in various combinations, with a course characterised by exacerbations and remissions. On the basis of symptoms, patients can often be subdivided into groups; there is some evidence that these subgroups may be pathophysiologically distinct entities, and subgroups 1 to 3 can be collectively termed the *functional bowel disorders*:

1. chronic or recurrent abdominal pain with an accompanying alteration of bowel habit (spastic colon). This is the most common subgroup, and some authorities now restrict the definition of IBS to this subgroup. Alternating diarrhoea and constipation, or a predominance of one or the other, is the usual pattern of altered bowel habit;
2. chronic painless diarrhoea (*functional diarrhoea*);
3. chronic constipation without significant abdominal pain (*functional constipation*);
4. Chronic or recurrent abdominal pain without an accompanying alteration of bowel habit (*chronic functional abdominal pain*).

The abdominal pain in IBS varies from mild to severe, is either dull or cramping in nature and is usually situated in the lower abdomen or in the periumbilical region (see Figure 9.2, p. 226). It is often eased by defecation and the passage of flatus, and may be accentuated by aerophagy (see below). In most cases, *diarrhoea* consists of loose or watery stools and associated urgency; daily stool weights are within the normal range. It usually does not waken the patient, and may occur mostly after breakfast ('morning rush syndrome'). *Constipation* consists of hard or scybalous and/or infrequent stools that may be accompanied by excessive straining. Other descriptions include pellet-like or ribbon-like stools.

Additional symptoms that make the diagnosis of IBS more likely include looser or more frequent stools at the onset of pain, a sensation of incomplete evacuation, abdominal distension or flatulence and the passage of rectal mucus.

Upper gastrointestinal symptoms, such as heartburn, nausea and early satiety are also frequent, as are symptoms of fatigue and migraine headache.

Diagnosis

This consists of awareness of the various clinical syndromes and the characteristic symptom clusters, and the exclusion of organic disease. Important features in the history include general good health, long-standing and often intermittent symptoms, and the slowness or absence of progression. Weight loss, fever, rectal bleeding, or features of steatorrhoea are not consistent with IBS. Physical examination, including rectal examination, is usually normal, although at times the colon is palpable and tender, especially in the left iliac fossa.

Further investigations will depend on the age of the patient, the length of the history, and the clinical syndrome. If the patient is over forty years of age, and symptoms are of recent onset, colonoscopy (with random mucosal biopsy) is the preferred investigation to rule out colorectal neoplasia. Other radiological studies may be necessary to exclude intermittent partial bowel obstruction.

If diarrhoea predominates, inflammatory bowel disease (especially Crohn's disease), coeliac disease, lactase deficiency, hyperthyroidism, giardiasis, purgative abuse, collagenous colitis and microscopic colitis should all be considered and excluded where appropriate. If constipation predominates, systemic disorders such as hypothyroidism, and depressive states should be excluded. In all cases, drug-induced constipation or diarrhoea must be sought (see Table 8.1).

Treatment

The major focus of therapy for all patients is a full explanation of the disorder, and reassurance of the absence of serious underlying disease, especially cancer. Mechanisms by which symptoms can arise in a structurally normal gastrointestinal tract should be described. A careful history should be aimed at identifying possible precipitating or contributing factors.

A high residue diet, that is, an increase in the intake of fibre-rich foods or the addition of unprocessed wheat bran (4–8 g/d) or one of the semi-synthetic bulking agents (e.g. methylcellulose, isphaghula husk, psyllium, sterculia) is effective in many patients, especially those with predominant constipation. In this latter group, the prolonged use of stimulant laxatives, such as senna extract, should be avoided. Lactulose or magnesium salts are often effective in restoring and maintaining a normal bowel habit. The role of novel prokinetic agents such as cisapride is yet to be determined.

For patients in whom diarrhoea is predominant, loperamide or aluminium hydroxide gel are effective. For patients with significant abdominal pain, although the precise mechanisms of action are still uncertain, antispasmodic agents may produce at least short-term improvement in abdominal pain. Such drugs usually should be employed in the short term only, and the dose adjusted to the timing and severity of symptoms. In refractory cases, a trial of low dose tricyclic antidepressant therapy may produce significant improvement in symptoms, even in the absence of overt psychological features.

Other modalities such as psychotherapy, hypnotherapy or relaxation therapy have been suggested to be helpful in IBS patients resistant to other forms of therapy, although further controlled studies are needed. With adequate treatment and follow-up, the prognosis of IBS is reasonably good; the patient may have to be encouraged, however, to live with some residual symptoms.

Aerophagy

Aerophagy strictly refers to the phenomenon of repetitive air swallowing and belching to relieve a sensation of abdominal distension or bloating. After belching, the patient may obtain some relief but soon develops the urge to repeat the process. The term is also sometimes used to describe the various syndromes that result from an apparent excess of gas within the gastrointestinal tract, where the cause is not due to obstructive gastrointestinal lesions. Some causes are:

1. *more frequent swallowing,* as is caused by chewing and drinking rapidly, chewing gum, smoking, excess salivation or a dry mouth, the presence of a naso-gastric tube or tracheostomy, or psychological factors;
2. *certain foods,* especially carbohydrates and some fruit juices and softdrinks, which may produce excess intestinal gas if incompletely absorbed in the small intestine. Specific foods such as beans and effervescent drinks are well known to result in excessive gas;
3. *malabsorption,* bacterial overgrowth of the small intestine and short bowel syndrome, which may be associated with the production of excess gas;
4. *disordered gastrointestinal motility,* which appears to play a role in some patients by preventing the normal co-ordinated propulsion of gas through the gastrointestinal tract.

In addition, in some patients with symptoms of excess gas, there may be a *heightened pain response to bowel distension,* as such patients do not appear to have greater volumes of intestinal gas than normal persons, when gas is measured by isotopic methods.

Clinical syndromes

Any of the following may dominate the symptom complex but usually several are present concurrently; an alteration of bowel habit often co-exists—part of the overlapping spectrum of irritable bowel syndrome.

1. *oesophageal belching;*
2. *abdominal distension syndrome,* resulting in epigastric discomfort and distension, worse after meals and towards the end of the day, the symptoms subsiding during the night. Acute dilatation of the stomach is a separate entity which may occur after major surgery;
3. *excess borborygmi;*

4. *splenic flexure syndrome*, that is, left hypochondrial discomfort if gas is trapped or localised in the splenic flexure region;
5. *hepatic flexure syndrome*, that is, right hypochondrial discomfort if gas is trapped or localised in the hepatic flexure region;
6. *excess rectal flatus.*

Diagnosis

This depends upon awareness of the clinical syndromes; essential features are a long and non-progressive course. Relevant organic syndromes that may cause similar discomfort, such as peptic ulcer, cholelithiasis, ischaemic heart disease and colonic disease may need to be excluded.

Treatment

The patient should be reassured of the genuine nature of his or her disability, and the mechanisms of symptoms explained. Advice should be given not to induce belching, to avoid chewing gum, drinking effervescent and softdrinks, smoking, and eating beans and certain fruits such as apples, grapes, raisins and bananas. Other carbohydrate restriction may also be helpful. Therapy for irritable bowel syndrome (see p. 217), if present, may be helpful.

With this advice the symptoms of most patients are improved; the remainder of patients live in symbiosis with what they now accept as a benign malady. There is no substantial evidence that the so-called gas absorbents and antiflatulents have a beneficial effect.

Functional (non-ulcer) dyspepsia

Dyspepsia may be defined as any form of discomfort, episodic or persistent, related or unrelated to meals, and referrable to the abdomen, in the absence of jaundice, dysphagia or gastrointestinal bleeding. Functional or non-ulcer dyspepsia may be defined as dyspepsia in which panendoscopy has excluded organic disease such as peptic ulcer, oesophagitis or malignancy, and in which clinical evaluation and basic laboratory tests have failed to reveal an obvious structural or metabolic cause for the symptoms.

In most cases, the symptoms are either due to irritable bowel syndrome or gastro-oesophageal reflux or both; a lesser proportion are due to aerophagy, and a small number due to cholelithiasis or rare disorders. In the remainder, the cause of symptoms is not well defined. It is likely, however, that disturbed upper gastrointestinal sensorimotor function is important. Delayed gastric emptying of solids and/or liquids (idiopathic gastroparesis), postprandial antral hypomotility and antroduodenal inco-ordination, gastric myoelectrical arrhythmias and dysfunction of visceral afferents are the major alterations which have been described. Chronic psychological stress may also play a role by altering upper gut motility.

Symptoms such as nausea, vomiting, early satiety and bloating, worse postprandially, and present on most days, may be a clue to the presence of gastric dysmotility, but at times episodes may be paroxysmal with marked nausea and vomiting which subsides spontaneously. Isotopic scintigraphy, using radiolabelled meals, can be used to confirm the presence of gastroparesis. If gastroparesis is present, the various secondary causes such as diabetes mellitus, connective tissue disorders, thyroid disease and the postvagotomy state should be excluded.

Management is based on reassurance of the patient of the genuine nature of his symptoms and of their benign nature. Dietary manipulation, for example, low fat, more frequent smaller meals, may be helpful. Prokinetic agents appear to be useful as short-term medical therapy in some patients. These medications may be particularly useful in patients with documented gastroparesis.

Severe idiopathic constipation

Most patients with constipation where there is no organic disease of the anus, rectum or colon, or no systemic disease associated with constipation, have either simple (primary) constipation, due to a deficiency of dietary fibre or fluid intake, or constipation associated with the irritable bowel syndrome (see p. 214). A small group, however, suffer with a far more severe form of functional constipation, sometimes termed severe idiopathic constipation or *slow transit constipation.* This disorder occurs almost exclusively in females, the onset of symptoms often dating from adolescence. Defecation may not occur spontaneously for weeks or more. Digitation of the rectum or vagina by the patient is sometimes needed to aid defecation. Barium enema reveals a normal-sized colon. Assessment of colonic transit, using radio-opaque shapes and abdominal x-ray, or radio-isotope labelling of ingested food, demonstrates a prolonged, often grossly delayed, transit time.

In addition, physiological tests of defecatory functions demonstrate disordered defecation in some patients, with paradoxical contraction of the voluntary anal sphincter occurring during straining. Treatment is difficult; osmotic laxatives such as magnesium sulphate or lactulose are usually the most effective. Suppositories or enemas are often needed to maintain an empty rectum. Surgical treatment (various forms of colectomy) may produce improvement in some patients, but a good response cannot be predicted beforehand.

Adult megacolon, where the diameter of the rectum or colon is increased on x-ray examination, is a rare disorder associated with constipation. It is due either to Hirschsprung's disease presenting for the first time in adult life, or to an inherited or acquired defect in nerve or muscle of the colonic wall (enteric neuropathy or myopathy). This latter disorder is part of the spectrum of *chronic idiopathic intestinal pseudo-obstruction.* Acquired cases may be due to the prolonged ingestion of stimulant laxatives, or associated (reversibly) with the use of antidepressant, antipsychotic, or anti-Parkinsonian drugs.

SUGGESTED FURTHER READING

Drossman, D. A., The functional gastrointestinal disorders, in Sleisenger, M. H., Fordtran, J. S., Scharschmidt, B. F., and Feldman, M. (eds), *Gastrointestinal Disease*, 5th edn, W. B. Saunders, Philadelphia, 1993.

Drossman, D. A., Thompson, W. G. and Talley, N. J. et al., Identification of subgroups of functional gastrointestinal disorders, *Gastroenterology International*, 1990; 3:159–72.

Lynn, R. B. and Friedman, L. S., Irritable bowel syndrome, *N. Engl. J. Med*, 1993;329: 1940–5.

Smout, A. J. P. M. and Akkermanns, L. M. A., *Normal and Disturbed Motility of the Gastrointestinal Tract*, Wrightson Biomedical Publishing Ltd, Petersfield, 1992.

Snape, W. J. Jr (ed.), *Pathogenesis of Functional Bowel Disease*, Plenum Publishing Corporation, New York, 1989.

Wingate, D. L., Disorders of motility, in Weatherall, D. J., Ledingham, J. G. G. and Warrell, D. A. (eds), *Oxford Textbook of Medicine*, 2nd edn, Oxford University Press, 1987.

CHAPTER 9

Common symptoms

N. D. Yeomans

Individual symptoms originating from the gastrointestinal system are dealt with under specific diseases in other chapters. Here, the common symptoms are brought together with an indication of the pathophysiological mechanisms responsible for them.

Oesophageal symptoms

The main symptoms that can arise from the oesophagus are heartburn, pain and dysphagia.

Heartburn

This is a very common symptom. The mechanism is almost certainly stimulation of mucosal pain fibres by refluxed gastric acid. The main features are:

1. discomfort in the middle of the chest, substernally;
2. usually described as 'burning' or 'acidic' in quality;
3. relieved by antacids, and aggravated by events that increase reflux (e.g. smoking, recumbency, alcohol, fatty foods).

Pain

As this is very similar in site to cardiac pain, differentiation can be difficult. The pain is central in the chest; tight, knot-like or constrictive; and may radiate to the teeth, jaws or arms. Its mechanism is usually high-pressure oesophageal contraction (spasm). It is sometimes provoked by swallowing or is associated with dysphagia—features which, if present, help in differentiating it from cardiac pain at rest.

Pain or burning discomfort during the swallowing of a bolus is termed *odynophagia*. It is commonly provoked by acid foods (e.g. orange or tomato juice) in patients with reflux oesophagitis, the pain being caused by the passage of food over the inflamed oesophagus.

Dysphagia

This is the sensation of sticking or obstruction after swallowing a bolus of food or drink. The site of hold-up may or may not be accurately identified by the patient. The mechanisms are either simple mechanical obstruction from a stricture or tumour, an arrest in the progress of the liquid or solid bolus because of disordered motility pattern (spasm, failure of lower sphincter relaxation); or neurological disease. The causes and classification of dysphagia are given in Chapter 1 (p. 4).

Abdominal symptoms

Abdominal pain

The terms used by patients to describe abdominal pain vary. Some refer to pain, others to discomfort, fullness, heartburn or indigestion. Also, individual response to pain varies: what some patients refer to as agonising pain is apparently trivial to others.

Mechanisms of production of abdominal pain

These include:

1. abnormal motility due to distension of hollow organs, obstruction or increased motility as seen in the irritable bowel syndrome (p. 214);
2. stretching of the capsules of solid viscera (e.g. the liver in hepatitis, or congestion);
3. acid and pepsin acting on nerve fibres in the base of a peptic ulcer;
4. inflammation, especially if acute;
5. malignant invasion of nerves.

The more rapidly distension is produced, the greater the pain. This is especially the case in the distension of hollow organs and the stretching of the capsules of solid viscera. Distension of the gallbladder due to cystic duct obstruction or a gallstone produces severe pain, whereas distension caused by obstruction by cancer of the head of the pancreas produces little or no pain.

Types of pain

Usually patients can tell whether pain is superficial or deep in character. Superficial pain may arise from lesions in the abdominal wall or hernial sac, but may also represent referred pain, from disease in intra-abdominal or thoracic viscera. Referred pain is usually felt in the dermatomal area corresponding to the spinal segment(s) innervating the deeper structure that gives rise to the painful afferents.

Deep pain may arise from the viscera themselves or from involvement of the parietal peritoneum (somatic pain) by the disease processes. Characteristics of these types of pain are indicated in Table 9.1.

Table 9.1 *Characteristics of different types of abdominal pain*

Viceral	*Somatic (parietal)*[a]	*Referred*[b]
Dull	Sharper or aching	Sharper or aching
Midline	Lateralised	Lateral or bilateral
Poorly localised	Roughly localised	Roughly localised to somatic dermatome
Often nausea/sweating	Worse on movement	

[a] Somatic pain indicates involvement of the peritoneum.
[b] Referred pain usually occurs when the painful stimulus in the viscera is more intense.

Characteristics of pain from different organs

Stomach and duodenum (spinal cord segments T7–T9)

Refer to Figure 9.1.

1. Site usually epigastric and midline and initially localised: may be situated to the right or left of midline and occasionally anywhere between nipple level and umbilicus (see Fig. 9.1(a)).
2. As pain becomes more severe, it becomes more diffuse anteriorly and radiates to the back to the interscapular region (i.e. T7–T9 segments) posteriorly.
3. Radiation to the back in the upper lumbar region (L1) indicates penetration of ulcer or tumour into the pancreas (see Fig. 9.1(b)).
4. Ulcer pain is often:
   (a) eased by food or antacids (or sometimes vomiting), consistent with the concept that low pH is important in its genesis in most patients;
   (b) sometimes awakens the patient at night (at about 1 am when pH is lowest);
   (c) subject to remissions and exacerbations (as ulcers heal and relapse spontaneously).

Pancreas (segment T12)

1. Pain is usually felt in the epigastrium, but may be anywhere between the nipples and inguinal ligament (see Fig. 9.1(a)).
2. Pain is usually felt posteriorly in the T12 region as well.
3. The site of pain roughly indicates the region of pancreas affected: left of midline, tail; midline, body; right of midline, head.
4. There is occasionally radiation to the shoulder tip (C3) due to involvement of the diaphragm.
5. Pain is often severe if due to pancreatitis, but may be mild.

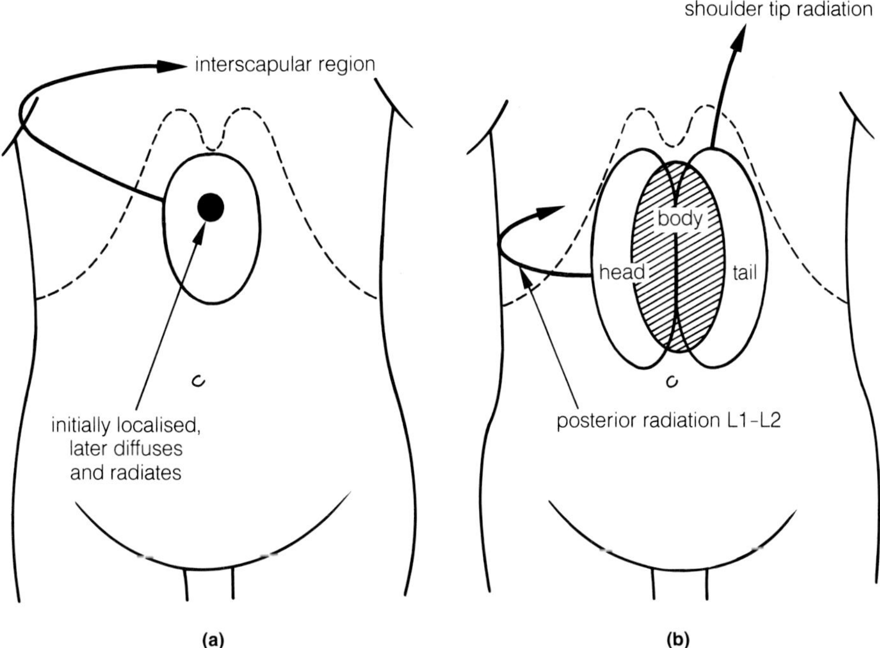

Fig. 9.1 *Localisation of* **(a)** *gastric or duodenal ulcer pain,* **(b)** *pancreatic pain*

Biliary tree (segments T6–T10, chiefly T9)

Biliary pain:

1. is located in the midline in epigastrium (see Fig. 9.2(a));
2. radiates to the right scapular, and interscapular region in T9 segment;
3. is usually constant, and of rapid onset and severe if due to gallstones;
4. tenderness develops in the right hypochondrium if the gallbladder becomes inflamed (Fig. 9.2(a)).

Small intestine (segment T10)

1. Pain is usually central (periumbilical).
2. Pain is colicky if due to obstruction, but otherwise constant (inflammation, irritable bowel syndrome).
3. Pain may lateralise if the parietal peritoneum is involved.

Colon (segments T8–T12)

1. Pain is usually lower abdominal and central.
2. Often the segment of colon involved cannot be predicted, but sometimes it can: for example, ascending colon, to right of umbilicus; transverse and sigmoid, hypogastrium; descending colon, to left of umbilicus; rectum, over sacrum (Fig. 9.2(b)).

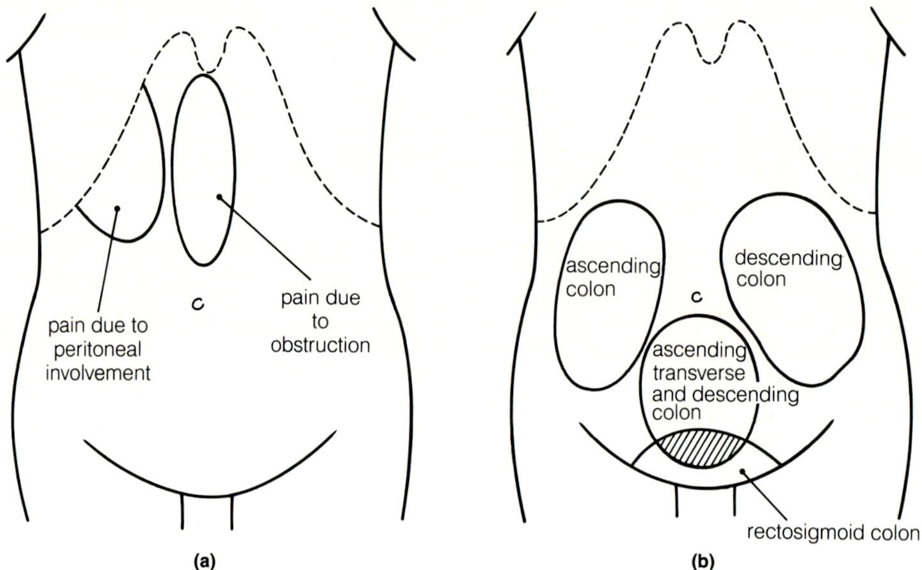

Fig. 9.2 *Localisation of* **(a)** *biliary pain,* **(b)** *colonic pain*

3. Pain may be eased by defecation or passage of flatus.
4. Pain may be colicky.
5. There may be other pointers to colonic disease (e.g. passage of blood or mucus).

Guiding principles in diagnosis of abdominal pain

Acute abdominal pain ('acute abdomen')

1. Detailed history and examination (including rectal exam and often pelvic exam) should be performed.
2. Body temperature and white cell count are helpful (but not always reliable) as indicators of infection/inflammation.
3. Serum amylase should help exclude acute pancreatitis (p. 112).
4. Plain x-ray should be taken to exclude perforated ulcer or intestinal obstruction (p. 26).
5. Microurine should help exclude renal disease.
6. Remember that one of the most common causes of acute abdomen is acute appendicitis.
7. If in doubt, review history and signs in two hours when results of tests should be available.
8. If still in doubt, operate.

Chronic abdominal pain

1. By detailed history, define the organ and disease process most probably involved.
2. By appropriate diagnostic tests, exclude or confirm the likely diagnoses.
3. If still no diagnosis, consult with colleagues.
4. If still in doubt, see and investigate during an acute exacerbation of symptoms.
5. Be mindful of the fact that:
   (a) pain is almost never purely psychogenic, but malingering may be encountered;
   (b) chronic pain may have a devastating psychological effect;
   (c) relief from a placebo injection occurs in 30% of patients with organic pain syndromes;
   (d) most cases of obscure chronic abdominal pain are ultimately found to be due to the irritable bowel syndrome or similar motility disturbances.
6. Utilise, as appropriate, ultrasonography and CT scanning.
7. Ultimately, check for rare causes listed in major textbooks. (In patients with chronic abdominal pain, if a diagnosis cannot be made using available techniques, laparotomy almost invariably yields no diagnosis.)

Dyspepsia

Dyspepsia is very common. In a recent population study it was found to be by far the most common gastrointestinal symptom in adults, and was exceeded only by backache, tiredness and irritability.

Dyspepsia is defined as any pain, discomfort or nausea referable to the upper alimentary tract, which may be intermittent or continuous, related or unrelated to meals, has been present for longer than one month, is not precipitated by exertion, and is not relieved within five minutes by rest. Patients with jaundice, dysphagia or bleeding are excluded.

Non-ulcer dyspepsia This is defined as dyspepsia in which clinical evaluation and basic laboratory tests fail to reveal an obvious structural cause for the symptoms, and in which panendoscopy has excluded acute or chronic peptic ulceration, oesophagitis and malignancy. This broad definition includes patients with symptoms of gastro-oesophageal reflux, but without macroscopic oesophagitis or other definable disorders such as cholelithiasis and the essential dyspepsia subgroup. The common causes of non-ulcer dyspepsia are the irritable bowel syndrome (p. 214), oesophageal reflux (p. 2, 7) and aerophagy (p. 218). Gallstones are a rare cause (p. 175). About 25% of cases have no cause, and are classified as essential dyspepsia (p. 228).

Essential dyspepsia This is defined as non-ulcer dyspepsia in which biliary tract disease has been excluded radiologically, irritable bowel syndrome and gastro-oesophageal reflux have been excluded by objective clinical criteria, and there is no evidence of other gastrointestinal diseases that would explain the dyspepsia. As it remains uncertain whether chronic gastritis, duodenitis or both cause dyspepsia, patients with these mucosal lesions are included in this group. The term 'essential' is provisionally used in a fashion analogous to its use in describing hypertension without demonstrable cause.

Aetiology

Smoking and the ingestion of alcohol, coffee, tea, aspirin and antiarthritic drugs, and psychosomatic factors are not convincingly associated with dyspepsia. Anticholinergic drugs, on the other hand, relax the lower oesophageal sphincter, and can cause reflux and dyspepsia. Included in this group are not only conventional anticholinergic drugs, but also drugs such as the tricyclic antidepressants and antihistamines.

Those who should be investigated at initial presentation include:

- patients over forty years of age;
- patients with severe symptoms, especially if not previously investigated;
- patients with other significant symptoms or signs (e.g. weight loss, fever, night pain, periodicity of pain or abdominal mass);
- patients with abnormal screening laboratory investigations (e.g. anaemia, elevated ESR).

Diarrhoea and constipation

Definition of these terms is difficult as the normal pattern varies enormously; defecation can occur twenty-three times daily to two times weekly. What matters clinically is a change in the bowel movement pattern, because this may be the first sign of an organic disease. Diarrhoea is said to be present when the motions become unduly frequent or soft, constipation when the motions become unduly hard or infrequent. Normal stool volume is 1000 mL(g) per day; so that a working definition for diarrhoea, for use when patients are on a bowel chart while being investigated in hospital, is that diarrhoea exists if stool output is more than 300 g per day.

Diarrhoea

Pathophysiologically, diarrhoea can be divided into four groups.

1. In *osmotic diarrhoea*, unabsorbed or unabsorbable solutes retain water as they progress down the gut lumen—as when saline purgatives are used, in general malabsorption (p. 46), or in selective malabsorption such as lactase deficiency (p. 52).

2. In *secretory diarrhoea*, the small and/or large intestine, instead of absorbing water and electrolytes, switches to net secretion (see Fig. 4.1, p. 73). This reversal of function may be induced by such agents as bacterial toxins, anthroquinolone purgatives, prostaglandins. In the colon, malabsorbed bile acids or fatty acids are potent inducers of secretory diarrhoea. The mechanism of action is by stimulation of cyclic-AMP in the intestinal mucosa cell. The diarrhoea is often profuse and watery, and persists when the patient fasts.
3. The third kind, *exudative diarrhoea*, is seen in mucosal inflammation (e.g. ulcerative colitis or neoplasms), where there is an outpouring of serum, blood and mucus.
4. Finally, *altered intestinal motility* is seen in hyperthyroidism, carcinoid syndrome and irritable bowel syndrome.

The pathophysiological classification, however, is not very useful in many clinical circumstances, as several mechanisms may be involved: for example, in Crohn's disease there may be an osmotic diarrhoea due to malabsorption, an exudative diarrhoea due to inflammation, and increased motility stimulated by a high volume load caused by the osmotic and exudative mechanisms. When a patient with chronic diarrhoea is seen, it is often practical to note, in order, the answers to the following questions:

1. Is evidence of inflammatory bowel disease present (e.g. exudative diarrhoea characterised by the passage of blood and mucus)?
2. Is evidence of malabsorption present (e.g. anaemia, vitamin B or folic acid deficiency)?
3. Is there a history of current or past drug ingestion (i.e. antacids, antibiotics)?
4. Is there evidence of systemic disease (e.g. thyrotoxicosis, carcinoid syndrome)?
5. Is the diarrhoea severe (e.g. incontinence, night diarrhoea)? (If severe, it is more likely to be organic.)

The initial steps in the diagnosis include sigmoidoscopy: if the bowel is inflamed, it is investigated as stated earlier, with microscopy for pathogens, culture and biopsy. If melanosis coli is present, purgative abuse is probably the cause. If sigmoidoscopy is normal, the other causes are investigated and excluded *seriatim*. A low serum potassium level suggests laxative abuse (p. 70), but it may be caused by other diarrhoeal states.

The common causes of chronic diarrhoea are irritable bowel syndrome, inflammatory bowel disease, drug-induced diarrhoea and, in many countries, *Giardia lamblia* infestation (p. 188).

Constipation

Constipation, like diarrhoea, may be acute or chronic. The essential feature is reduction of the water content of the faeces, which is usually secondary to slow transit. Acute constipation may complicate any illness, including acute inflammatory intra-abdominal disease (e.g. acute appendicitis), the confinement of a patient to bed or the administration of drugs (e.g. analgesics, narcotics, antacids).

Chronic constipation may be caused by:

1. local intestinal disease (e.g. painful perianal disease), intestinal tumours, focal inflammatory disease such as diverticulitis, descending perineum syndrome (p. 102);
2. chronic disorders of motility, as in the irritable bowel syndrome, intestinal pseudo-obstruction (p. 114);
3. systemic disease, such as depressive states, hypothyroidism, hyperparathyroidism, porphyria and diabetes mellitus;
4. drugs such as aluminium-containing antacids, anticholinergic drugs (including tricyclic antidepressants), opiates, analgesics and hypotensive agents;
5. neurogenic causes, such as diseases of the spinal cord, peripheral nerves, plexuses within the intestinal wall (Hirschsprung's disease).

As in the case of diarrhoea, investigations depend upon age, duration and cause of the symptoms. Sigmoidoscopy is always indicated in chronic constipation and, if in the cancer age group, barium enema examination or colonoscopy may also be indicated. Systemic disease and drug-related causes should be considered before embarking on extensive and expensive investigations.

Miscellaneous symptoms

Nausea and vomiting

While these can be provoked by a variety of non-gastroenterological mechanisms, which act directly on the brain stem vomiting centre or chemoreceptor trigger zone, they often arise from afferent stimulation that originates in the upper gut. Major local stimuli are:

1. gut obstruction (either mechanical or motility disorder);
2. inflammation (e.g. gastroenteritis, peptic ulcer);
3. luminal irritants (e.g. alcohol, copper sulphate).

Vomiting may also be a symptom of acute pancreatitis or acute biliary tract disease (e.g. biliary colic).

Flatulence and bloating

These common symptoms often go together. Flatulence refers to the patient's perception that he or she is passing excessive flatus or belching more than normal. Bloating refers to abdominal distension, either real or perceived.

On average, the human gut contains about 100 mL of gas at any one time. The major gases are nitrogen, oxygen, carbon dioxide, hydrogen and methane; trace amounts of other gases are responsible for the characteristic odours of flatus.

Increased belching is usually due to excessive swallowing of air (aerophagy). At times this seems to become a habit, and patients may be able to be trained out of it, but the pathophysiology is not well understood. Some patients genuinely produce excessive flatus. There are some indications that this is a consequence of having more gas-producing flora in their gut. Food composition is also important: beans and high-fibre diets are good substrates for colonic bacteria and increase flatulence.

Bloating may be due to an increased gas content in the gut. It is an important symptom of partial or complete bowel obstruction, and this diagnosis should be considered, especially if the onset is abrupt and there is associated vomiting and/or constipation. Bloating is also a very common symptom in the irritable bowel syndrome. There is controversy over whether this is really due to more gas in the intestine (perhaps compartmentalised differently because of segments of spasming gut) or whether the bloating is merely due to an accentuated lumbar lordosis, perhaps in an attempt to reduce abdominal wall pressure on tender bowel.

Jaundice

Classifications of jaundice have changed as knowledge and technology have advanced. A classification based on bilirubin metabolism divides jaundice according to whether the bilirubin is:

1. predominantly unconjugated (lesions occurring before hepatic microsomal conjugation of bilirubin with glucuronide); or
2. predominantly conjugated (lesions occurring after conjugation) (see Fig. 9.3).

Unconjugated hyperbilirubinaemia is characterised by the absence of bilirubin in the urine—sometimes with excess urobilinogen—and normal values for liver enzymes in serum. The most common causes are haemolytic disorders (increased bilirubin production) and Gilbert's syndrome (reduced hepatocyte uptake/conjugation of bilirubin) (see p. 173).

Conjugated hyperbilirubinaemia reflects liver dysfunction, either hepatocellular (characterised by jaundice, bilirubinuria, pale stools, malaise, moderately or markedly raised serum transaminase levels) or cholestatic due to stasis of bile flow (characterised by jaundice, pale stools, bilirubinuria, pruritus and raised serum levels of hepatic alkaline phosphatase, bile salts and cholesterol) (see p. 178). The serum transaminase level reflects the extent of continued cell

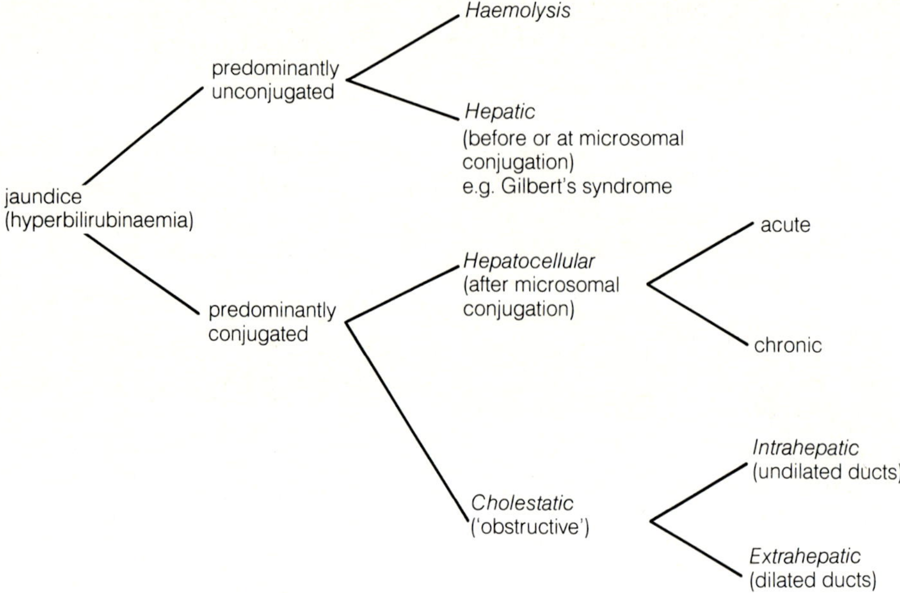

Fig. 9.3 *The causes and classification of jaundice*

damage, and in inactive cirrhosis the level may be normal or only slightly elevated.

Cholestasis may result from the interference of bile flow anywhere distal to the microsomal conjugating enzymes within the hepatocyte. Extrahepatic causes include gallstones, bile duct stricture and carcinoma. Extrahepatic cholestasis is usually associated with hepatomegaly and dilated bile ducts, whereas with intrahepatic cholestasis the liver size is variable but bile ducts are of normal size.

Diagnosis

With modern technology, especially organ imaging, the specific diagnosis of the causes of jaundice has been greatly simplified; however, the importance of a careful history and physical examination with the intelligent assessment of laboratory tests cannot be stressed too strongly. The inappropriate use of multiple diagnostic procedures often leads to misinterpretation, potential risks and unnecessary expense. A flow chart for the diagnosis of causes of jaundice is given in Figure 9.4, and the specific diagnostic techniques are discussed in more detail on p. 177.

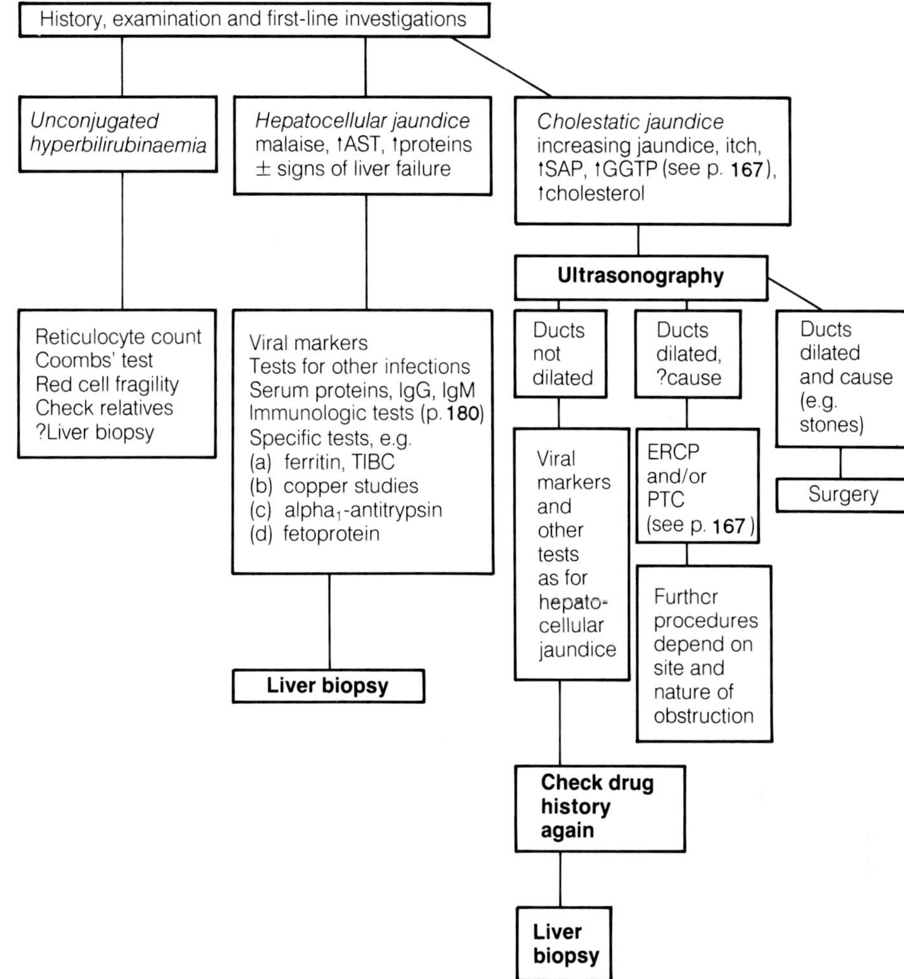

Fig. 9.4 *Diagnosis of the jaundiced patient*

SUGGESTED FURTHER READING

Gazzard, B. and Theodossi, A. (guest eds), Symptoms in gastroenterology, in *Clinics in Gastroenterology*, Vol. 14, No. 3, W. B. Saunders, London, 1985.

Sleisenger, M. H. and Fordtran, J. S., *Gastrointestinal Disease: Pathophysiology, Diagnosis and Management*, 5th edn, W. B. Saunders, Philadelphia, 1993.

Self-assessment workbook: questions

CHAPTER 1

Mouth, pharynx and oesophagus

Question 1

A fifty-year-old woman complains of a lower retrosternal and epigastric pain, ill-defined in character, but noticeably worse after eating a large meal and aggravated also by stooping or lying flat. It is associated sometimes with regurgitation of gastric contents into the mouth and recently with increasing dysphagia. Physical examination reveals the presence of obesity but no other abnormality. Investigation shows that there is a microcytic hypochromic anaemia. The most likely diagnosis is:

1. achalasia of the oesophagus
2. gastric ulceration with incompetence of the lower oesophageal sphincter
3. sideropenic dysphagia (Plummer-Vinson syndrome)
4. reflux oesophagitis
5. rolling hiatus hernia

Answer: *Text ref. pp. 7, 10*

Question 2

Which of the following therapeutic measures often improve(s) symptoms associated with a sliding hiatus hernia?

1. weight reduction
2. elevation of the head of the bed at night
3. cessation of smoking
4. metoclopramide
5. iron therapy

Answer: *Text ref. pp. 10, 12*

Question 3

The initial treatment of choice for achalasia of the oesophagus is:

1. anti-cholinergic drugs
2. sedation
3. passage of a bougie
4. pneumatic dilation of the lower oesophageal sphincter
5. bethanechol

Answer: *Text ref. p. 13*

Question 4

Which of the following is/are causally associated with recurrent aphthous ulcers of the mouth?

1. coeliac disease
2. iron-deficiency anaemia
3. Crohn's disease of the colon
4. oral candidiasis (moniliasis)
5. corticosteroid therapy

Answer: *Text ref. pp. 53, 59, 79*

Question 5

A forty-six-year-old patient presents with progressive dysphagia and heartburn over five years; the dysphagia has become almost complete. A history consistent with peptic ulcer has been present for ten years and one uncle died after a haematemesis. The most likely diagnosis is:

1. peptic ulcer of the oesophagus
2. 'Barrett's oesophagus'
3. peptic oesophagitis and stricture
4. cancer of the oesophagus
5. a large, rolling hiatus hernia

Answer: *Text ref. pp. 8, 9, 10, 15*

Question 6

Large rolling hiatus hernia without reflux may be causally related to which of the following?

1. heartburn
2. oesophageal stricture
3. pain in epigastrium
4. dyspnoea
5. macrocytic anaemia

Answer: *Text ref. pp. 5, 10, 222*

Question 7

Which of the following is/are causally related to achalasia?

1. stress
2. gastric stasis
3. increased sensitivity of the lower oesophageal sphincter to gastrin
4. reflux oesophagitis
5. loss of ganglion cells in the body of oesophagus

Answer: *Text ref. pp. 7, 12*

Question 8

A patient presents with symptoms suggestive of oesophageal reflux which have been present intermittently for ten years. Which of the following would make you suspect oesophagitis and request endoscopic examination?

1. the presence of dysphagia
2. a long history
3. the presence of a coexisting gastric ulcer
4. weight loss
5. retrosternal pain waking the patient up at night

Answer: *Text ref. pp. 4, 8, 222*

Question 9

Which of the following is/are true concerning carcinoma of the oesophagus?

1. It is more common in the lower third than in the upper third of the oesophagus.
2. An adenocarcinoma may arise in the columnar epithelium in the oesophagus.
3. Alcohol and cigarette-smoking are predisposing factors.
4. Haematemesis is the usual predisposing factor.
5. Weight loss is uncommon.

Answer: *Text ref. p. 15*

Question 10

Oral lesions, if persistent, should lead the astute clinician to the possibility of a systemic disease. Which of the following lesions is/are correctly matched with the corresponding systemic disease?

1. glossitis—vitamin B12 deficiency
2. oral pigmentation—Peutz-Jeghers syndrome (hereditary intestinal polyposis)
3. Koplik's spots—Addison's disease
4. hyperplastic gingivitis—phenytoin therapy
5. aphthous ulcers—scleroderma

Answer: *Text ref. p. 3*

Question 11

Of the following, which is/are causes of dysphagia?

1. oesophageal webs
2. hiatus hernia of rolling type
3. Schatzki ring
4. bronchial cancer
5. microcytic anaemia

Answer: *Text ref. pp. 4–7*

Question 12

Endoscopy is usually preferred to barium swallow examination for the definitive diagnosis of oesophageal disorders. Which of the following lesions is best diagnosed by barium swallow?

1. sliding hiatus hernia
2. Schatzki ring
3. oesophageal webs
4. oesophageal stricture
5. Mallory-Weiss tear

Answer: *Text ref. pp. 10, 14*

CHAPTER 2

Stomach and duodenum

Question 1

The pain of peptic ulcer is due to:

1. spasm
2. gastric distension
3. acid and pepsin acting on the nerve fibres in the base of the ulcer
4. a high acid secretory rate
5. oesophageal reflux

Answer: *Text ref. p. 22–5*

Question 2

A patient aged forty years has had his duodenal ulcer healed with H^2-receptor antagonists. What plan of treatment is indicated in his long-term management, albeit initially?

1. intermittent therapy
2. cimetidine maintenance therapy
3. Billroth I gastrectomy
4. maintenance therapy with colloidal bismuth suspension
5. highly selective vagotomy

Answer: *Text ref. p. 28*

Question 3

The usual indications for surgery in chronic duodenal ulcer in a person over fifty years of age are:

1. large ulcer
2. complications not responsive to medical measures
3. slow healing of initial ulcer
4. fear of malignancy
5. frequent attacks of ulcer dyspepsia

Answer: *Text ref. p. 29*

Question 4

Surgery is indicated in the emergency treatment of a bleeding chronic gastric ulcer if:

1. the patient is over sixty years of age;
2. the ulcer is chronic;
3. the bleeding is recurrent or continuous;
4. the patient has had severe disability from the ulcer;
5. a coexistent chronic duodenal ulcer is present.

Answer: *Text ref. p. 30*

Question 5

Gastric ulcer can be distinguished from duodenal ulcer by the fact that:

1. pain is always after meals in duodenal ulcer;
2. vomiting is less common in duodenal ulcer patients;
3. the response to treatment is more prompt in duodenal ulcer;
4. the age of onset is earlier in duodenal ulcer;
5. none of the above.

Answer: *Text ref. p. 25*

Question 6

Which of the following statements is/are correct regarding chronic gastritis?

1. In autoimmune chronic gastritis, the antrum is not involved.
2. In type B, the body of the stomach is not involved.
3. Environmental gastritis is multifocal and diffuse.
4. Type A gastritis is a premalignant condition.
5. Intestinal metaplasia is not seen in autoimmune and environmental gastritis.

Answer: *Text ref. p. 34*

Question 7

Which of the following increase the risk of gastric cancer?

1. atrophic gastritis

2. a close family history of gastric cancer
3. a small, pedunculated polyp
4. membership of certain racial groups
5. the presence of gastric ulcer

Answer: *Text ref. pp. 26, 35*

Question 8

Radiology is an unreliable way to diagnose chronic duodenal ulcer because:

1. it is difficult to fill the duodenum with barium;
2. scarring from previous ulceration may leave the duodenum deformed, and this deformity is indistinguishable from the deformity due to an active ulcer;
3. it is difficult to distinguish the prepyloric gastric ulcer from the duodenal ulcer;
4. cancer is common in the duodenum and can cause deformity that is indistinguishable from the deformity due to an ulcer;
5. the barium does not adhere well to the duodenal mucosal wall.

Answer: *Text ref. p. 21–5*

Question 9

A patient with a known gastric ulcer is found to have gastric cancer. Which of the following explanations is/are likely to be correct?

1. The ulcer underwent malignant change.
2. There was an error in diagnosis, an ulcerating cancer being confused with a benign gastric ulcer.
3. If there is coexistent duodenal ulcer, the risk of gastric cancer is increased.
4. Gastric cancer is more common in patients with gastric ulcer than would be expected by chance.
5. With modern diagnostic procedures the differentiation of ulcer from cancer is almost 100% accurate.

Answer: *Text ref. p. 26*

Question 10

A patient with pernicious anaemia diagnosed fifteen years previously presents with epigastric discomfort and anaemia. She has received vitamin B12 injections every four weeks since diagnosis, and her last haemoglobin concentration six months ago was 137 g/L. On this occasion the haemoglobin concentration is 98 g/L and x-ray examination after barium meal shows a prepyloric gastric ulcer which appears benign. Which of the following statements is/are relevant to this patient?

1. If the diagnosis of pernicious anaemia was correct, the diagnosis of benign gastric ulcer is wrong.

2. The treatment of her pernicious anaemia resulted in a return of acid secretion and subsequent peptic ulcer.
3. The diagnostic criteria for pernicious anaemia should be reviewed.
4. The more recent anaemia was due to blood loss and not to vitamin B12 deficiency.
5. The next step in the diagnosis is gastric biopsy.

Answer: *Text ref. pp. 22, 35*

Question 11

A sixty-seven-year-old patient presents with a two-year history of ulcer-like dyspepsia, and barium meal shows an apparently benign gastric ulcer which a gastroscopy performed at a provincial hospital confirms. Relevant to the patient's diagnosis, which of the following statements is/are correct?

1. The patient has a 10% chance of having an ulcerating gastric cancer.
2. The patient should be assessed by his or her response to a period of medical treatment based on the assumption that the ulcer is benign.
3. Gastric biopsy should be performed.
4. If cancer is present, the biopsy, in skilled hands, will be indicative of cancer in 95–99% of cases.

Answer: *Text ref. pp. 19, 26, 36*

Question 12

The following points have to be considered in a patient with duodenal ulcer refractory to H_2-receptor blocker:

1. heavy smoking
2. excessive use of alcohol
3. excessive use of spicy foods
4. the possibility of carcinoma
5. the possibility of gastrinoma

Answer: *Text ref. pp. 22, 28, 124*

Question 13

Which of the following is/are an indication for surgery for duodenal ulcer?

1. nocturnal pain
2. remission and exacerbations
3. radiation of the pain to the back
4. no relief by H_2-receptor blocker
5. none of the above

Answer: *Text ref. p. 28*

Question 14

Which of the following statements on ulcer epidemiology are correct?

1. Gastric ulcers occur in body mucosa.
2. Duodenal ulcer is more common than gastric ulcer.
3. Ulcer disease seems to be increasing in frequency in most parts of the world in association with a rise in living standards.
4. Gastric ulcer patients tend to be older than duodenal ulcer patients.
5. Duodenal ulcer may be associated with excessive NSAID intake.

Answer: *Text ref. p. 21–3*

Question 15

Concerning peptic ulcer disease, which of the following statements is/are correct?

1. Hunger often brings on ulcer pain.
2. Acute stress may cause ulcer.
3. Ulcers are a common cause of chronic blood loss.
4. Smoking delays ulcer healing.
5. Co-morbidity influences ulcer death rates.

Answer: *Text ref. pp. 24, 32*

Question 16

Regarding gastritis:

1. The diagnosis involves gastric biopsy.
2. Endoscopic gastritis causes symptoms in 80% of cases.
3. Histological gastritis causes symptoms in 80% of cases.
4. Acute ulcers can cause major gastrointestinal haemorrhage.
5. Acute ulcers often result from the use of anti-inflammatory drugs.

Answer: *Text ref. p. 24, 33, 34*

Question 17

A patient has recently returned from the Far East and for the first time in his life has complained of diarrhoea. He inquires whether this could be due to omeprazole which he is taking for a refractory duodenal ulcer. Which of the following statements are correct in explaining this patient's problem?

1. Omeprazole is a powerful anti-secretory agent.
2. The anacidity induced by omeprazole may lead to an increased risk of gastro-intestinal infections due to the absence of the sterilising effect of acid gastric juice.
3. Other causes of a hyposecretory state include pernicious anaemia and following gastric resection.

4. In any patient who has ulcer dyspepsia and diarrhoea, one must exclude the ingestion of magnesium-containing antacids as a cause of his diarrhoea.
5. All of the above statements are correct.

Answer: *Text ref. pp. 20, 21, 27*

Question 18

The rate of gastric emptying is relevant to the time of action of certain drugs. Which of the following statements are correct?

1. Gastric emptying is slowed by non-isotonic fluids.
2. As a rule, liquids empty from the stomach more rapidly than solids.
3. The half-life of liquids in the stomach is approximately twenty minutes and that of a mixed meal approximately 100 minutes.
4. The major determinant of gastric emptying is the activity of the peristaltic waves of the gastric antrum.
5. All of the above statements are correct.

Answer: *Text ref. pp. 18, 19*

CHAPTER 3

Small intestine

Question 1

Concerning intestinal fluid and electrolyte absorption, which of the following statements is/are true?

1. The colon is the major site of water reabsorption in the intestinal tract.
2. In the jejunum, passive water flow created by monosaccharide absorption is the major mechanism for water and sodium absorption.
3. The small intestine has a mechanism for sodium absorption that is stimulated by actively transported glucose and amino acids.
4. About 7–9 L of fluid enter the intestinal tract every twenty-four hours.
5. The normal adult stool volume is about 500 mL.

Answer: *Text ref. pp. 39–45, 68*

Question 2

Concerning dietary fats and their digestion, which of the following statements is/are correct?

1. Fats represent up to 50% of the caloric intake in the Western diet.
2. About 50% of dietary fat comprises long-chain triglycerides.
3. Cholesterol and fat-soluble vitamins require bile salts for adequate absorption.

4. Specialised carrier proteins transport fatty acids and monoglyceride across the intestinal epithelial cell membrane.
5. Triglycerides are resynthesised from fatty acids and monoglyceride in the intestinal epithelial cell.

Answer: *Text ref. p. 41*

Question 3

Which of the following statements is/are true about digestion?

1. Carbohydrates are digested in the intestinal lumen by pancreatic amylase into monosaccharides.
2. Brush border peptidases hydrolyse oligopeptides into amino acids, dipeptides and tripeptides.
3. Hydrolysis of long-chain triglycerides into fatty acids and monoglyceride is essential for their absorption.
4. Cholecystokinin induces an enzyme-rich pancreatic secretion.
5. Cholecystokinin causes the gallbladder to contract, releasing its bile salts and phospholipids into the duodenum.

Answer: *Text ref. pp. 41–8*

Question 4

Which of the following statements is/are true about bile salts?

1. They are reabsorbed by sodium-coupled active transport in the terminal ileum.
2. The total bile salt pool is about 2–4 g.
3. The total bile salt pool circulates through the enterohepatic circulation four to twelve times per day.
4. About 5% of the bile salt pool is lost with each enterohepatic circulation.
5. Bile salt secretion is increased in haemolytic anaemia.

Answer: *Text ref. pp. 41–6, Fig. 3.5*

Question 5

You are consulted by a twenty-one-year-old man who was diagnosed and treated for coeliac disease in childhood. A small bowel biopsy at the age of five years revealed a flat mucosa (subtotal villous atrophy), but the biopsy returned to normal appearance after twelve months of dietary gluten exclusion. For the past eight years he has eaten a normal diet and has remained asymptomatic and well in all respects. Which of the following abnormalities might you expect to find?

1. an abnormal result on ^{14}C-glycine bile acid breath test
2. an abnormal result on jejunal biopsy
3. an abnormal D-xylose excretion
4. a low plasma vitamin B12 assay
5. a low serum folate assay

Answer: *Text ref. pp. 46–50*

Question 6

In isolated intestinal lactase deficiency:

1. an increase in blood glucose of less than 1.5 mmol/L occurs after ingestion of 100 g of lactose;
2. steatorrhoea is commonly found;
3. the histology of intestinal mucosa is normal;
4. there is an increased prevalence in Asians;
5. galactose absorption is normal.

Answer: *Text ref. pp. 50, 52*

Question 7

Excessive loss of serum protein into the gut may occur in which of the following diseases?

1. nephrotic syndrome
2. regional enteritis (Crohn's disease)
3. gastric cancer
4. coeliac disease
5. ulcerative colitis

Answer: *Text ref. p. 63*

Question 8

As a result of internal injuries received in a car accident, a thirty-year-old woman has 100 cm of lower ileum removed, including the ileocaecal valve. Which of the following statements is/are correct?

1. Colonic bacteria will probably proliferate in the small intestine.
2. Prophylactic therapy with iron and folic acid should be given.
3. A Schilling test will give abnormal results.
4. A bile acid breath test will give normal results.
5. Watery diarrhoea is likely to occur.

Answer: *Text ref. pp. 39, 44, 47, 49, 51*

Question 9

Surgical resection of the terminal ileum will significantly reduce the absorption of which of the following?

1. iron
2. vitamin B12
3. folic acid
4. bile salts
5. vitamin C

Answer: *Text ref. pp. 39 (Fig. 3.1), 46 (Fig. 3.5)*

Question 10

A fifty-five-year-old home worker complains of diarrhoea of six months' duration. The stools have been loose, watery and without blood. She has also suffered from recurrent lower abdominal pain, which is frequently worse after meals, and has lost 5 kg in weight during this time. Physical examination reveals a slightly tender, ill-defined mass in the right iliac fossa, but no other abnormality. Rectal examination and sigmoidoscopy are normal. Which of the following diagnoses is/are likely in this patient?

1. carcinoma of the ascending colon
2. Meckel's diverticulum
3. Whipple's disease
4. Crohn's disease of the terminal ileum
5. diverticulosis of the small intestine

Answer: *Text ref. pp. 59, 79*

Question 11

Which of the following statements is/are true of medium-chain triglycerides (MCTs)?

1. They are absorbed intact by small bowel mucosa in significant amounts.
2. They are rapidly hydrolysed by pancreatic lipase to glycerol and free medium-chain fatty acids.
3. The medium-chain fatty acids are absorbed via lymphatics after re-esterification to MCTs in the mucosal cell.
4. They are water-soluble, unlike most dietary triglycerides.
5. They are an appropriate dietary supplement following massive intestinal resection.

Answer: *Text ref. pp. 43, 46, 57, 58*

CHAPTER 4

Colon, rectum and anus

Question 1

Compare Crohn's disease of colon with ulcerative colitis considering the following features:

Features	Crohn's colitis	Ulcerative colitis
1. Small intestine involvement		
2. Rectal disease (nature and frequency)		
3. Anal lesions		
4. Histological findings		
5. Colonic cancer as complication		
6. Barium enema findings		
7. Response to drug treatment		
8. Surgical treatment		

Answer: *Text ref. pp. 59, 79*

Question 2

A twenty-five-year-old woman is admitted to hospital after two weeks of severe bloody diarrhoea. She was treated for five days with amoxycillin for a respiratory infection three to four weeks before onset of symptoms. Her weight has fallen by 13 kg, and she has a peripheral blood haemoglobin of 90 g/L, tachycardia (120/min) and fever (39.5°C). Abdominal examination reveals tenderness over the colon and some abdominal distension. Sigmoidoscopy shows a friable, oedematous mucosa throughout the rectum. Which of the following investigations are required urgently?

1. barium enema
2. plain x-ray of the abdomen
3. serum electrolytes
4. stool microscopy and culture
5. stool examination for *C. difficile* toxin
6. colonoscopy

Answer: *Text ref. pp. 72, 197, 198*

Question 3

Which of the following statements are true regarding the use of sulphasalazine in the treatment of chronic idiopathic colitis?

1. In the acute attacks it is less effective than corticosteroids.
2. Its chief use is in the prevention of relapses in the maintenance therapy of chronic ulcerative colitis.
3. The active constituent is 5-aminosalicylic acid, which is formed from the parent compound by bacterial action in the colon.
4. It is more effective in Crohn's disease than in idiopathic ulcerative colitis.
5. In acute attacks it carries the risk of precipitating toxic megacolon.

Answer: *Text ref. pp. 72, 197, 198, 219*

Question 4

An eighty-four-year-old woman has had a myocardial infarction. Two days after admission she develops abdominal pain and diarrhoea with the passage of blood. Plain x-ray of the abdomen shows distended intestine but no fluid levels. Her serum amylase level is slightly elevated and mild fever is present. The most likely diagnosis is:

1. ulcerative colitis
2. acute pancreatitis
3. ischaemic colitis
4. diverticulitis
5. phenindione-induced colitis

Answer: *Text ref. p. 85*

Question 5

A twenty-five-year-old man complained of passing small amounts of bright red blood in his stools associated with mild constipation, occasional rectal urgency and discomfort. These symptoms had been present for over six weeks. Previously his bowel habit had been normal. X-ray studies of the small and large intestine with barium showed no abnormality. Sigmoidoscopy on several occasions showed a uniformly friable mucosa with pinpoint bleeding erosions extending 8 cm above the anorectal line. The mucosa above that level appeared normal. The most likely diagnosis is:

1. carcinoma of rectum
2. idiopathic ulcerative proctitis
3. rectal prolapse
4. intestinal tuberculosis
5. giardiasis

Answer: *Text ref. p. 74*

Question 6

A fifty-year-old woman with a five-year history of active ulcerative colitis has developed jaundice and itching. She has noted periodic short attacks of vague right upper quadrant discomfort without local tenderness; her temperature is normal. Laboratory studies show a serum AST level twice the upper limit of normal and a serum alkaline phosphatase level nearly five times the upper limit of normal. Bilirubin is found in her urine. Of the following diseases, which would most probably cause jaundice?

1. carcinoma of the ampulla of Vater
2. sulphasalazine-sensitivity hepatitis
3. active chronic hepatitis
4. sclerosing cholangitis
5. primary biliary cirrhosis

Answer: *Text ref. pp. 75, 163*

Question 7

An eighteen-year-old youth is admitted with fulminant ulcerative colitis. If he dies in the first week of admission, the most likely cause(s) of death is/are:

1. potassium depletion
2. perforation of the colon
3. liver failure
4. carcinoma of the colon
5. drug complications

Answer: *Text ref. pp. 74*

Question 8

A twenty-five-year-old man with a strong family history of colonic polyps presents to you with intermittent bright rectal bleeding. On examination and investigation, he is found to have hundreds of polyps in the colon and rectum. Which of the following is appropriate advice for this patient?

1. Proctocolectomy is advisable now.
2. Proctocolectomy is advisable in five years.
3. Ileoanal anastomosis with creation of a pelvic reservoir is contraindicated in this disease.
4. His wife should be examined for polyps.
5. His five-year-old son should be examined for polyps.

Answer: *Text ref. p. 92*

Question 9

Which of the following is/are risk factors for the development of colorectal cancer?

1. increasing age
2. adenomatous polyps
3. ulcerative colitis
4. diverticular disease of the colon
5. positive family history of colon cancer

Answer: *Text ref. pp. 89, 91 (Table 4.2)*

Question 10

Which of the following statements concerning colorectal carcinoma is/are true?

1. The incidence is decreasing in Western societies with improved medical care.
2. The prognosis is related to the duration of the patient's symptoms.
3. The most common sites are the rectum and sigmoid colon.
4. Cancer of the left and right colon have quite different modes of presentation.
5. Faecal occult blood tests (slide guaiac test) performed at home by the patient on a meat-free diet are a useful screening device.

Answer: *Text ref. pp. 91–6*

Question 11

Concerning colonic epithelium, which of the following statements is/are true?

1. Proliferative cells are distributed evenly throughout the crypt and surface cells.
2. Products of fermentation of fibre provide the principal metabolic substrates.
3. Radiation-induced damage is followed in the short term by a rapid, reparative increase in proliferation.

4. Radiation damage in the long term is due, at least in part, to vasculitis.
5. Patients with large bowel cancer have a higher rate of proliferation than normals.

Answer: *Text ref. pp. 68, 87*

Question 12

Concerning the patient who presents for the first time with acute, severe bloody diarrhoea, which of the following is/are true?

1. Giardiasis could be the cause.
2. Sigmoidoscopy and biopsy are useful in helping to ascertain the cause.
3. Plain abdominal x-ray has no value in management.
4. Non-specific anti-diarrhoeal medication (e.g. loperamide) should not be prescribed.
5. Diverticular disease could be the cause.

Answer: *Text ref. pp. 185*

CHAPTER 5

Pancreas

Question 1

Stimulation of pancreatic acinar cells by CCK involves all of the following except:

1. mobilisation of calcium from intracellular stores
2. activation of protein kinases
3. increased formation of cAMP
4. increased breakdown of membrane phosphoinositides

Answer: *Text ref. pp. 106–8*

Question 2

Which of the following play a role in pancreatic fluid secretion?

1. chloride ion
2. carbonic anhydrase
3. cystic fibrosis transmembrane conductance regulator
4. secretin
5. cAMP

Answer: *Text ref. pp. 105, 106*

Question 3

In acute pancreatitis:

1. vomiting is infrequent;
2. abdominal rebound tenderness is often observed;

3. bowel sounds are increased;
4. fever is uncommon;
5. none of the above.

Answer: *Text ref. pp. 110–11*

Question 4

Which of the following can be of value in the management of acute pancreatitis?

1. fasting the patient
2. glucagon
3. pethidine
4. both 1 and 3 are correct
5. all are correct

Answer: *Text ref. pp. 113*

Question 5

Regarding acute pancreatitis, which of the following is/are correct?

1. A normal serum amylase excludes the diagnosis.
2. Bluish discoloration around the umbilicus occurs in 30% of cases.
3. Erythema nodosum may be observed.
4. Hypercalcaemia is an adverse prognostic sign.
5. Anti-cholinergic drugs are contraindicated.

Answer: *Text ref. pp. 109, 113*

Question 6

All of the following are associations of chronic pancreatitis, except:

1. alcohol abuse
2. protein deficiency
3. gallstones
4. hyperparathyroidism
5. hypertriglyceridaemia

Answer: *Text ref. pp. 114–15*

Question 7

Which of the following is the most sensitive test of exocrine pancreatic function?

1. ERCP
2. duodenal intubation and secretin stimulation
3. bentiromide test
4. serum pancreatic isoamylase
5. three-day faecal fat excretion

Answer: *Text ref. pp. 116–19*

Question 8

Pancreatic cancer:

1. affects men and women equally;
2. usually involves the tail of the gland;
3. arises from alcoholic pancreatitis;
4. often causes vomiting in its early stages;
5. should usually be managed by resection and postoperative radiotherapy.

Answer: *Text ref. pp. 120*

Question 9

Abdominal ultrasonography is of *particular* value in the diagnosis of:

1. gallstones
2. acute pancreatitis
3. pancreatic pseudocyst
4. 1 and 3 are correct
5. all are correct

Answer: *Text ref. pp. 113, 121, 176*

Question 10

A seventy-two-year-old man presents with a five week history of progressive painless jaundice, pruritus and weight loss. Physical examination reveals jaundice, hepatomegaly, a palpable gallbladder and bilirubinuria. The most likely diagnosis is:

1. carcinoma of the pancreas
2. hepatitis
3. chronic pancreatitis
4. multiple hepatic metastases
5. obstructive jaundice due to gallstones

Answer: *Text ref. pp. 120*

Question 11

A forty-eight-year-old alcoholic man presents with intermittent central abdominal pain radiating through to the back, weight loss and steatorrhoea. Plain abdominal x-ray indicates the presence of diffuse pancreatic calcification. Abdominal ultrasound reveals a solitary gallbladder calculus. A fasting blood glucose level is 50 mmol/L. Which of the following is correct?

1. He will require large doses of insulin in order to control his diabetes.
2. A cholecystectomy will relieve his pain and lessen the steatorrhoea.
3. Serum amylase may be normal during attacks of abdominal pain.
4. The calcification is parenchymal rather than intraductal.
5. Continued alcohol abuse will not influence the prognosis.

Answer: *Text ref. pp. 112*

Question 12

A twenty-eight-year-old multiparous woman presents with abdominal pain. The pain is periumbilical in location, radiates through to the back and is associated with nausea and vomiting. Abdominal examination reveals slight guarding and diminished bowel sounds. Serum amylase is 1200 IU/L. Abdominal ultrasound reveals calculi in the gallbladder but the pancreas is obscured by bowel gas. Over the next thirty-six hours, the patient becomes hypotensive and hypoxaemic. Serum calcium concentration is low. All of the following are appropriate therapeutic measures, except:

1. nasogastric suction
2. admission to an intensive care unit with ventilatory and circulatory support
3. urgent cholecystectomy
4. urgent ERCP
5. blood transfusion

Answer: *Text ref. pp. 113*

Question 13

A forty-five-year-old factory worker with a history of alcohol abuse is recovering three weeks after an attack of pancreatitis. He complains of persistent abdominal pain. Physical examination reveals mild abdominal tenderness. Serum amylase is elevated (four times the upper limit of normal). The most appropriate next investigation is:

1. serum lipase
2. ERCP
3. abdominal CT scan
4. abdominal ultrasound
5. secretin stimulation test

Answer: *Text ref. pp. 111*

Question 14

A mother presents with her six-year-old son. She has recently noticed that he has been passing pale, offensive and bulky stools. The child has suffered from recurrent respiratory infections since infancy. On examination, the boy is short for his age. A course of tinidazole fails to correct the stool abnormality. The most likely diagnosis is:

1. giardiasis
2. Schwachman's syndrome
3. nutritional pancreatitis

4. cystic fibrosis
5. coeliac disease

Answer: *Text ref. pp. 115, 119*

Question 15

A fifty-two-year-old man presents with a six-month history of abdominal pain. The pain is described as constant and sometimes radiates to the back. The patient reports that the pain interferes with his sleep and that there has been an associated 10 kg weight loss. Diabetes was diagnosed three months earlier and is being managed with diet and an oral hypoglycaemic agent. Abdominal ultrasound reveals multiple stones in the gallbladder. Abdominal CT scan reveals a 4 cm mass in the body of the pancreas. Which of the following should you now advise?

1. referral to an oncologist
2. cholecystectomy
3. exploratory laparotomy
4. fine-needle aspiration under CT guidance

Answer: *Text ref. pp. 120–3*

Question 16

A forty-seven-year-old heavy drinker suffers from persistent epigastric pain which radiates through to the back. Endoscopic pancreatography reveals the changes of chronic pancreatitis. Abdominal ultrasound examination indicates the presence of a solitary 3 cm calculus in the gallbladder. Which of the following is true?

1. A cholecystectomy is likely to ameliorate the abdominal pain.
2. Serum amylase is likely to be elevated.
3. Abstinence from alcohol is associated with a better prognosis.
4. Both 1 and 3 are correct.
5. All are correct.

Answer: *Text ref. pp. 116–20*

Question 17

Pancreatic islet cell tumours:

1. are easy to localise;
2. always secrete hormones;
3. are always benign;
4. may secrete multiple hormones;
5. can be inherited.

Answer: *Text ref. pp. 124*

CHAPTER 6

Liver and biliary tract

Question 1

Contrast hepatocellular jaundice with cholestatic jaundice due to extrahepatic bile duct obstruction considering the following features:

Features	*Hepatocellular jaundice*	*Cholestatic jaundice*
Presence of anorexia and lethargy		
Presence of severity of pain		
Pruritus		
Xanthomata		
Splenomegaly		
Palpable gallbladder		
AST level		
Alkaline phosphatase level		
Ultrasonography findings		
Bile duct cannulation (ERCP) findings		

Answer: *Text ref. pp. 167, 232*

Question 2

Which of the following is/are recognised complications of hepatitis B infection?

1. erythema nodosum
2. polyarteritis nodosa
3. chronic persistent hepatitis
4. primary hepatocellular carcinoma
5. cirrhosis of the liver

Answer: *Text ref. pp. 133*

Question 3

Which of the following statements about chronic hepatitis is/are correct?

1. It is more common in men.
2. It may follow hepatitis A.
3. It is improved by corticosteroid therapy if it is due to hepatitis B.
4. In some patients the disease is drug-induced.
5. It is accompanied by a significant incidence of serum autoantibodies to body tissues.

Answer: *Text ref. p. 142–5*

Question 4

All except one of the following are frequently seen in patients with acute alcoholic hepatitis. The one exception is:

1. intracellular hyaline deposits

2. total bilirubin 100 μmol/L serum
3. serum alkaline phosphatase level 100 IU
4. fatty infiltration of the liver
5. AST 2000 U/mL

Answer: *Text ref. p. 166*

Question 5

Each of the following clinical histories describes a patient with a hepatic problem. For each clinical history choose the appropriate disease entity:

A. acute viral hepatitis
B. acute cholecystitis
C. chronic active hepatitis
D. primary biliary cirrhosis
E. haemochromatosis

1. jaundice, pruritus, xanthomata, hepatosplenomegaly, elevated serum alkaline phosphatase and cholesterol levels
2. anorexia, nausea, vomiting, jaundice, tender liver, high transaminase and normal alkaline phosphatase levels
3. jaundice, hepatosplenomegaly, elevated serum transaminase levels, hypergammaglobulinaemia, positive smooth muscle antibody
4. hepatomegaly, diffuse skin pigmentation, diabetes mellitus, testicular atrophy
5. jaundice, right upper quadrant pain and tenderness, leukocytosis

Answer: *Text ref. pp. 138, 147–9, 161–4*

Question 6

All except one of the following are commonly accompanied by cirrhosis of the liver. The one exception is:

1. Wilson's disease
2. haemochromatosis
3. infectious mononucleosis
4. alcoholic hepatitis
5. chronic active hepatitis

Answer: *Text ref. pp. 151, 161–4*

Question 7

Which of the following statements concerning gallstones is/are true?

1. Gallstones are found incidentally in 10% of autopsies in Western countries.
2. Gallstones located in the gallbladder usually cause no symptoms.
3. In 10% of patients the gallstones are radio-opaque.

4. Cholecystectomy is advisable when gallstones are discovered, even in asymptomatic subjects.
5. Chenodeoxycholic acid is effective therapy only when there are radiolucent stones in a functioning gallbladder.

Answer: *Text ref. p. 174*

Question 8

A nineteen-year-old university student had an episode of anorexia, fatigue and jaundice six months ago, which was diagnosed as hepatitis. The jaundice cleared and she has been back at class for three months. Nevertheless, she still complains of fatigue and diminished appetite. Physical examination reveals numerous spider naevi on the arm and neck, and the liver and spleen are both palpably enlarged. The following test results are obtained: serum total bilirubin 35 μmol/L, direct reacting (conjugated) bilirubin 30 μmol/L, AST 250 IU/L, serum alkaline phosphatase 80 IU/L, total serum globulin level 48 g/L (IgG 32 g/L). Tests for hepatitis A and B antigens and antibodies all show negative results, but tissue autoantibodies are detected in high titre. Which of the following is/are likely to be correct?

1. The patient probably has chronic hepatitis.
2. Autoimmune hepatitis is most likely.
3. The previous jaundice was probably due to hepatitis C.
4. Tests for Epstein-Barr virus infection will be positive.
5. Liver biopsy will probably lead to a firm diagnosis.

Answer: *Text ref. pp. 135–8*

Question 9

A fifty-year-old childless home worker is admitted to hospital because of fatigue, progressive weakness, mild anaemia and fever (38°–39°C) for one month. She has numerous psychological problems and was prescribed diazepam (5 mg three times a day) one month ago. Her husband left her six months ago. The liver is palpable 4 cm below the costal margin with a total span of 18 cm on percussion, and it is tender. The spleen is not definitely palpable. Investigations reveal: serum total bilirubin 50 μmol/L (3 mg%), AST 250 IU/L, serum alkaline phosphatase 105 IU/L, peripheral blood haemoglobin normal, but white cell count 15 000/mm^3 (80% neutrophils). Which of the following diagnoses should be seriously considered?

1. acute cholangitis (complicating gallstones)
2. diazepam-induced liver disease
3. chronic active hepatitis
4. acute alcoholic hepatitis
5. acute hepatitis B

Answer: *Text ref. p. 166*

Question 10

A twenty-year-old female student complains of nausea, jaundice and generalised itching of two weeks' duration. Physical examination reveals no definite abnormality other than icterus. She began taking oral contraceptives two months ago. Two of her friends were jaundiced two and four months ago, respectively. Relevant investigations are: serum bilirubin 250 mmol/L (12 mg%), AST 100 IU/L, serum alkaline phosphatase 350 IU/L. Which of the following statements is/are correct?

1. Cholestatic jaundice due to the 'pill' is likely.
2. If her friends were female, steroid-induced cholestasis was the probable cause of the jaundice.
3. This illness is compatible with hepatitis B infection.
4. This illness is compatible with hepatitis C infection.
5. An ERCP should be performed.

Answer: *Text ref. p. 167*

Question 11

A forty-five-year-old waterside worker complains of lethargy, weight loss and polyuria. Examination reveals a palpable liver and spleen and abdominal collateral veins. The serum bilirubin level, AST and serum alkaline phosphatase are normal but BSP retention is prolonged. Glycosuria is discovered on examination of the urine. Which of the following is/are likely causes?

1. alcoholic hepatitis
2. compensated cirrhosis
3. haemochromatosis
4. malignant hepatoma
5. fatty liver due to diabetes mellitus

Answer: *Text ref. p. 161–2*

Question 12

Which of the following drug/liver damage associations are correct?

1. methyltestosterone	cholestasis
2. methyldopa	chronic active hepatitis
3. benzene derivatives	predictable centrizonal necrosis
4. chlorpromazine	cholestatic hepatitis
5. halothane	hepatitis resembling viral hepatitis

Answer: *Text ref. p. 169*

Question 13

Primary liver cancer (hepatocellular carcinoma):

1. seldom metastasises;
2. is often due to hepatitis A;

3. has a higher incidence in patients with haemochromatosis than alcoholic cirrhosis;
4. is frequently associated with levels of alpha-foetoprotein greater than 500 μg/L;
5. occurs predominantly in association with cirrhosis in Western societies.

Answer: *Text ref. p. 172*

Question 14

Hepatic encephalopathy is likely to be aggravated by:

1. high-calorie diet
2. smoking
3. constipation
4. lactulose therapy
5. gastrointestinal bleeding

Answer: *Text ref. pp. 150, 158*

Question 15

Which of the conditions listed below have been correctly linked with the investigatory procedure most appropriate to its diagnosis?

1. chronic active hepatitis	liver biopsy
2. Wilson's disease	serum ferritin estimation
3. gallstone with bile duct obstruction	ultrasonography
4. hydatid cyst of the liver	computerised tomography
5. carcinoma of the intra-hepatic bile ducts	percutaneous transhepatic cholangiography

Answer: *Text ref. pp. 135, 161–4, 166*

Question 16

Which of the following statements about bilirubin and bile salt metabolism is/are true?

1. Bilirubin is formed exclusively from the destruction of senescent red cells in the RE system.
2. Unconjugated bilirubin is water-insoluble, it is transported in the plasma bound to albumin, and it is not filtered by the renal glomeruli.
3. The uptake of unconjugated bilirubin at the hepatocyte is shared by other organic ions but not bile acids.
4. Bile acids are absorbed specifically in the jejunum and undergo entero-hepatic circulation.
5. Elevated serum bile acid levels are diagnostic of cholestatic liver disease.

Answer: *Text ref. p. 131*

Question 17

Concerning hepatitis C, which of the following is/are correct?

1. Serological evidence for HCV infection can be detected in 60–90% of cases of transfusion-associated hepatitis.
2. The risk for IV drug users who have been using more than two years is over 90%.
3. Chronic HCV infection is a common cause of chronic hepatitis and cirrhosis.
4. The progression of HCV-induced liver disease is usually slow.
5. Alpha-interferon therapy is effective in some patients with HCV-induced chronic hepatitis.

Answer: *Text ref. p. 135, 137, 147*

CHAPTER 7

Infectious diseases of the gastrointestinal tract

Question 1

Which of the following pathogens occur with increased frequency in patients with AIDS and enterocolitis?

1. cytomegalovirus
2. *Cryptosporidium parvum*
3. *Aeromonas hydrophila*
4. *Vibrio parahaemolyticus*
5. *Salmonella* (non-typhi)

Answer: *Text ref. pp. 188, 194, 195, 203 (Table 7.2)*

Question 2

Rotavirus:

1. is the most common cause of infantile gastroenteritis;
2. infection is associated with lactose intolerance;
3. causes disease by increasing mucosal fluid and electrolyte secretion;
4. cannot be cultured in the laboratory;
5. causes nosocomial outbreaks of gastroenteritis.

Answer: *Text ref. pp. 187, 199*

Question 3

Abdominal pain and eosinophilia are prominent features of:

1. giardiasis
2. strongyloidiasis
3. *Taenia saginata* infection

4. *Enterobius vermicularis* (pinworm) infestation
5. ciguatera poisoning

Answer: *Text ref. p. 204–5*

Question 4

Features characteristic of enterotoxin-mediated diarrhoea include:

1. fever
2. leukocytes in the stool
3. reduced absorption of fluid and electrolytes in the small intestine
4. flatulence
5. tenesmus

Answer: *Text ref. p. 184*

Question 5

Which of the following pathogenic organisms induce diarrhoea by the secretion of enterotoxins?

1. staphylococci
2. *Clostridium difficile*
3. *Escherichia coli*
4. *Campylobacter* species
5. *Entamoeba histolytica*

Answer: *Text ref. pp. 184, 189, 190, 196, 199*

Question 6

Which of the following are commonly associated with pseudomembranous colitis?

1. amoxycillin
2. ampicillin
3. vancomycin
4. clindamycin
5. doxycycline

Answer: *Text ref. p. 196*

Question 7

Which of the following procedures is/are likely to establish a diagnosis of amoebiasis in a patient with diarrhoea who has recently emigrated from South-East Asia?

1. examination of a fresh specimen of faeces for cysts or trophozoites
2. rectal biopsy
3. barium enema
4. routine stool culture
5. ultrasonography

Answer: *Text ref. p. 198*

Question 8

All except one of the following intestinal infestations are diagnosed readily by careful examination of faeces for characteristic ova or larvae. The one exception is:

1. ascariasis
2. giardiasis
3. tapeworm infestation
4. enterobiasis
5. hookworm infestation

Answer: *Text ref. pp. 188, 190, 204–5*

Question 9

Examination of the faeces of a recent immigrant from Asia with recurrent mild diarrhoea reveals cysts of *Entamoeba histolytica.* Which of the following statements is/are true?

1. Family members should have their stools tested for *Entamoeba histolytica.*
2. It can cause hepatic abscess.
3. If the diarrhoea settles spontaneously, the patient is not a potential source of transmission of the disease.
4. It is a cause of traveller's diarrhoea.
5. Treatment with metronidazole is indicated.

Answer: *Text ref. pp. 197–9, 202*

Question 10

Within six hours of attending a banquet, about 10% of the participants develop severe nausea, vomiting, abdominal cramps and diarrhoea. In the majority the disorder subsides spontaneously but several subjects are admitted to hospital because of dehydration. The most likely cause is:

1. *Salmonella* food poisoning
2. botulism
3. staphylococcal food poisoning
4. giardiasis
5. *Clostridium perfringens* food poisoning

Answer: *Text ref. pp. 189–90*

Question 11

The most common cause of traveller's diarrhoea is:

1. *Shigella* species
2. *Campylobacter jejunii*
3. *Giardia lamblia*
4. Enterotoxigenic *E. coli*
5. *Salmonella enteritidis*

Answer: *Text ref. pp. 202*

CHAPTER 8

Motility and functional disorders of the gastrointestinal tract

Question 1

In relation to the normal patterns of motility in the gastrointestinal tract, which of the following statements is/are true?

1. Receptive relaxation of the proximal stomach occurs in response to swallowing during ingestion of a meal.
2. A special pattern of contractions occurs in the small intestine after feeding.
3. Migrating motor complexes are regular cycles of contractile activity occurring every few hours in the fasting stomach and small bowel.
4. Colonic transit accounts for about 50% of the transit time through the entire gastrointestinal tract.
5. Distension of the rectum by faeces produces relaxation of the internal anal sphincter.

Answer: *Text ref. pp. 212, 213*

Question 2A

A woman aged forty-seven years presents with epigastric and right hypochondrial pain, worse after meals, worse towards the end of the day and associated with epigastric distension and excess rectal flatus. Her gallbladder has been removed for these symptoms, but without relief and without gallstones being found. Her symptoms have been present for seven years and they have been present every day to a variable extent. Which of the following is the most likely diagnosis?

1. peptic ulcer
2. aerophagy
3. biliary tract pain
4. biliary tract pain and postcholecystectomy syndrome
5. chronic pancreatitis

Answer: *Text ref. pp. 218*

Question 2B

Before this diagnosis was finally accepted, which of the following should be excluded?

1. peptic ulcer
2. carcinoma of the caecum
3. choledocholithiasis
4. depression
5. Crohn's disease

Answer: *Text ref. pp. 219*

Question 3

A man aged forty-one years complains of intermittent diarrhoea and abdominal pain which seriously interrupts his social and working life, and which has been present for at least eight years. The stools are semi-formed and mucoid but he has not noticed blood. The pain is felt diffusely over the abdomen and is eased by defecation. Colonoscopy shows a few diverticula. Which of the following is the most likely diagnosis?

1. early cancer of the colon
2. irritable bowel syndrome
3. ulcerative colitis
4. chronic diverticulitis
5. idiopathic proctitis

Answer: *Text ref. pp. 216*

Question 4

A women aged sixty years has complained of diarrhoea for ten years. This has at times been associated with incontinence but she has not noticed the passage of blood or mucus, and denies purgative ingestion. Positive findings include a normal physical examination, a serum potassium of 2.1 mmol/L, and sigmoidoscopy which shows melanosis coli. Which of the following is the most likely diagnosis?

1. polyposis coli
2. purgative-induced diarrhoea
3. WDHA syndrome
4. irritable bowel syndrome
5. Zollinger-Ellison syndrome

Answer: *Text ref. pp. 126, 214, 217, 228*

Question 5

Which of the following may cause constipation?

1. hypothyroidism
2. iron tablets
3. irritable bowel syndrome
4. depression
5. duodenal ulcer

Answer: *Text ref. pp. 21, 214, 217, 229*

Question 6

A woman aged forty-six years complains of alternating attacks of constipation and diarrhoea with urgency but no blood. The diarrhoea does not occur at night and is worse in the morning after breakfast. The duration of symptoms is ten years with slight progression in severity. Sigmoidoscopy and barium enema reveal no abnormality and her general health is satisfactory. The most likely diagnosis is:

1. idiopathic proctitis
2. ulcerative colitis
3. carcinoma of the colon
4. depression
5. irritable bowel syndrome

Answer: *Text ref. pp. 74, 91–7, 214*

Question 7

Which of the following features help one differentiate diarrhoea of functional origin from diarrhoea due to organic gastrointestinal disease?

1. diarrhoea wakes the patient at night
2. the passage of blood and mucus
3. weight loss
4. the presence of anaemia
5. all of the above

Answer: *Text ref. pp. 74, 216, 228*

Question 8

Which of the following disorders may cause function (non-ulcer) dyspepsia?

1. gastro-oesophageal reflux
2. aerophagy
3. irritable bowel syndrome
4. gastroparesis
5. all of the above

Answer: *Text ref. pp. 218, 219, 227*

Question 9

Which of the following conditions can be associated with delayed gastric emptying?

1. diabetes mellitus
2. cigarette-smoking
3. vagotomy
4. Hirschprung's disease
5. anorexia nervosa

Answer: *Text ref. pp. 212, 214*

CHAPTER 9

Common symptoms

Question 1

Which of the following are typical symptoms of heartburn?

1. aggravated by fatty foods
2. aggravated by alcohol
3. eased by lying down
4. described as burning
5. eased by gastric neutralisation

Answer: *Text ref. pp. 222*

Question 2

Which of the following are correct innervations of the corresponding organ?

1. small intestine (T6)
2. stomach and duodenum (T7–T9)
3. pancreas (T12–L2)
4. biliary tree (T9)
5. colon (T8–T12)

Answer: *Text ref. pp. 224–6*

Question 3

Which of the following are common causes of chronic constipation?

1. depression
2. irritable bowel syndrome
3. tricyclic anti-depressant drugs
4. hypoparathyroidism
5. hyperthyroidism

Answer: *Text ref. pp. 230*

Question 4

Which of the following features are suggestive of diarrhoea due to large bowel pathology?

1. tenesmus
2. large, bulky stools
3. passage of blood and mucus
4. suprapubic pain
5. nocturnal diarrhoea

Answer: *Text ref. pp. 74, 216*

Question 5

Which of the following are suggestive of haemolytic jaundice?

1. dark faeces
2. deep jaundice
3. absence of bilirubin in urine
4. abdominal pain
5. pruritus

Answer: *Text ref. pp. 231*

Question 6

Essential dyspepsia is defined as dyspepsia where:

1. essential hypertension is present
2. oesophageal and gastric disease has been excluded
3. non-ulcer dyspepsia is present
4. all known causes have been excluded
5. the dyspepsia is due to oesophageal flux

Answer: *Text ref. pp. 219, 227*

Self-assessment workbook: answers

Chapter 1

1. 4
2. 1, 2, 3, 4
3. 4
4. 1, 3
5. 3
6. 3, 4
7. 5
8. 1, 2, 4, 5
9. 1, 2, 3
10. 1, 2, 4
11. 1, 3, 4, 5
12. 1, 2, 3, 4

Chapter 2

1. 3
2. 1
3. 2
4. 1, 2, 3
5. 5
6. 1, 2, 3, 5
7. 1, 2, 4
8. 2, 3
9. 2, 5
10. 1, 3, 4, 5
11. 1, 3, 4
12. 1, 5
13. 5
14. 2, 4
15. 1, 4, 5
16. 1, 4, 5
17. 5
18. 5

Chapter 3

1. 2, 3, 4
2. 1, 3, 5
3. 2, 3, 4, 5
4. 1, 2, 3, 4
5. 2, 3, 5
6. 1, 3, 4, 5
7. 2, 3, 4, 5
8. 1, 3, 5
9. 2, 4
10. 1, 4
11. 1, 2, 4, 5

Chapter 4

1. see text
2. 2, 3, 4
3. 1, 2, 3
4. 3
5. 2
6. 4
7. 1, 2
8. 1
9. 1, 2, 3, 5
10. 2, 3, 4, 5
11. 2, 3, 4, 5
12. 2, 4

Chapter 5

1. 3
2. 1, 2, 3, 4, 5
3. 5
4. 4
5. 5
6. 3
7. 2
8. 3
9. 4
10. 1
11. 3
12. 3
13. 4
14. 4
15. 4
16. 3
17. 4, 5

Chapter 6

1.

Features	*Hepatocellular jaundice*	*Cholestatic jaundice*
Presence of anorexia and lethargy	+	−
Presence of severity of pain	−	+
Pruritus	−	+
Xanthomata	−	+
Splenomegaly	+	+
Palpable gallbladder	−	+
AST level	high	−
Alkaline phosphatase level	−	high
Ultrasonography findings	normal	dilated ducts
Bile duct cannulation (ERCP) findings	normal	dilated ducts

2. 2, 3, 4, 5
3. 4, 5
4. 5
5. 1D, 2A, 3C, 4E, 5B
6. 3
7. 2, 3, 5
8. 1, 2, 5
9. 1, 4
10. 1, 3, 4
11. 2, 3
12. 1, 2, 3, 4, 5
13. 3, 4, 5
14. 3, 5
15. 1, 3, 4, 5
16. 2, 3
17. 1, 2, 3, 4, 5

Chapter 7

1. 1, 2, 5
2. 1, 2, 5
3. 2
4. 3
5. 1, 2, 3
6. 1, 2, 4
7. 1, 2
8. 2
9. 1, 2, 4
10. 3
11. 4

Chapter 8

1. 1, 2, 3, 5
2A. 2
2B. 1, 3
3. 2
4. 2
5. 1, 2, 3, 4
6. 5
7. 5
8. 5
9. 1, 2, 3, 5

Chapter 9

1. 1, 2, 4, 5
2. 2, 3, 4, 5
3. 1, 2, 3, 4
4. 1, 3, 4, 5
5. 1, 3
6. 2, 3, 4

Index

abetalipoproteinaemia, 58
abscess
  liver, amoebic, 185
  pancreatic, 103
  pericolic, 76
abdominal pain, 223
absorption
  carbohydrates, 39, 40
  D-Xylose, 48
  fats, 43
  protein, 43
  tests, 48
acetaminophen, 156
achalasia, 5, 12
achlorhydria, 20
acid secretion, peptic ulcer and, 16
adenoma
  large bowel, 89
  tubular, 89
  villous, 89
adult respiratory distress syndrome, 102
aerophagy, 218
alcohol, 152
  cirrhosis and, 152
  fatty liver and, 152, 165
  gastritis and, 29
  hepatitis and, 153
  liver disease and, 151, 165
  pancreatitis and, 108
  peptic ulcer and, 109
alcoholic cirrhosis, pancreatitis and, 92
alkaline phosphatase, 178
alpha foetoprotein, 172
$alpha_1$-antitrypsin deficiency, 149, 163
amoebiasis, 184, 197
  colitis and, 66
  hepatic, 184
  serological tests, 198
  treatment, 200
amoebicides, 200
amoeboma, 200
ammonia, serum, 166
ampulla of Vater, carcinoma of, 82
amylase, 105
  iso-enzymes, 105
  pancreatitis and, 107
  renal clearance, 105
  serum, 105
anabolic steroids, hepatic injury and, 167
anal
  abscess, 99
  fissure, 98
  fistula, 99
  haematoma, 99
analgesics, peptic ulcer and, 33
ancylostomiasis, 200
anaemia
  carcinoma of colon and, 85
  carcinoma of oesophagus and, 15
  coeliac disease and, 53
  hiatus hernia and, 10
angina, abdominal, 85
angiodysplasia, 97
angiography
  coeliac, 26
  ischaemic colitis and, 96
  mesenteric, 96
anorectal abscess, 99
antacids, peptic ulcer and, 24
anthraquinone drugs, 24
anticholinergic drugs
  functional bowel disease and, 215
  irritable bowel syndrome and, 215
antigens, hepatitis B, 138
antinuclear factor, 180
antrum, excluded, 199
anus, imperforate, 71
aphthous ulcers, 2
aprotinin, pancreatitis, use in, 112
arthritis, ulcerative colitis and, 76
ascariasis, 190
ascites, 159
ascitic fluid examination, 187
aspirin
  gastritis and, 20
  peptic ulcer and, 23
azathioprine
  Crohn's disease of colon: use in, 80
  hepatic injury and, 168

bacillary dysentery, 183
barium enema, 94
  colonic carcinoma, 94
  diverticulosis, 84
  ischaemic colitis, 85
  ulcerative colitis, 72
barium meal
  gastric carcinoma, 35
  gastric ulcer, 26
  peptic ulcer, 26
barium swallow, 8
  carcinoma of oesophagus, 15
  hiatus hernia, 10
  oesophageal webs, 14
  Schatzki ring, 14
Barrett's oesophagus, 8
  Behcet's syndrome, 4
bethanechol, 9
bile acid breath test, 46
bile salts, 39
  malabsorption, 46
  diarrhoea and, 46
  enterohepatic circulation, 44
  fat absorption, 43
biliary
  colic, 176
  tract disease, 175
bilirubin
  serum, 178
  urine, 178
biopsy
  gastric carcinoma, 35
  gastric ulcer, 26
  jejunal,
    coeliac disease, 53
    liver, 182
    small intestine, 53
blind loop syndrome, 51
  see also stagnant loop syndrome
botulism, 199
bran
  diverticular disease and, 85

bran *(continued)*
irritable bowel syndrome and, 214
breath test
bile acid, 49
stagnant loop syndromes and, 49
brush border
defects, 47
enzymes, 47

calcific pancreatitis, 114
Campylobacter pylorus, 194
(*see Helicobacter*)
C-ampylobacter jejum, 194
cancer, *see* carcinoma
candidiasis, 4
carbohydrate absorption, 39
carcinoid
syndrome, 64
tumour, 64
carcinoma ,
colonic, 88, 94
ulcerative colitis and, 77
gastric, 35
diagnosis, 36
early, 35
symptoms and signs, 36
treatment, 36
hepatocellular, primary, 172
oesophageal, 15
pancreatic, 120
rectal, 94
carriers
amoebic, 198
hepatitis B, 139
Shigella, 194
caeruloplasmin, 179
Chagas' disease, 13
chenodeoxycholic acid, 42
cholangiography
endoscopic, 187
intravenous, 187
oral, 187
transhepatic, 187
cholangitis, 176
cholecystectomy, 177
cholecystitis
acute, 174
chronic, 175
cholecystrogram, 176
cholecystokinin, 106
cholelithiasis, 174
cholera,
pancreatic, 116
cholereic enteropathy, 53
cholestasis, 167
causes, 167
drug-induced, 167
hepatitis and, 135, 139
cigarette-smoking, peptic ulcer and, 22
ciguatera, 210
cimetidine,
peptic ulcer, use in, 21
cirrhosis, 148
alcohol and, 149
ascites and, 159
cryptogenic, 149
hepatitis and, 149
malabsorption and, 46
portal hypertension and, 154
primary biliary, 163
renal failure and, 161
secondary biliary, 164
special types, 149
clonorchiasis, 161
clostridium
botulinum, 199
difficile, 196
perfringens, 195
coeliac
disease, 53
Society, 55
colic, biliary, 228
colitis, 85
collagenous, 87
Crohn's, 79
ischaemic, 79
gangrenous, 76
radiation, 79
ulcerative, 72
classification, 72
complications, 74
diagnosis, 73
prognosis, 74
treatment, 79
colon
carcinoma of, 88, 94
irritable, 214
polyps, 89
premalignant lesions, 89
spastic, 214
coma, hepatic, 150
computed tomography (CT)
hydatid cyst of liver, 187
liver, 187
pancreatitis and, 187
constipation, 220
contraceptive steroids,
hepatic injury and, 171
copper, serum, 179
corkscrew oesophagus, 12
Courvoisier's sign, 121
Coxsackie virus, hepatitis and, 132
Crohn's disease
of colon, 79
of small bowel, 59
of large bowel, 80
Cullen's sign, 108
cyst, pancreatic, 113
cystic fibrosis of pancreas, 115
cytomegalic virus, hepatitis and, 135

Dane particle, 135
dermatitis herpetiformis, 53
descending perineum syndrome, 102
diabetes, pancreatic carcinoma and, 117
diarrhoea
cholera and, 183
drug-induced, 185
gastroenteritis and, 64
secretory, 64
traveller's, 202
diet, peptic ulcer and, 21
diffuse oesophageal spasm, 13
disaccharides, 40
diverticular disease
colon, 81
acute, 81
chronic, 82
complications, 8
haemorrhage and, 83
Meckel's diverticulum, 63
diverticulosis
colon, 81
small intestine, 49
DNA polymerase, 134
drug-induced liver damage, 168
Dubin-Johnson syndrome, 174
Dukes' classification of colonic cancer, 94
duodenal ulcer, 21
Zollinger-Ellison syndrome
and *see also*
peptic ulcer
duodenum, 43
D-Xylose absorption test, 46
dysentery
amoebic, 197
bacillary, 183
dysphagia, 1
dyspepsia, non-ulcer, 219
essential, 227

emetine, in amoebiasis, 184
empyema, gallbladder, 176
encephalopathy, hepatic, 150
endoscopic
examination, 181
papillotomy, 181
retrograde
cholangiopancreatography (ERCP), 181
extrahepatic biliary obstruction
focal pancreatic lesion, 117
gallstones, 181
pancreatic carcinoma, 119
pancreatitis, 115
sphincterotomy, 181
ultrasonography, 187
enema, barium *see* barium enema
enema, small bowel, 49
Entamoeba histolytica, 197
enterohepatic circulation, 45

enteritis, 183
radiation, 62
regional, 59
see also Crohn's disease
Enterobius, 204
enteric fever, 192
Epstein-Barr virus, 132
erythema
multiforme, 3
nodosum, 3

Faecal incontinence in rectal prolapse, 100
familial adenomatous polyposis, 92
Fasciola hepatica, 207
fat
absorption, 43
necrosis, 108
fat, faecal
digestion and absorption, 43
excretion, 43
fatty
acid absorption, 43
liver, 165
ferritin, 179
fetor hepaticus, 1, 150
fibrocystic disease of pancreas, 115
fistulae
anorectal, 88
Crohn's disease and, 86
diverticulitis and, 86
flatulence, 230
flukes
liver, 207
intestinal, 207
focal nodular hyperplasia, 172
folic acid, serum, 48
food poisoning
botulism, 209
cholera, 190
Clostridium perfringens, 200
Salmonella, 191
staphylococcal, 189
traveller's diarrhoea, 202
functional disease of the gastrointestinal tract, 211
fundoplication, 16

Galactosaemia, 149
gallbladder, bile ducts and, 174
gallstones, 176
complications, 176
pancreatitis and, 176
treatment, 177
gamma glutamyl transpeptidase, 178
gastric
carcinoma, 35
erosions, 21
function tests, 34
inhibitory peptide, 126
outlet obstruction, 31
secretion, 17
peptic ulcer and, 21
Zollinger-Ellison syndrome and, 124
gastrin,
Zollinger-Ellison syndrome and, 124
gastrinoma, 124
gastritis
acute, 33
autoimmune, 34
chronic, 34
hypersecretory, 34
environmental, 33
erosive, 34
giant hypertrophic, 34
pernicious anaemia and, 34
gastroenteritis, acute, 183
gastrointestinal haemorrhage
occult, 25
gastroscopy
gastric carcinoma, 35
gastric ulcer, 25
Giardia lamblia, 188
giardiasis, 188
Gilbert's syndrome, 173
gingivitis, 3
globulin
gamma, 179
serum, 179
globus hystericus, 4
glossitis, 3
glucagon, 124
glucagonoma, 124
glucocorticoids
see corticosteroids
glucose tolerance test, 112
gluten enteropathy, 53
granuloma, amoebic, 200
Grey Turner's sign, 108
gynaecomastia, 151

Haematemesis
gastric ulcer and, 25
gastrointestinal, 25
management, 30
see also haemorrhage
haemochromatosis, 161
ferritin and, 162
haemorrhage, gastrointestinal, 30
diverticulitis and, 83
Meckel's diverticulum, 63
ulcerative colitis, 72
varices, caused by, 157
haemorrhoids, 98
halitosis, 2
halothane
hepatic injury and, 171
hepatitis and, 171
heartburn, 222
Heller's cardiomyotomy, 15
Helicobacter pylori, 21
hepatitis
A, B, non-A, non-B, 135
acute alcoholic, 165
acute viral, 135
amoebic, 198
antibodies, 135
antigens, 133
carrier, 136
chronic, 142
chronic active, 142
chronic persistent, 142
complications, 138
fulminant, 147
immune complex disease, 139
non-A, non-B, 136
relapsing, 139
subacute, 118
viral, 135
hepatocellular
failure, 150
carcinoma, 172
hepatolenticular degeneration, 162
hepatoma, malignant, 172
hepatorenal syndrome, 161
hereditary haemorrhagic telangiectasia, 4
hiatus hernia, 10
Hirshsprung's disease, 71
histocompatibility antigens
haemochromatosis and, 161
hookworm, 204
hormonal gastrointestinal disease, 124
hydatid cyst, 181
hyperbilirubinaemia
congenital, 173
hyperparathyroidism, 109
multiple endocrine, 124
adenomatosis, 124
hypertension, portal, 154
hypoalbuminaemia, 152
hypokalaemia
purgative-induced diarrhoea and, 124
villous papilloma and, 89
WDHA syndrome and, 126
Zollinger-Ellison syndrome and, 124

Ileal resection, 59
ileitis
regional, 59
terminal, 60
immunodeficiency, 65
immune
complex disease, 139
serum globulin, 141
immunoglobulin A deficiency, 64
immunological tests, 178
immunology
and the intestine, 64
and the liver, 178
imperforate anus, 97
infectious mononucleosis, 132

insulinoma, 124
intrinsic factor, 124
iron, serum
  haemochromatosis and, 161
  malabsorption, 46
irritable bowel syndrome, 214
ischaemic colitis, 85
islet cell tumours, pancreatic, 124
isoniazid
  hepatic injury and, 168

jaundice, 231
  pancreatitis and, 108
jejunal biopsy, 53

Kayser-Fleischer rings, 162
Koplik's spots, 3
Kupffer cells, 127

lactase deficiency, 52
lactose
  intolerance, 52
lactulose, 40
laparoscopy, 182
LE cells, 146
leuconychia, 152
lipases, 41
lipolytic phase of fat absorption, 43
liver
  biopsy, 182
  copper concentrations, 178
  function tests, 178
  scan, 178
  transplantation, 153
liver disease
  alcoholic, 156
  drug-induced, 168
loperamide, 21
lymphagectasia, intestinal, 63
lymphoma, 49
  intestinal, 49

malabsorption, 46
  classification, 48
  investigation, 55
Mallory bodies, 166
Mallory-Weiss tear, 15
malignant hepatoma, 172
maltose, 44
Manometry, oesophageal, 2
Meckel's diverticulum, 63
medium-chain triglycerides, 42
edullary carcinoma, thyroid, 64
megacolon, toxic, 72
Melanosis coli, 79
melena, 30
  see also haemorrhage, gastrointestinal
Menetriere's disease, 34
mesenteric arterial insufficiency, 63
methotrexate
  hepatic injury and, 168
methylcellulose, 219
methyldopa
  hepatic injury and, 168
micelles, 43
microvillus, 38
migrating myoelectric complex, 211
milk alkali syndrome, 21
mitochondrial antibodies, 178
moniliasis, 3
monoamine oxidase inhibitors
  hepatic injury and, 168
monoglycerides, 43
motilin, 215
mucocele, gallbladder, 177
multiple endocrine adenomata, 124
myasthenia gravis, 124
myotomy, 14

neomycin, 150
neonatal hepatitis, 149
non-alcoholic steatosis, 165
non-steroidal anti-inflammatory drugs and ulcers, 21
non-ulcer dyspepsia, 219
nutrition, tests of, 50

obstruction, acute large bowel, 97
occult bleeding
  blood tests for, 88
odynophagia, 1
oesophageal
  carcinoma, 15
  dilatation, 10
  dysmotility, 2
  manometry, 6
  pain, 1
  reflux, 2
  regurgitation, 2
  ring (Schatzki),6
  spasm, diffuse, 13
  sphincter, 2, 11
  stricture, 14
  varices, 156
  webs, 14
oesophagitis
  reflux, 8
opistorchis (liver flukes), 207

pain
  abdominal, 223
  biliary, 225
  colonic, 225
  pancreatic, 223
  ulcer, 21
pancreas
  abscess, 115
  ascites, 117
  carcinoma, 120
  cyst, 113
  disease, diagnosis, 112
  function tests, 112
  islet cell tumours, 124
  polypeptide, 106
  steatorrhoea, 109
  tumours of, 120
pancreatitis
  acute, 108
  acute relapsing, 108
  aetiologic factors, 110
  alcohol-induced, 109
  calcific, 110
  chronic, 114
  chronic relapsing, 115
  complications, 116
  cysts, 117
  diabetes and, 117
  drug-induced, 110
  fulminant, 112
  gallstones and, 111
  haemorrhagic, 112
  oedematous, 112
  risk factors, 110
  steatorrhoea, 117
  treatment, 119
pancreozymin, 116
papilloma, villous, 89
paracentesis in cirrhosis, 159
paracetamol, 168
parenteral nutrition in pancreatitis, 110
Paterson-Kelly syndrome, 14
penicillamine, 162
pepsin, 8
peptic ulcer, 21
  chronic, 21
  Meckel's diverticulum and, 63
  treatment, 21
  see also duodenal, gastric ulcer
peptide
  gastric inhibitory, 126
  vasoactive intestinal, 126
percutaneous cholangiography, 173
perforation
  carcinoma of colon, 94
  diverticulitis, 96
  peptic ulcer, 32
  ulcerative colitis, 75
perianal haematoma, 101
pericholangitis
  ulcerative colitis and, 75
peritonitis, diverticulitis and, 82
pernicious anaemia, gastric carcinoma and, 35
Peutz-Jeghers syndrome, 3
phenothiazines, hepatic injury and, 168
phenylbutazone, hepatic injury and, 168
pig bel, 190
pigmentation, mouth, 3
piles, 98
pinworm, 204
Plummer-Vinson syndrome, 14

Pneumatosis coli, 98
polyarteritis, hepatitis B and, 136
polypectomy, 94
polyps
  adenomatous, 92
  colonic, 94
  familial, 92
  villous, 89
  polyposis, 94
polyvinylchloride
  hepatic injury and, 168
portal hypertension, 154
  management, 158
  presinusoidal, 158
  postsinusoidal, 158
  prognosis, 159
primary biliary cirrhosis, 163
proctitis, 100
prolapse of rectum, 100
proliferative glomerulonephritis
  hepatitis and, 136
prostaglandins
  peptic ulcer and, 21
protein absorption, 43
protein-losing enteropathy, 63
proteinases, 43
proteolytic enzymes, 43
pruritus
  ani, 100
  cholestasis and, 167
  primary biliary cirrhosis and, 163
pseudomembranous enterocolitis, 99
psychogenic vomiting, 211
purgative abuse, 211
pyloric stenosis
  adult hypertrophic, 28
  infantile hypertrophic, 27
pyoderma gangrenosum, ulcerative
colitis and, 72

Q fever, 138
quantitative test of liver function, 182

radiation enteritis, 62
radiology, small intestine, 59
ranitidine, in peptic ulcer, 21
rectum
  carcinoma, 96
  prolapse, 100
  ulcer, 102
reflux oesophagitis, 2
regional enteritis, 59
Reiter's syndrome, 4
rota virus, 187
rotor syndrome, 174

sacroleitis
  ulcerative colitis and, 72
salicylates
  hepatic injury and, 168
  peptic ulcer and, 21
Salmonella food poisoning, 191
scan, radioisotope, liver, 181
Schatzki ring, 14
Schilling test, 49
schistosomiasis, 206
scintiscanning, hepatic, 181
scleroderma, 48
sclerosing cholangitis, 164
secondary biliary cirrhosis, 164
secretin, 106
secretin test, 106
secretin-pancreozymin test, 106
sedation
  peptic ulcer and, 22
Sengstaken-Blakemore tube, 158
sentinel loop
  acute pancreatitis, 109
serological tests
  amoebiasis, 197
serotonin, 107
serum
  albumin, 178
  ceruloplasmin, 179
  cholesterol, 179
  copper, 178
  ferritin, 179
  globulin, 141, 179
  iron, 179
  protein, 180
serum sickness-like syndrome, 135
serum transaminases, 178
Shigella, 193
shigellosis, 193
  acute, 193
  carriers, 194
  chronic, 194
short bowel syndrome, 56
Sjogren's syndrome, 3
small intestine
  biopsy, 54
  function, 39
    assessment, 46
smoking
  peptic ulcer and, 21
smooth muscle antibodies, 178
solitary ulcer of the rectum, 102
somatostatin, 157
spastic colon, 214
sprue, tropical, 56
stagnant loop syndrome, 51
staphylococcal food poisoning, 183
steak-house syndrome, 14
steatophepatitis, 165
steatorrhoea
  bacterial overgrowth and, 51
  cholestasis and, 167
  coeliac disease and, 53
  liver disease and, 167
  management, 46
  pancreatic, 110
  pancreatitis, 112
steatosis, 165
stenosis
  adult, 8
  para-pyloric, 31
  pyloric, 8
Stevens-Johnson syndrome, 3
stomach, hourglass, 22
stomal ulcer, 21
stomatitis, 4
stool
  examination, 177
  fat determination, 43
stress and peptic ulcer, 21
strongyloidiasis, 190
subtotal villous atrophy, 59
sucralfate, and peptic ulcer, 24
sulphasalazine, use in Crohn's disease
  of colon, 79
  ulcerative colitis, 72
sulphonamides, hepatic injury and, 168
sweat sodium, 115
sweat test, 115

tapeworm infestation, 208
telangiectasia, hereditary haemorrhagic, 3
terminal ileitis, 59
tetracycline, hepatic injury and, 168
threadworms, 204
thrush, 4
transaminase, serum, 178
transplantation, hepatic, 153
traveller's diarrhoea, 202
triglycerides, 39
tripotassium dicitrato bismuthate, 24
tropical sprue, 56
tuberculosis, 201
tumour *see* specific organs
typhoid fever, 192

ulcer
  acute, 20
  analgesics and, 21
  corticosteroids and, 21
  Cushing's syndrome and, 21
  hyperparathyroidism and, 22
  multiple adenomatosis and, 21
ulcer equation, 21
ulcerative colitis, 72
  treatment, 73
ulcers
  aphthous, 3
  duodenal, 22
  gastric, 21
  jejunal, 23
  malignant, 25
  oral, 21
  peptic, 21
  rectal, 102
  stomal, 32

ulcers *(continued)*
  stress, 21
  treatment of peptic, 27
ultrasonography, 187
ultrasound examination, 187
  extrahepatic bile duct
    obstruction
  gallstones, 187
urobilinogen, 178
uveitis, ulcerative colitis, 72

vagotomy, peptic ulcer and, 21
varices, oesophageal, 154
vasoactive intestinal peptide, 124
villus, 38
Vincent's angina, 3
VIPoma, 126
viral hepatitis *see* hepatitis
vitamin B12 absorption test, 49
vitamin deficiency
  coeliac disease and, 58
  stomatitis and, 3
vomiting
  peptic ulcer and, 21
  perforation and, 28
  psychogenic, 21

WDHA syndrome, 126
whipworm, 205
Whipple's disease, 57
Whipples triad, 125
Wilson's disease, 162

xanthoma
  cholestasis and, 163
  primary biliary cirrhosis and,
    163
xerostomia, 3
xylose absorption test, 46

yersinia enteritis, 195

Zollinger-Ellison syndrome, 124